Lighting Up a Hidden World

CFS and ME

Valerie Free

What Readers Are Saying About
Lighting Up a Hidden World: CFS and ME

"Ms. Free's goal in writing this book was to help the general public understand what it is like to deal with ME/CFS, a severe, common and often-overlooked chronic condition. She accomplishes her goal by sharing her personal journey in Section 1 and featuring vignettes from members of the ME/CFS community in Section 2. The book blends science, information, caring, wisdom and humour. As a fellow Canadian, I am very proud of Ms. Free's contribution to lighting up this hidden world. Everyone will find insight into ME/CFS through the tapestry of stories found in this important and informative book."

—Margaret Parlor, President, National ME/FM Action Network (Canada)

"There is truth in this inspiring book, which shares the heroic stories of individuals with ME/CFS who have battled stigma, discrimination and persecution in their search for appropriate care. This moving account of what Valerie and others have done is a must read and ultimately provides hope for us all that the status quo can be transformed through social action."

—Leonard A. Jason, PhD, Professor at DePaul University, Director of the Centre for Community Research, and author of Principles of Social Change, Oxford University Press (2013) (IL, U.S.)

"This book's creative setup, blending poetry with science, is what first gained my attention. With Valerie's encouragement, I started reading and discovered it told a story I wanted to learn more about: In 2012, during my third year of university, a healthy, vibrant, and active friend suddenly vanished. I was told by those closest to her that she had contracted CFS and could no longer participate in the things she was doing just weeks earlier. I had never even heard of CFS before, but I thought if this disease could take a young woman like her and confine her to a bed and a wheelchair, it must be truly awful.

Fast forward to *Lighting Up A Hidden World: CFS and ME.* The stories horrified me as I read about people who have been reduced to a fraction of their former selves and the callousness of those in power who have done little to help them. Yet, reflecting on these stories is also motivational. I hope that *Lighting Up A Hidden World: CFS and ME* will get people fired up to move ME/CFS from the sidelines and bring about real change for those who are suffering."

—Bryan Sandberg, BA in Communications (AB, Canada)

"Valerie Free has managed the nearly impossible. She has brought together descriptions and patient stories that convey what the world has refused to believe – that ME/CFS is not only real, but it is a nightmare that rivals hell itself and continues to be dismissed as a trivial neurosis by educated physicians who should have moved beyond this twenty years ago."

—David Bell MD, FAAP (U.S.)
Author of: A Doctor's Guide to Chronic Fatigue Syndrome: Understanding,
Treating and Living with CFIDS

"I was shocked to discover how little I knew about this devastating, widespread disease before I read Val's story! Her story, and the others shared in this book, brought to light just how appallingly ignorant and dismissive most of us, and especially medical professionals, have been with respect to people with ME/CFS.

I would urge everyone to read these captivating stories and become conscious supporters of their quest for a cure."

—Mary McGrath, Book collaborator and friend (CO, U.S.)

"*Lighting up a Hidden World: CFS and ME* is hybridized life writing that uses storytelling to blend illness narrative, a wealth of knowledge and resources about ME/CFS, with a call to action. Author Valerie Free generously shares her personal journey with a baffling illness that takes her into places of darkness and despair, including into a medical labyrinth that has yet to figure out how best to support people with ME/CFS. Free's searingly honest and gently humourous memoir uses the insights of her personal journey, as understood through art and poetry, to speak powerfully to patients, practitioners and advocates."

—*Tara Hyland-Russell, PhD, Professor of English (Life Writing) and Vice-President Academic at St. Mary's University (Calgary, AB, Canada)*

"Valerie's personal story, conveyed in the form of an engaging poem/song, along with the testimony of other ME/CFS patients and advocates, provides much-needed support and validation. It is a valuable information source for those of us who are struggling with this isolating, life-limiting illness within an indifferent medical establishment. I am encouraged by her call for meaningful change, delivered in a gentle but determined voice, infused with intelligence and hope.

So many of us are unable to function as advocates for change, either individually or as part of a group. We feel frustrated and inadequate. By sharing this book with family and friends, we can increase understanding and empathy as well as our personal sense of empowerment."

—*Carol Lefelt, ME/CFS patient since 1999 (NJ, U.S.)*

"This book takes us on a flyover journey through the 30-year history of CFS and ME, with touchdowns along the way so readers can jump out and explore. It gathers resources that Val and her collaborators have spent years collecting, and it is full of life experiences. *Lighting Up a Hidden World: CFS and ME* is a "one-stop shop" for people new to this hidden world, as well as for those who have been here for a while. Every time I pick up this book, I come across something interesting that is either new to me or a rediscovery – either in Val's story or in the amazing contributions from others.

By exposing and exploring the past and showing the possibility of a brighter future, Val's fervent hope is that everyone, including the public and the illness community, can hold one focus – resolution for ME/CFS and other complex illnesses. It is my hope too."

—*Maureen MacQuarrie, Book collaborator, ME/CFS patient since 2001 (ON, Canada)*

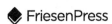 FriesenPress

Suite 300 – 990 Fort St
Victoria, BC, V8V 3K2
Canada

www.friesenpress.com

ISBN
978-1-4602-8050-8 (Paperback)
978-1-4602-8051-5 (eBook)

1. HEALTH & FITNESS, DISEASES, CHRONIC FATIGUE SYNDROME

Distributed to the trade by The Ingram Book Company

TABLE OF CONTENTS

ILLUSTRATIONS

These illustrations are by Simon Glassman, AB, Canada.

Foreword to Lighting Up a Hidden World: CFS and ME
by Toni Bernhard

When I was diagnosed with Chronic Fatigue Syndrome in 2001, I wish I'd had this book. With it in hand, I could have known it wasn't my fault that I didn't recover from a seemingly harmless viral infection. I could have felt compassion for myself instead of blame when I was forced to give up my 20-year career as a law professor. And, I could have understood that doctors who turned their backs on me did so out of ignorance and misinformation.

Most importantly, I would have had an invaluable resource to turn to again and again for help in my ongoing efforts to be treated with dignity, despite the trivializing name given to my illness.

Chronic fatigue syndrome is more currently known as myalgic encephalomyelitis/chronic fatigue syndrome (ME/CFS). It has left me mostly housebound and often bed-bound. I describe it as the flu without the fever: the aches and pains; the dazed, sick feeling; the low-grade headache; the inability to stand or sit up for long. It cost me my career. It cost me friendships. It cost me the ability to be active in my community and in the lives of my children and grandchildren.

Lighting Up a Hidden World: CFS and ME is of critical importance and arrives not a moment too soon. It is a book for everyone. Not only will those with an ME/CFS diagnosis feel validated when they read it, the book will also serve as a powerful resource for educating family, friends, doctors, and the general public about this debilitating illness.

Valerie is the perfect person to have written this book. She's suffered from ME/CFS since 1990. She tells her story with honesty, clarity, and compassion—and, as an added bonus, with artwork and poetry. The book gives readers a rare glimpse into what it's like to live day-to-day with this illness.

In addition, Ms. Free has done her homework. The book contains an astonishing array of resources, ranging from essays by fellow-sufferers to critical information from doctors and researchers who've devoted their professional lives to solving the mystery of this illness.

Lighting Up a Hidden World offers both a compelling personal story and a comprehensive, up-to-date review and analysis of the issues that need to be addressed before progress can be made in understanding and effectively treating ME/CFS.

I expect this book to have a worldwide impact and to inspire everyone, including the ME/CFS community, health care professionals, and government agencies to multiply their efforts toward finding a solution.

I'm indebted to Valerie Free for her courage, her hard work, and her determination to shine a bright light on this life-disrupting illness.

Toni Bernhard
Davis, California
March, 2016

Toni is the author of *How to Be Sick: A Buddhist–Inspired Guide for the Chronically Ill and Their Caregivers; How to Wake Up: A Buddhist–Inspired Guide to Navigating Joy and Sorrow;* and *How to Live Well with Chronic Pain and Illness: A Mindful Guide.*

ACKNOWLEDGEMENTS

MY FAMILY AND FRIENDS: Thank you to my husband David for taking care of life even more than usual as I focused on this project; and to my daughter Jenna for supporting and encouraging me not to give up when the going got tough. Also to my mom, dad, close family and friends who were patient with me, as this has been the topic of most of our conversations for some time.

ILLUSTRATOR: Simon Glassman – Alberta, Canada. It was always exciting working with Simon to create the illustrations for this book. It was a creative process that I really enjoyed.

CONTRIBUTORS: There was a wealth of material to draw from for this book as you will see in Section 2. Thank you to everyone who wrote original stories or who gave permission for their published work to be included. It was a pleasure to work with you and to get to know you.

There were others who shared their precious material with me, but due to space limitations, their work does not appear in this book. I want to express my appreciation to the almost 300 of you who did so: Your outstanding original stories, important blogs, and other published articles all contributed to the development of this project. I believe that if you continue to share your perspectives, your input will play a big part in finding the answers that we, ME/CFS patients, so desperately desire.

EDITORS AND/OR JOURNALISTS: Charlene Petitjean – New York, USA; Laura Orsini – Arizona, USA; and Rhonda Hayter – FriesenPress.

ASSISTING EDITORS: Edward Sweet – Arizona, USA; John Willis – Alberta, Canada; Tina Tidmore – Alabama, USA; Doris Fleck – Alberta, Canada; and Tami Dait – Alberta, Canada.

COLLABORATORS: This book could not have been completed without hours and hours of collaboration with many people over the years. Maureen MacQuarrie of Ontario, Canada was one. Maureen volunteered her time doing research, editing, and offering guidance and support. She was a practicing lawyer until she became ill with ME/CFS in 2001. With some improvement in her health over the years, the support of her husband, and the free time accorded to her after their teens had grown, she became involved as an ME/CFS advocate in Canada. I am so grateful she chose to take such an important role on this project and that we have become very good friends.

The other major collaborator was Randy Warner of Alberta, Canada, whom I have known for many years. Despite being largely bedbound with ME/CFS, Randy was involved in this project from the beginning when I sang the first verse of my story. He has helped with computer technology and trouble-shooting, day or night. I needed his skills because it was my first computer in over a decade. He also participated in most editing decisions. As we proceeded, he provided irreplaceable support and friendship.

Other important collaborators are Jenna Free – Alberta, Canada; Mary McGrath – Colorado, USA; Bonnie Coolum – Arizona, USA; Carol Lefelt – New Jersey, USA; Terri Warning – Illinois, USA; Debbie Lueers – Alberta, Canada; and Lisa Wolfe (deceased) – Alberta, Canada (Carol and Lisa's stories are in Section 2).

OTHERS WHO HAVE ASSISTED IN VARIOUS WAYS (Reading, brainstorming, encouragement): My sisters, Carole Scheetz and Vicki Fritz – Alberta, Canada; Laurie Scheetz – Alberta, Canada; Terry Rasko – Alberta, Canada; Valerie Fritz – Alberta, Canada; Andi Bell – Arizona, USA; Valerie Larsen – Alberta, Canada; Deanne and Jason Mansfield – Alberta, Canada; Terri Harris – Alberta, Canada; Mary Logan – Colorado, USA; Linda McLaughlin – Alberta, Canada; Corinne Blandino – Arizona, USA; Brenda McKay – Alberta, Canada; and Bryan Sandberg – Alberta, Canada.

Many others contributed hours for proofreading and feedback. Thank you all.

As I worked on this book, it was lovely to reconnect with friends and colleagues who are still in the court-reporting field. Some of them volunteered their time to transcribe audio material for me and I thank them. Until I faded away into the world of ME/CFS, I had many good friends made in my fifteen-year career as a court reporter. I still miss them.

ORGANIZATIONAL LEADERS: Thank you to those who have continually guided and inspired me. There are simply too many to mention. But special thanks to: Margaret Parlor (National ME/FM Action Network); Denise Lopez-Majano (Speak Up About ME); Cort Johnson and writers (Health Rising); Staff and writers (Phoenix Rising); Staff and writers (ProHealth); and Staff and writers (Invest in ME Research).

PROFESSIONALS WHO ENCOURAGED WRITING FOR SOCIAL CHANGE: Chris Carruthers, PhD – Alberta, Canada; Tara Hyland-Russell, PhD – Alberta, Canada; Arthur W. Frank, Professor Emeritus and author of *The Wounded Storyteller* – Alberta, Canada; David S. Bell, MD – New York, USA; Patricia Fennell, MSW, LCSW-R – New York, USA; Leonard A. Jason, PhD – Illinois, USA; Kenneth J. Friedman, PhD – New Jersey, USA; and Eleanor Stein, MD FRCP(C) – Alberta, Canada.

FINANCIAL SUPPORT: David Free – Alberta, Canada; and Debbie Lueers – Alberta, Canada.

PUBLISHER: Thank you to the team at FriesenPress who guided me through the self-publishing process. It has been quite a learning experience.

FOREWORD: A special thanks to author, Toni Bernhard, for taking the time and having the interest to write the Foreword for this book.

DEDICATION

To those with serious chronic illness who remain off the grid
of care and cure and for those who support them.

A PERSONAL THANK YOU

I would like to extend a personal thank you to my meaningful others: my husband and daughter, my parents and family, my friends, and the clinicians who have witnessed my ongoing illness experience firsthand, have held steady, and have cared for me unconditionally.

I know it is not always easy – in fact, maybe never easy.

They have allowed me an exceptional quality of life that would otherwise have been impossible. There are no words to express how deeply I love and appreciate them. I pray for their continued support – and that I can continue to support them in some ways – as I explore my future with the challenges and unpredictability that myalgic encephalomyelitis/chronic fatigue syndrome creates in all of our lives.

This gratitude extends to my many friends who also live with ME/CFS and other chronic illness, as well as my fellow advocates, for their encouragement, friendship, and input for this book.

Last but not least, thanks to you, the readers, for your interest in taking this guided tour of our hidden world.

Best,
Valerie Free

AUTHOR'S NOTE

Throughout the body of this work, I use the terms myalgic encephalomyelitis (ME), chronic fatigue syndrome (CFS), and myalgic encephalomyelitis/chronic fatigue syndrome (ME/CFS) interchangeably; and I am referring to these terms as defined by the Canadian Consensus Criteria (Appendix A).

INTRODUCTION
Breaking Ground

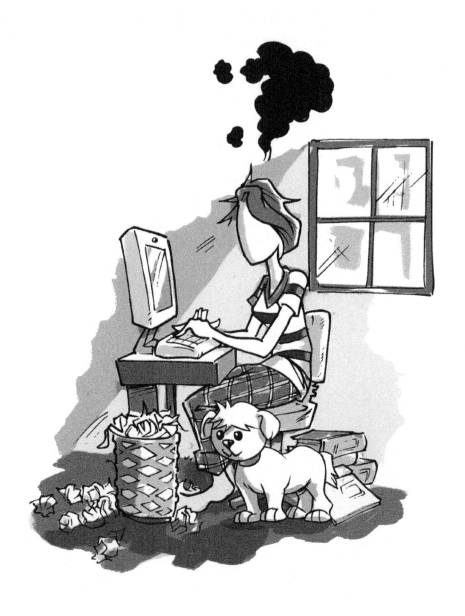

Setting the Stage

Valerie Free

"Memory is a responsibility because as it is told
it becomes witness and reaches beyond the individual
into the consciousness of the community."

Arthur W. Frank
The Wounded Storyteller: Body, Illness, and Ethics

It was 12:00 p.m. on March 23, 2013. I was resting in my bed in Arizona – a holiday place to escape the Alberta Canadian winters – propped up by pillows. I was experiencing the second day of a bad relapse – a very real part of the illness I'm going to tell you about in this book.

My spine felt like a wet noodle, unable to hold me up. My brain hurt from pressure, while somehow feeling like mush at the same time. My muscles ached and were so weak that walking and standing were simply not options for me. I couldn't help but remember one of the initial labels for my illness – Raggedy Ann syndrome – as I melded into the bed like a limp doll. Despite the fact that this label had only been briefly used in the late 'eighties, it was still a rather apt description of how I felt.

I looked out my window and saw my good friends drive away to a local fair. My husband had gone for a motorbike ride and was planning to attend a car show later on. Earlier, a neighbor down the street had told me about the seven-mile hike she had taken with her dog. As life went on around me, I quietly watched, listened, and reflected on the fact that I had just turned down an invitation to ride above the mountains of Arizona in a small plane. I had to say "no" to life so many times.

To prevent self-pity from taking over, I reminded myself that I loved all the wonderfully active people around me. Their vigor and enthusiasm enhanced my life, whether I participated or not. I settled for a bath and a little writing, hoping that I wouldn't feel so weak and miserable for much longer.

This particular relapse had been the result of "pushing myself" the week before. All I had done during that entire seven-day period was to visit with a nearby neighbor, spend brief periods on the computer, watch some of my favorite TV shows, make two meals, go out once for a quick supper, and walk my beloved dog while I rode my scooter. Most people can take these activities for granted, but I was paying dearly for daring to experience a few of my favorite things in the lovely Arizona warmth.

I Didn't See It Coming

Imagine a healthy, happy thirty-year-old woman. She's a loving wife and the mother of a darling baby girl. She's active, strong, and hardworking. Interested in and curious about life, she loves to have fun and keep busy. Being part of a large, extended family, having lots of friends, and living on a beautiful acreage in Alberta, Canada fill this woman's life. She has a fulfilling career as a court stenographer, but has recently cut it down to part-time to make motherhood a priority. Everything is in its place to enter a new chapter of her life.

You've probably figured out that the woman I'm describing is me. In July 1990, at age thirty, I came down with a sudden, flu-like sickness. Several months later I was diagnosed with chronic fatigue syndrome (CFS), which was later to be understood as myalgic encephalomyelitis (ME) or ME/CFS, and I've been living with it ever since.

It Can Happen to Anybody

ME/CFS is a serious, chronic illness that affects many parts of the body, including the brain, nervous system, and immune system, as described in the Canadian Consensus Criteria (Appendix A). There's no single known cause, no universally-accepted treatment plan, and no cure – even though the disease has affected people around the world for many decades.

Very little effort for research, care, or prevention has been made by governmental health agencies, so millions of people worldwide – including at least one million Americans and more than 400,000 Canadians – are suffering from this debilitating disease, often without medical help. It's difficult to pin down an exact number, because studies indicate that fewer than twenty percent of people with the condition have been properly diagnosed.

Like many diseases, ME/CFS is an "equal opportunity" condition. Anyone, regardless of age, race, or social status, can end up in its grip.

Many people with ME/CFS can appear perfectly normal and healthy at times. This gives others the impression that we're over it, or that we're somehow faking the condition when it suits us, or that we're suffering primarily from mental problems, not neurological ones that span body and brain.

On top of it all, we have to deal with the very undermining label of "chronic fatigue syndrome." This name presents the illness as a lamb, but it is a wolf disguised in a benign and misleading title. Chronic fatigue syndrome glosses over the fact that ME/CFS is an aggressive, life-altering, life-threatening, and often progressive illness. Would anyone call Parkinson's disease "chronic shaking syndrome?" Or refer to multiple sclerosis as "chronic numbness syndrome?" I hope not. A primary symptom can't describe the whole picture, and it muddies the waters because almost everyone experiences "chronic fatigue" at one time or another. Calling the condition "chronic fatigue syndrome" has slowed the acceptance of it as a legitimate and serious illness that requires funding, support, and research for effective treatment and cure. The name has been, and continues to be, a barrier to progress.

The invisibility and silence that come with ME/CFS prevent meaningful change. When people do reach out to the public or to medical advisors, they're often met with criticism, disbelief, or minimization. Our families and friends have a hard time coping with the illness because they don't know how to deal with the altered lives of their loved ones long-term.

An Important Breakthrough

As part of the first generation of people living with ME/CFS in North America, I felt pretty helpless until 2003. At that time, international experts gathered in Canada to link CFS with a disease identified in Europe in 1959, which is called myalgic encephalomyelitis (ME). Symptoms include acute onset (meaning that it occurs suddenly), infectious onset, headache, myalgia or muscle pain, numbness, muscle weakness and fatigability, central nervous system problems, and symptom fluctuation, as well as fluctuating emotions.

The name myalgic encephalomyelitis means "inflammation of the brain and spinal cord with muscle pain," and the description resonates with me and many other patients. Today, CFS and ME are widely used interchangeably and together as ME/CFS. As previously noted, throughout this book, I'll use all three to mean the illness described in the Canadian Consensus Criteria (CCC) (Appendix A).

The linking of ME and CFS in the CCC was a breakthrough that had a positive effect on my view of the illness and my experience with it. It led me to a greater understanding of my signs and symptoms. It's given me the clarity and confidence I need to communicate with my doctors and request laboratory testing to rule other disorders in or out. And it has helped me manage my long-term disability claim.

I found some new roots as well and began to feel very connected to a worldwide problem. Prior to that I felt mine was a fairly isolated experience.

An Illness Without a Home

People with ME/CFS are still waiting for objective evidence to get the attention of the medical establishment. Mainstream laboratory blood work and other tests are often not helpful, as a specific biological marker has yet to be identified (although researchers are getting closer). Even when we feel like we're at death's door, our mainstream lab reports can come back showing a clean bill of health.

Private research labs are working on new tests that show promise. These tests reveal pathologies in the areas of immunity, neurology, brain function, hormones, energy production, infectious agents, and genetics. Unfortunately, many people with ME/CFS don't have access to this testing because of its cost or location.

The condition is taught in very few medical schools and is not handled very well in hospitals, clinics, or private practices. Compared to a disease such as HIV/AIDS, which engaged the scientific and medical communities due, in part, to its potential terminal and contagious nature as well as to conclusive test results, ME/CFS languishes.

At present, no medical specialty is "home" for patients with the illness. Only a handful of doctors have developed a special interest and expertise in ME/CFS and related illnesses.

The Problem with Public Sentiment

ME/CFS remains disconnected from politics and the media. In the United States, the Chronic Fatigue Syndrome Advisory Committee (CFSAC) provides advice to the U.S. Secretary of Health and Human Services, but it seems the secretary rarely heeds its recommendations. National organizations are working to rally people around our cause: for example, in Canada, the National ME/FM Action Network; in the United States, the Solve ME/CFS Initiative; and in the U.K., Invest in ME. There are many more working internationally, nationally, and locally. We've got a long way to go before the general population fully appreciates the gravity of the situation, how widespread ME/CFS really is, and how costly it can be to individuals and society as a whole.

Abraham Lincoln once said, "Public sentiment is everything. With public sentiment, nothing can fail; without it, nothing can succeed." I couldn't agree more, and I believe the biggest challenge facing people with ME/CFS is for the illness to get some appropriate recognition all the way from political leaders to the general population.

As I struggled with my symptoms year after year, I wanted to know why ME/CFS was not being addressed in a more serious fashion. I found some answers in a research project led by Charles Salmon called "Mobilizing Public Will for Social Change."[1]

---

1   www.ncdsv.org/images/mobilizingpublicwillsocialchange.pdf (accessed July 10, 2016).

> Why are some social problems defined in terms of "poor behavioral choices" of individuals while other problems are blamed on the unhealthy business practices of companies that manufacture harmful products or the governmental agencies that regulate them?…Their answers tend to rest less with the objective characteristics of social problems themselves and more with the power, resources, and skills of those who seek to mold public sentiment about them.

This holds true for ME/CFS. This community of patients, because it is fragmented and continually diminished in many ways, doesn't have the kind of power, resources, or skills with which to mold public sentiment in a productive way. However, I am happy to report that this ability is growing, in part, due to social media.

It's fascinating to me that my condition has been so ignored, especially when one knows about the unique circumstances of its discovery in North America. In the mid 1980s, multiple outbreaks of a strange and unknown illness occurred in different locations including Incline Village, Nevada, US; Lyndonville, New York, US; and Montreal, Quebec, Canada. Each of these epidemics affected hundreds of people and some centered around schools and hospitals. The U.S. Centers for Disease Control and Prevention (CDC) were called in to investigate, but eventually all that came from it was the label "chronic fatigue syndrome" and a broad definition of its signs and symptoms.

Most media didn't pay attention to the outbreaks. If they did, it was often with inaccurate information. You'd think that such a mystery would have generated huge media interest, but when there was no conclusive evidence as to what the illness was or why it happened, reporters moved on. The ME/CFS story lacked some critical elements that the media requires to build a story, including a happy ending or some conclusion.

According to "Mobilizing Public Will for Social Change," the media will only approach a subject when the public is already partially on board. And since no one was really interested in these strange outbreaks, which had occurred in a few isolated communities, governmental health agencies and the media kept quiet and fed the "spiral of silence" that kept ME/CFS in the shadows, where it still resides in 2016. Until there's a large sway in public opinion on the subject, like there was with the civil rights movement and the movement for women's rights, supportive media will never hit critical mass.

A Call to Action

While the linking of ME with CFS – and the definition for it proposed in the CCC – was personally meaningful, I didn't know what I could do to help except to follow developments as they occurred.

In the summer of 2009, Canada's National ME/FM Action Network newsletter *Quest* revealed statistics from the 2005 Canadian Community Health Survey (CCHS). It outlined the number of Canadians who reported being diagnosed with CFS, FM (fibro-myalgia syndrome), and/or MCS (multiple chemical sensitivities). The CCHS showed that in Canada, there were over one million people with one or more of these conditions (over 300,000 with CFS). These were high ratios as Canada had just over thirty-two million people at that time. The survey was repeated in 2010 and a breakdown of the results for the two years are reflected in Appendix B.

Margaret Parlor, a statistician and the president of the National ME/FM Action Network in Canada, analyzed the data which demonstrated that people with these conditions were among those with the highest unmet needs compared to those with other serious illnesses[2] (Appendix C).

I had been part of the 2005 CCHS survey and this was a synchronicity I could not ignore. My answers to the survey were the same as many others who had ME/CFS, and this illustrated that I was not alone.

I'll never forget that day in the summer of 2005. As I was sitting peacefully on the swing on our deck, the phone rang. When I picked it up, a friendly man on the other end asked me if I wanted to participate in a survey about Canadian community health.

"Sure, why not?" I said. It was my resting time, so there really wasn't much else I could be doing.

He asked me if I'd ever been diagnosed with a number of different illnesses. I couldn't believe it when he said, "chronic fatigue syndrome."

"Yes!" I exclaimed.

He continued to ask pertinent and important questions: "How are you doing socially and financially?… What is your level of disability?" He even asked about suicidal thoughts and feelings.

Wow. This anonymous survey taker was asking me better questions than most doctors had in more than fifteen years. At the time, I was struggling to find a family doctor who would accept a patient with ME/CFS, so the fact that I was finally being heard gave me a much-needed boost.

Shortly after the 2005 statistics from the CCHS were published, Ms. Parlor published in *Quest* 82 how little research funding ME/CFS, FM, and MCS were receiving from the Canadian Institutes of Health Research (CIHR) relative to other illnesses.[3] I took all of this information and the injustice it exposed as a call to action.

---

2   National ME/FM Action Network spring/summer 2009 Quest 80. "Profile and Impact of 23 Chronic Conditions in the 2005 Canadian Community Health Survey." This survey was repeated in 2010 and the results are in Spring/Summer Quest 88. Find a list of all the newsletters at www.mefmaction.com/index.php?option=com_content&view =article&id=157&Itemid=208 (accessed July 12, 2016).

3   National ME/FM Action Network, Winter 2009/2010, Quest 82, "CIHR Funding for Research into 15 Chronic Illnesses." www.mefmaction.com/images/stories/quest_newsletters/Quest82winter2009.pdf (accessed July 15, 2016). An excerpt of the table is included in this book at Part V, Stanza 43 Notes, "Fund the Research."

The Power of Narrative Medicine

As I met or learned about some professionals who were to become so influential to me, the universe started to feel in sync with my goal to take action.

I read about Chris Carruthers, PhD in a local newspaper. She had recovered from ME/CFS after seven years. When I contacted her, she encouraged me to journal each day, to help process the many feelings and thoughts I had about this relentless and unpredictable illness. She knew what she was talking about.

The focus of her doctoral research was how "Expressive Writing about Personal Trauma" had positive health benefits. She told me that journaling has been proven to provide an opportunity for healing by clearing the past and reconciling what has happened in our lives. Achieving some sort of closure on past events can make it easier to cope with the present, even if challenges are ongoing. Chris went on to say that sharing my story with others who have similar circumstances could be beneficial – offering validation and connection – and that the personal stories of patients serve a valuable role in informing medical care professionals about illness experiences and how to better respond to them.

You can read more about Chris in Chapter 8 – Recovery, Improvement and Hope.

I began journaling every day. Remembering how it all started was very emotional, stirring up shock, grief, and sadness, but it was also liberating because it gave me a chance to validate my feelings. Before long, the journaling exposed all kinds of threads, taking me into areas I didn't even know were waiting and ready to be unraveled.

Next, I met Tara Hyland-Russell, PhD, a professor of English, literature, and life writing at St. Mary's University in Calgary. Tara kindly came to visit me at my home, because I was very ill and unable to go to her. We talked about writing and its purpose, and she introduced me to the concept of blending literature and social justice. Tara explained the importance of bearing witness to the history of an oppressed group – and that storytelling can be used to mobilize social change.

It was a life-altering conversation, and I felt my heart light up when she reminded me that many traditions and cultures have storytelling circles for all of these reasons.

Things were starting to make sense in a whole new way, and my motivation, understanding and confidence grew.

In 2010, Tara referred me to a wonderful book by Arthur W. Frank, *The Wounded Storyteller: Body, Illness, and Ethics*. It became another resource for me, clarifying the process and outcomes of writing stories about illness. Dr. Frank was Professor Emeritus of Sociology at the University of Calgary, and he tells of his own illness journey:

> As wounded, people may be cared for, but as storytellers, they care for others. The ill, and all those who suffer, can also be healers ... Because stories can heal, the wounded healer and wounded storyteller are not separate, but are different aspects of the same figure. But telling does not

come easy and neither does listening. Seriously ill people are wounded not just in body but in voice. They need to become storytellers in order to recover the voices that illness and its treatment often take away...[4]

Arthur Frank's words about acting as a witness to an illness, instead of simply surviving it, encouraged me: "My first choice as a designation is 'witness.'" He continues:

Survival does not include any particular responsibility other than continuing to survive. Becoming a witness assumes a responsibility for telling what happened. The witness offers testimony to a truth that is generally unrecognized or suppressed. People who tell stories of illness are witnesses, turning illness into moral responsibility.[5]

I later came to learn of this as Narrative Medicine, which has become a large field of its own in recent years.

The Writing Process

Before I began to write this book, I was under the impression that authors work on their books. But I now understand that is not the case – it is quite the opposite; I had a book working on me. On many days – though I was very sick, bedbound, and foggy-minded – ideas would flow, so I'd always keep pen and paper close by. Numerous times, I would write without lifting my head from the pillow because I just couldn't. This left me with a lot of gibberish to decipher the next day.

Later, I mentioned this to an editor, telling her that, in those moments, I was very aware that my brain was unable to "think" in any rational way (due to the extreme symptoms I was experiencing), and that this writing was coming from some place other than my brain. It seemed to be streaming out of my body somewhere – from a place I could not identify. As an experienced author, she acknowledged this phenomenon and said, "That is the place writing comes from."

This project seems to have a mind and life of its own, regardless of my health status. There is no doubt that my determination to write this book surprised even me and was a calling of its own.

---

4   Frank, Arthur W. "The Wounded Storyteller: Body, Illness, and Ethics." 1995. xii.

5   Frank, Arthur W. "The Wounded Storyteller: Body, Illness, and Ethics." 1995. 137.

Momentum for Change

And this is where we are today. Through my own story, and the dozens of others featured in these pages, my hope is to generate greater awareness of ME/CFS and accelerate progress toward better care, a cure, and prevention. I want to reach beyond the ME/CFS community to a new audience who will see our hidden world maybe for the first time. I know that it's possible because, during my writing process, I've seen again and again that people care for others who are suffering and have an honest interest in this matter. Once they gain knowledge and understanding, they're naturally inclined toward compassion and action.

The work of people like renowned author, Laura Hillenbrand, who has spoken out about ME/CFS, also inspires me. Laura is the author of the award-winning books *Seabiscuit* and *Unbroken* which have both become major motion pictures. She has written beautifully on the subject of her health struggles in her essay, "A Sudden Illness," and a story about her is in Chapter 7: The Good Fight.

But the voices of those who speak up are few and far between. People with ME/CFS rarely have the wellness, stamina or time available to do so. They either become too sick to do it and fade away into the background, or they're not willing to risk the disdain that may befall them if they do. Many of us have a limited time to influence anything because we are just not well enough to sustain our efforts.

A recent development is the extensive 2015 evidenced-based report on ME/CFS by the esteemed Institute of Medicine (IOM) in the United States – a report that recognizes the seriousness and multi-systemic nature of the disease. I am happy to see the attention it is garnering in medical and research circles. But even with this effort, there are issues for the ME/CFS professional and patient community to deal with to ensure the best outcome for the future.

I hold out great hope for improvement in my health and for the health of all of us, including for future generations. I want to be part of the change that makes it possible.

A Well Person's Glimpse into ME/CFS

Laura Orsini | May 2012

Before Valerie invited me into her life as her editor and collaborator for this book, I knew two things about Myalgic Encephalomyelitis/Chronic Fatigue Syndrome (ME/CFS):

- I knew it was a real illness that professionals in the healthcare industry often dismissed and/or did not take seriously.

- I knew it was chronic – that most people who had it suffered with it long-term.

What I have learned from Valerie and from the process of working on this book has been eye-opening, but my real wake-up call – in spite of all the academic, philosophical, and empathetic knowledge about the illness I've been amassing – is the head cold I'm just getting over… again.

The first bout came on suddenly about a month ago on a Wednesday evening. I was fine during the day, but by the evening my head was cloudy, my nose was running, and I was developing a severe headache. By the next morning, I felt pretty awful. This was in no way life-threatening, mind you; just symptomatic enough to deplete my energy and make me feel like someone was taking a punching bag to my sinuses.

Saturday came and I was extremely frustrated to realize I was still ill and had to skip a book-marketing conference I had very much wanted to attend. I slept some more. I spent Sunday catching up on work from Thursday and Friday instead of sleeping. But that meant I was back in bed on Monday. Tuesday was the first day I finally started to feel well enough to get up and move normally.

I had, at this point, only been down for *one week*, yet I felt severely incapacitated and was already way behind on my work.

I recovered, but it took two weeks to feel completely well again. The thing is, I knew all along I was getting better – in fact, I took it for granted. Although I have to admit, because of what I now know from my work on this book, I did have the fleeting thought, *I am going to get better, **right**?*

Val had told me that many cases of ME/CFS begin after a person has had a bad cold, flu, or a bout of mono or pneumonia – but instead of getting better, they get sicker. This is important knowledge to have. For one thing, it's a reminder to listen to our bodies, particularly if we're not healing as we usually do. The best time to take care of any illness is at its onset, as soon as you know your body is not behaving as it should.

My husband managed not to get my cold, but a couple weeks later, he went out and found his own cold, brought it home, and shared it with me. So exactly a month later, I went down with round two. The good thing is that the second bout was much less severe than the first; more or less gone after just a few days. Today as I write this, I'm just about symptom-free, the headache and runny nose finally, and blessedly, having taken a hike.

I told Valerie yesterday, "I can't even imagine what you must go through if these stupid colds even remotely resemble how you feel when you're experiencing this illness." And I can't. I can't even imagine knowing that the lousy feelings of a cold like this could hit again at any moment, even if I just recovered a day or two ago.

As I understand it, ME/CFS patients rarely recover to their pre-illness health, and when they do improve, they may not recover in the way that I, a healthy person, understand wellness. Improvement after any worsening or relapse for an ME/CFS patient means recovering "all the way back up" to their personal highest level of functioning within the illness, which may be only thirty percent of that enjoyed by someone in good health.[6]

Think about living the *rest* of your life with cold and flu-like symptoms coupled with low blood pressure, migraines, nausea, and sleep disturbances, as people with this illness do. Yesterday you were healthy, but today you are ill and struggling to function. On top of that, it may take a year or more to obtain the correct diagnosis. In the meantime, you have access to only some general medications that offer limited relief.

Most well people would be horrified to experience just one of the symptoms of ME/CFS. It's probably impossible for any healthy person to imagine living with all of them, plus more. People with ME/CFS face the very real need to adapt their lives around these and other symptoms just to survive.

It's frightening to imagine the consequences of living long-term with such debility – to consider the kind of havoc it would cause in a person's relationships or with their finances. When I was at my sickest during this common cold, my husband stepped up and managed dinner, the dishes, and caring for our five pets for nearly a week – this on top of his fifty to sixty-hour workweeks.

ME/CFS patients deal not only with long-term limitations and the subsequent reliance on family and friends for help, but this is all without the availability of a standard effective treatment or cure. Sometimes even basic medical care is inaccessible, and some patients end up on their own, isolated from the medical system, their families, and their community.

A small percentage of people with this illness do recover over time, but all live with the knowledge that while they may improve, they may also worsen or relapse into terrible levels of suffering that could cause them to be bedbound for life.

As a healthy person, I can't imagine routinely missing events because I just don't have enough energy to get dressed or go out. I can't imagine being unable to get my work

---

6   For a better understanding of this concept, you can look at the scale in Appendix H titled "Karnofsky Energy Rating Scale adapted for use in ME/CFS." This severity scale has a range from 10 percent to 100 percent. These guidelines describe 30 percent, for example, this way: "You can only perform one light task per day, as any extra physical movement makes you feel unwell. You have difficulty reading and writing."

done, or having to give up working entirely because I just don't have the strength to do it reliably anymore. I can't imagine pain, muscle weakness, and lack of stamina being my constant companions – never mind the brain changes and concentration losses that affect the ability to learn or do basic chores like balancing a checkbook.

Having too little energy to sit down at the dinner table or getting lost in my own neighborhood are pretty frightening things to contemplate.

I am fortunate to be healthy. My colds, as miserable as they were, were just colds – temporary conditions that resolved themselves fairly quickly.

❧

Think back to the last time you had a cold or the flu – recall how miserable you were and how you would have given anything to get better. And remember how good it felt to finally be on the mend.

Now imagine never fully recovering, or worsening and staying that way. Such a picture is great motivation, for those of us who are healthy, to put our energy behind this cause.

Although I may have been ahead of the curve because I was aware of ME/CFS before I met Valerie, my work with her has made it abundantly clear that we – the healthy – must take an active interest in finding a cure. Fundraising for increased research is something we can do to provide hope and support for this community. We must get involved because, whether we realize it or not, we have a stake in the cure. Every person suffering with this illness impacts the entire community. Not to mention that any one of us, or someone we love, could be afflicted in the future. Remember, that's how ME/CFS can work. You're well one day – then you experience a triggering incident like a personal trauma or the flu – and before you know it, you're in the midst of a debilitating illness without a clear path back to health.

As healthy people, we have the energy and strength to advocate for those who are too ill to do it for themselves. We have the ability to advocate for more research, medical education and better patient care so that future generations do not have to suffer and struggle like current and past ME/CFS patients have.

I'm happy to know I am making a difference. You can too. Easy ways to get involved are:

- Learning about this illness. Reading this book is a great first step.

- Educating those around you.

- Volunteering your time with organizations that work with the ME/CFS community.

- Talking to your local politicians and health policy makers regarding the needs of this population.

Before science caught up to them, most serious illnesses were once at the place where ME/CFS is today: largely unknown, completely misunderstood, and with very little support for those who were stricken with them.

Please join me in giving a voice to the people with ME/CFS so they can get the support and recognition they deserve.

SECTION 1
The Chronic-Call

My Story: Living With and Learning About ME/CFS

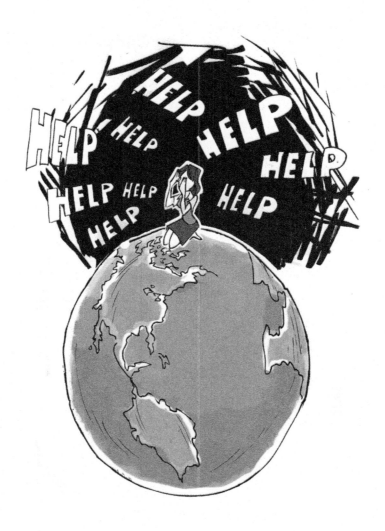

INTRODUCTION

"The Chronic-Call" is my story which spans over twenty years of being chronically ill with ME/CFS. It is written in verse and accompanied by explanatory notes. The symptoms and experiences I share are constantly changing, hour-to-hour and day-to-day. When awake, I am never symptom-free, at rest or otherwise. I have been adapting to the increasing limitations and restrictions that ME/CFS has imposed on my life for a long time and I feel I am progressively weakening. What has become stronger, however, is my longing for cure and resolution for myself and for everyone who struggles with this illness.

The song "**My Favorite Things,**" sung by actress Julie Andrews in the musical *The Sound of Music,* inspired the format and rhythm of my story in verse. It was not long after Christmas 2009 when I spontaneously started to sing my symptoms to the tune, and this continued for months until all had been told. I found out later that Julie Andrews' husband, the late, great Blake Edwards – who was the creator of many award-winning films such as *The Pink Panther* – also had ME/CFS.[7] In fact, he was one of its first vocal advocates in the North American celebrity world.

It was quite a synchronicity to be singing Mr. Edwards' symptoms to Ms. Andrews' tune. (Blake Edwards had passed on by the time this was all starting to unfold.)

Format

I wrote "The Chronic-Call" verses in order, as I remembered the events unfolding since 1990, using a timeline of five-year segments. The poem appears in its entirety first. Then I have broken it down into stanzas with accompanying notes. The notes help translate personal lines in the verse, fill in gaps, and provide facts and information about the world of ME/CFS. These notes were written looking back from the time of writing (2010 to 2016), so my sharing of what I have learned about ME/CFS in them is not always chronological.

---

7   "I Remember Me," a documentary film by Kim Snyder, (2000), features an interview with Blake Edwards. The full-length documentary is available at www.youtube.com/watch?v=401—WCB5dc (accessed July 20, 2016). Also see www.hollywoodreporter.com/news/blake-edwards-dies-88-60870 (accessed July 20, 2016).

The illustrations, which were created by Simon Glassman, have always been a priority for me. He and I would take hours for back-and-forth trials, perfecting each one to illustrate the message that I wanted to convey. A picture really can say a thousand words.

Some may prefer to read the poem alone while others may read just the notes. My goal is to include something for everyone, but if you combine the illustrations with the verses and the notes, the picture is more complete.

The Title

My original idea for the title was The Chronicle. This seemed fitting because the verse was a chronicle: a factual, written account of historical events in the order of their occurrence. Over time, The Chronicle began sounding to me like "The Chronic-Call."

"The Chronic-Call" fits both personally and universally. This primal call for solutions to regain my own health began as a response to my sudden ME/CFS onset in 1990. I'm still looking for those answers.

More universally, "The Chronic-Call" is a title suited to the larger, hidden world of ME/CFS. Lack of accurate knowledge, low research funding, and inadequate patient care continues despite over twenty-five years of calling out for political and medical help by patients, advocacy organizations, and dedicated professionals in the field.

Perhaps others with complex chronic illnesses might recognize some of my story as familiar to their own and be inspired to write a personal verse or two, making it unique to them. Despite the many obstacles and difficulties we still face with ME/CFS, the *one* thing we can take comfort in is that we are not alone so none of us should have to deal with our experiences solo.

THE CHRONIC-CALL

Poem

**This was created to the rhythm of
"My Favorite Things" from *The Sound of Music*.**

PART I
SUDDEN FLU-LIKE ONSET
(My age: 30-34)
July 1990-1994

Chinooks and low clouds and changes
in pressure,
Full moons and melting and things you
can't measure,
Perfumes and diesel and food allergies,
These are the things that bring me to
my knees.
Poor memory, no focus, and wrong
word retrieval,
Numbness and tingling, Bell's palsy –
sounds evil.
Sleep deprivation and low energies,
Blood pressure drops that bring me to
my knees.

>...When I stand up...
>...When I sit down...
>...When I walk a while...

Symptoms galore visit all of my self,
Leaving me slumped in a pile.

୬

Two or three weeks after getting a flu,
I was not any better so what should I
do?
I had symptoms of nausea, thirst,
hunger, weight loss,
Body-temp changes and blood
pressure drops.
It was only the flu so just how could
this be?
My anatomy books came in handy
to see,
That my brain is involved – it's the
master control.
When I told the docs, they gave their
eyes a roll.

>...Decades later...
>...Thru the research...
>...Was confirmed the piece...

That part of the brain can be harmed in
this way;
How did flu become complex disease?

୬

27

A career of fifteen years as a
court reporter,
Quick as a hummingbird –
solid as mortar.
Asleep now in the car after I'd get
to work,
Unable to keep up the shorthand
I took.
From someone who did teach aerobics
at lunch hour,
Who gardened and traveled – at hard
work did not cower,
Now my baby seems heavier – muscles
are weak,
Disoriented driving and it's hard
to speak.

    …Doc, what is wrong?…
    …Something serious…
    …My world is falling apart…

She said, "I think you have something
quite new:
Chronic fatigue syndrome, sweetheart."

❦

Bright lights and things that are too
stimulating,
Things that the healthy find
invigorating.
Nothing seems normal. How strange
can it be?
Sensory overload – back to my knees.
Temperature changes
and non-adaptation,
These are the things that
bring alienation.
Humbled and quiet, I'm forced
to withdraw,
Back to the place where I can feel it all.

…Petrifying…
…"Am I dying?"…
…"No, you'll stay alive"…

The doc told me this – but
it's overwhelming,
And all I can do is cry.

❦

In 1990, 'twas known as C-F-S,
"Chronic fatigue syndrome," the
diagnosis.
It's really not a name that tells how it is.
Until we know more, we are stuck with
a myth.
Unknown at the time other countries
had named this,
"My-al-gic En-ceph-a-lo-my-e-li-tis:"
The swelling of spinal cord and of the
brain,
Also including severe muscle pain.

    …What is the cause?…
    …We don't know yet…
    …Health destroyed; taken away…

By some mysterious force not
yet understood,
That could crush life all in one day.

❦

As someone who biked and who
camped in the woods,
And loved all of life, trying all that
she could,
"My body will heal. I'll just wait for
that day,
I know I'll be back my original way."
Over time I'm improving, although not
the same,

It will be okay and there's no one
to blame.
I'm sure I can fight this. I know that
I'm strong,
I've never been sick when it has
lasted long.

> …How could I know…
> …It would get worse?…
> …This was only the start…

Nothing prepared me for what was
to come…
Chronic illness that would break
my heart!

As a kid I ran behind the lawn mower,
Then jogged behind baby while pushing
the stroller,
So I thought it would help adding
exercise in;
But muscles were burning – slowed
my regimen.
Although I was able to keep
up part-time,
Physical effort is for me the worst kind.
Sitting and thinking – though different
– could do,
But walking or gardening, my
symptoms renew.

> …We did not know…
> …This could harm me…
> …No one said a thing…

In the early '90s, no one really knew,
No knowledge could anyone bring.

I thought a job change would be what
to do,
So I added to my plate a natural health
school.
I studied for three years to make myself
well,
But couldn't complete – down the
hallways I fell.
Now cognitive troubles, with numbers
a problem,
To read or multitask – not even
an option.
To balance a checkbook would make
my brain freeze,
I needed to know: "Who's watching
over me?"

> …It's Alzheimer's…
> …Or depression…
> …Or MS I fear…

These are the things that ran through
my poor mind,
Not CFS symptoms – severe.

PART II
MY RE-FLU, AND SEVERE CHRONIC ILLNESS
(My age: 35-39)
1995-1999

Zero to one hundred percent on
the scale,
To measure functioning, stronger or
frail.
An easy 100 when I was still well,
But on this re-flu, to 10 percent I fell.
People with CFS, they know "the
lingo,"
Healthy folk can't contemplate all
this jingle.
I hope that they know just how lucky
that is,
To not understand "it" means they
don't have THIS.

> …20 percent…
> …Maybe 30…
> …Oops, "flatlining" again…

This little engine that thought that
she could,
Her DRIVE and WILL could
not defend.

My brain is now tired, my stamina
gone.
Everything's slower, my thoughts take
too long.
Energy's draining right out from my
feet,
What odd sensations starting to repeat.
This herb – no, that med – oh, yes,
it is this one.

Oops, maybe not – I am worse now!
So not fun.
Time to pray harder and witness
it healed,
"They" say this is done in the large
Quantum Field.

> …When I exert…
> …When I think hard…
> …When I talk too long…

That's when I end up in bed
"paying back,"
Just wondering what went wrong.

Too sick to work after second flu onset,
Insurance for illness, a long fight to
get it.
Too ill to sort out all this crazy stuff,
With a union and doctor, it still felt
quite rough.
Never dreaming I'd need disability pay,
At age thirty-five; and still get to this
day,
For an illness I never had heard of
before.
On work and on play, it had closed all
the doors.

> …I am lucky…
> …To have had help…
> …And some financial aid…

And though one could never live
on that amount,
It has helped me along the way.

❧

Leaving professions and schooling
behind,
Leaving my social life – could I rewind?
Leaving the dreams and the goals that
I made,
These were the hardest of all to
have fade.
Some jobs were left for me so I was
grateful,
Still a mother and wife, though my
health had a big fall.
Parts of my life remained – they were
still there.
Thank God 'cause it helps with the
losses I bear.

    …Loving family…
    …A home and friends…
    …A CFS doctor, too…

These were the important things that
were left,
That always kept me moving through.

❧

Have to stop all exercise that I love now,
No physical working – spread two tasks
out somehow.
No dancing, no yard work, no biking,
no fun.
Walking is hard – never mind a
good run.
Stay connected to others, and share
their life stories,

Hear their celebrations, their bad times,
and glories.
Living vicariously I don't always mind,
But I hear my heart break when I must
stay behind.

    …When the pain strikes…
    …When my brain hurts…
    …With my muscles weak…

Leaving a mere shell of myself behind,
I have to continue to seek.

❧

Lab tests and blood work and alternate
care,
Resting and charting – Don't worsen a
flare!
Going against all that's natural for me,
How am I able to set myself free?
Denying, justifying, and rationalization,
Everything needing valid explanation.
Or how will the others know just what
I need?
Even with that, I don't always succeed.

    …Can I sit down?…
    …Can't stay too long…
    …Can we do it by phone?…

Needing to always excuse or defend,
I seek respite in my space at home.

❧

Fighting a war inside twenty-four/seven,
Hope it's relieving when I get to
Heaven,
'Cause the "Chronic" in CFS means 'til
I die.
Try to keep suffering low;
functioning high.

This is exhausting for all, you can see,
Including caregivers and my family.
I'm sorry to put them through all of
this stuff,
It has not been my choice – we've all
had enough.

>...Not a fair fight...
>...Erasing my life...
>...With what, we only guess...

But let it be hoped that the enemy
dissolves,
And that God can clean up the rest.

The body works well with two energy
systems,
Aerobic is one, using oxygen pistons.
It's used for sustaining long-term
energy,
But now it's not working – brings me to
my knees.
The other is called the Anaerobic
system,
Not needing oxygen; short, sharp
emission.
Like weights or the one-hundred yard
relay sprint,
Research reveals only this one is "mint."

>...Stairs a mountain...
>...Resting between...
>...Do things differently...

To have a relay for life's work and
demands,
I'd need 50 of me with ME.

Living in quicksand, I find
quite descriptive:
Try to crawl out and the symptoms
get vivid.
Stay in the zone where your energy's
best,
One small part of effort to three parts
of rest.
It sounds do-able, until one has to try it.
After one day, I'm sure you would
despise it.
Like quicksand it feels – doomed, if still
or in fits,
The harder one fights it, the deeper
it gets.

>...Limitations...
>...And restrictions...
>...Special needs galore...

How I wish I could feel solid ground
'neath my feet,
Which I took for granted before.

The payback is named "post-exertional
malaise."
It aggravates illness for months, weeks,
or for days.
It means ... after one exerts any way,
shape, or form,
New symptoms show up – old ones
worsen with scorn.
So instead of exertion that's making
us "stronger,"
The system is goofy – It's making us
"wronger."
Post-exertion relapse is one
diagnostic key,
And this type of relapse brings me to
my knees.

…Doomed if I do…
…Doomed if I don't…
…Doing this tightrope dance…

I try to stay grateful to struggle
each day,
Some illnesses don't get a chance.

∾

Orthostatic intolerance is a big
symptom,
It means all "signs" worsen in
upright positions.
The more I sit or stand, the more ill
I feel,
If pushing it, fainting or dizziness reel.
Neurological problems I cannot control,
Blood pressure, blood volume down,
heart rate that soars.
When upright my mind needs more
blood than supplied,
One symptom, hard – never mind the
whole pie.

　　…Keep your legs up…
　　…Keep your head down…
　　…Try some salt and meds…

How can I live life the way I was meant,
When lying on the floor instead?

∾

Another loud symptom is that of pain,
In Fibro 'n CFS, it makes many lame.
All kinds of pain are prominently there,
I have spine pain and bone pain and at
times my hair!
The treatment for pain is to give things
a test,
Small doses of this or that –
try to get rest.

Some need to use the most
powerful drugs,
Even morphine hardly gives theirs
a tug.

　　…We can't bear it…
　　…Always hurting…
　　…Why the chronic pain?…

Sometimes the chaos inside of ME,
Could drive a sound person insane.

∾

No cure, no treatment that's standard
for care yet,
Coping and pacing and
symptom management.
Finding new ways to conserve energy,
New choices in lifestyle – no "style" do
I see.
Things that I learned were unhealthy
to do,
Now all have changed – the CFS doc
knew:
Eat lots of salt, lots of protein from
meat,
Stop moving your body, and stay off
your feet.

　　…I'll just lie here…
　　…Resting my brain…
　　…Trying to heal this "mess"…

But even imagining a bird in flight,
Is putting me to the test.

PART III
TREATMENT, SETBACKS, POLITICS, AND FAMILY
(My Age: 40 to 44)
2000-2004

My immune system's different, not
working the same,
No more colds for me, no more flus
to tame.
Even when others around me get sick,
These are the things that I no
longer get.
Instead symptoms worsen, like
weakness and pain,
I have learned my body and brain
can inflame.
In our sick immune systems, markers
they find,
One more bit of proof that it's not in
our minds.

> …Where is the switch?…
> …Back to balance…
> …To work as it did before…

It's one neuro-endocrine-
immune disease,
Or N.E.I.D. for short.

∽

No bleeding, no bandages, no
broken bones,
Looking quite normal when out of
our homes.
A strange thing for all, invisible disease,
'Cause people can't believe how sick we
can be.

One patient wrote a book; the title
she picked,
I Have CFS But I Don't Look Sick,
Which shows how this frustrates the
patients galore,
For people to believe appearances more.

> …Looking okay…
> …Is a nice thing…
> …But does not mean we're well…

For all kinds of disease that this
applies to,
What's inside is hard to tell.

∽

I deal with doctors who still do not
get it,
And if they do, they might rather
dismiss it.
Nurses who still think that I am
just tired,
"No, I'm not loony or lazy – and you
should be fired."
Presenting and sharing the latest
in testing,
Hoping the doctors find it
worth investing.
The complexity and the difference
in views,
Every so often ends up in abuse.

...Educating...
...Can be deflating...
...But how else can they see?...

That's a big burden for someone unwell,
And it can bring me to my knees.

∽

IVs and needles and supplements to try,
I do things so that my health
doesn't decline.
Bedridden forever, I don't want to be,
I wish there was some form of
a guarantee.
Hot moxibustion and T.C.M. herbals,
This medicine helpful, getting over
hurdles.
Can't try them all at once or I'll break
the bank,
Have to try one by one, see how
they rank.

...This one's helpful...
...That one's doubtful...
...This one makes me worse...

I seem to be working hard just to exist,
How do we remove this CURSE?

∽

There were some treatments I was really
hurt from,
Experimental – they promised me
the sun.
Before we understood CFS at all,
I gave them a chance and I took some
bad falls.
They didn't care or take responsibility,
A near-death experience – no
accountability.

Others have had the same story as this,
Pushing me deeper into the abyss.

...More months in bed...
...Loss of progress...
...Have I lost my mind?...

If someone else asks me what I have
to lose,
The risk–benefit ratio they'll find.

∽

From toxins to mold spores, harmful
heavy metals,
MS to Lyme disease; where
trauma settles,
Coxsackie to Epstein, metabolic disease,
In circles we go – give us one
answer, please.
From body to psyche, from feelings
to karma,
Environment, genetics; don't let it
alarm ya.
This is the confusion that CFS brings,
No known cause or cure yet, so check
out all things.

...Doc, make your mind up...
...What should we treat?...
...Can't it be more clear?...

When dealing with illness with no end
in sight,
It's hard not to live with some fear.

∽

Some say: "What doesn't kill you will
just make you STRONGER."
This is one myth that I believe
no longer.
For ME/CFS, with this I concur:

"What does not kill you will just make
you STRANGER."
Some say: "God doesn't give you more
than you can handle."
Not what I see in the case of
this scandal.
I do think He leaves us with choices
to make,
But having CFS is not our mistake.

>   …Just ignore it…
>   …Just work through it…
>   …Change what's in your head…

A lot of advice like this just makes
no sense,
When suff'ring at home in your bed.

I love nature and music and yoga
and psychics,
Humor and beauty and sunshine in
the mix,
Angels and family and those who
can sing,
These are a few of my favorite things.
Chiropractic treatments and
myofascial release,
Massage and cranio and all kinds
of therapies,
Acupuncture needles that go up
my spine,
These are the things that help keep
me aligned.

>   …It is costly…
>   …Time-consuming…
>   …But it's nurturing too…

I know to be grateful to get such
a chance,
To help myself try to improve.

I think that I've been a good wife
and mother,
I've completely enjoyed all of our
time together.
To let them down is gut-wrenching
for me,
Please don't grow impatient –
it is a disease.
Phases and stages of illness
keep changing,
Just as in life, constantly rearranging.
It's odd how I'm happy for all the
good things,
But then it comes back, and grief is
what it brings.

>   …It's a relapse…
>   …No, a bad crash…
>   …Slow recoveries…

This illness "don't" care if I rest, work,
or play,
It still immobilizes me.

PART IV
ADAPTING TO LIFE WITH CHRONIC ILLNESS
(My Age: 45-49)
2005-2009

With scooters and wheelchairs for
getting around,
Oxygen helps – who knows why –
I have found.
Homebound, or bedbound,
or carbound I feel.
These are the things I wish were not
so real.
Mercury taken out of all my fillings,
Doing it properly, pulling and drilling.
"I'm sure you'll be better –
Oh darn, maybe not."
One more thing I learned that does not
cure this lot.

>...With the research...
>...With the conflict...
>...With the misinformed...

That's when I give up on healing myself,
But only until the next morn.

જી

A celiac diagnosis so many years later,
Wheat, rye, oats, and barley are grains
grown in nature.
An autoimmune disease triggered
by these,
Left me with no choice but a gluten-
free feast.
Reading the labels and learning
the jargon,
Gluten-free food, believe me, is
no bargain.

It's just one more thing making my
freedoms yield.
It wouldn't be difficult if I had healed.

>...I am still trapped...
>...CFS ruled...
>...No relief was had...

Just more cost and separation to
deal with,
How does one not get so mad?

જી

Try to ... stay independent;
prevent isolation,
Who wants to think like a CFS patient?
Stay self-sufficient as best as you can,
But 'til there's improvement, you'll need
a BIG HAND.
I need help in ways I never expected,
Cannot believe it – I once was perfected.
How could this happen just after a flu,
When 30 and healthy, and shiny
and new?

>...Humiliation...
>...And frustration...
>...A pot of emotional stew...

Grief, guilt and fear, anger,
jealousy too;
Disappointment, to name a few.

જી

I miss ... my power, my confidence,
trusting my body,
Learning new things like tai chi
and karate,
Planning and knowing that I will
be there,
Without all the hassles, without all
the care.
I miss ... finances and earning a good
solid dollar,
Traveling afar with my husband
and daughter.
I miss ... the feelings of fitness, well-
being, and strength,
A predictable day 'stead of one
moment's length.

    ...To feel solid...
    ...To feel steady...
    ...Strong in my own way...

Reliable, skillful, and organized too,
"It" disabled all these in one day.

Acceptance, I try to, but how can I
do that?
Affecting my loved ones, I hate what
that feels like.
Fear of leaving all I care for behind,
Makes it so hard to let go with
my mind...
Kindness and caring are soul food
for me;
Compassion and healing
with simplicity.
Slowly and gently I pace out my life,
Keep a loving perspective amidst all
the strife.

...Where it's honest...
...Where it's joyful...
...Where it's peaceful too...

That's where I do well to survive
my mess,
And where you might do well too.

I need... patience, and courage, more
stamina for bearing,
More faith in my spirit, to keep up
the caring;
More perseverance to press for a cure,
More insight to heal; love to keep my
heart pure.
I give friendship and nurturing, I help
where I can,
I'm happy, when able, to massage feet
or hands.
I share info and prayers and a meal now
and then,
Encouraging words to my family
and friends.

    ...Set just small goals...
    ...Value each step...
    ...Do simple things to please...

This is not what I expected at all,
But this illness brings humility.

I can do...light household tasks and
errands that are drive-thru,
Arrange things for others; make lists for
them to do,
Work on the computer for short spurts
of time,
Take care of "my healthcare" and make
these words rhyme.

Pay bills, chat on Facebook, do the
research needed,
Write articles 'bout things I think
should be heeded,
Shop in the mall; travel once in a while,
That wheelchair and scooter let me go
in style.

>...To worsen, easy...
>...To improve, hard...
>...Which way will it go?...

Take nothing for granted with CFS,
'Cause the future we do not know.

PART V
HIDDEN NO MORE
(My Age: 50+)
2010 to the Future

Who will clean the house and make
enough income?
Who will pay the bills and raise all
the children?
Who will take care of our
everyday lives,
While we're out of commission; trying
to survive?
It's easy to say:
"Only do what you can,"
But who does the rest until we take
a stand?
People don't need any more on
their plates,
Who is to take care of us all with
this fate?

  …No place for it…
  …Need to get well…
  …What's the other choice?…

Most do not think 'bout how this life
would be,
Until we all give it a voice.

∾

This hidden illness, its enculturation
Is taking too long and is hurting
the patients.
The functional, bedbound, and a
restored few,
Each has a story worth listening to.

Teens who cannot school and adults
who can't work;
Mothers who can't lift the children they
have birthed.
People from complications who
have died;
And some who took their lives from
suffering denied.

  …Where's the media?…
  …Affecting millions…
  …Needing social change…

No proper care, and few doctors
who know,
There is so much to rearrange.

∾

To each person I've met, I have asked
the same question:
"What do I do with this
suffering damnation?"
I'd get "the look" and not much would
be said.
I thought, "Someone must know this."
No comfort was led.
Years later, I heard the answer to
my query.
It came from inside me, not from
Madame Curie;
"To change things for you and for the
others too,
You use the suffering as a source
of fuel,

...For speaking out...
...Awareness Day...
...Advocacy times"...

The next generation depends on us now,
Not to fight for them would be a crime.

❧

So, I'm telling my story at twenty
years ill.
Child grown, husband travels, gives me
time to kill;
Writing and research when "on"
and awake,
Gives purpose for me when my health is
at stake.
This illness community, global
and strong,
It needs so much help but I'm glad
to belong.
Thank you to everyone working
so hard;
Many are ill, but they still hold
these cards;

...Choosing action...
...And compassion...
...Connecting ME to you...

I believe there is a voice that you can
hear now;
The outcome will be what we do.

❧

The public, the systems, the funding
too slow;
Cost to society? Billions, you know.
You're meeting patients from all walks
of life,
At different stages and phases of strife.

So now that you know the "new" illness
on the block,
And know some people who have to
"walk the talk,"
If everyone can move toward the
same goal,
Better outcomes, a cure, and some rest
for our souls.

...A worthy cause...
... Justifiable...
... Money, time, energy...

Underdog no longer with you by
our sides,
We will have a winning team.

❧

With science and politics
working together,
An official apology to help remember,
That research, education, and good
patient care,
Can follow our efforts: Speak up if
we dare.
There's so much more now that
is understood,
About why we're ill and what's under
our hoods.
With your help and ours,
in cooperation,
The future is hopeful for all of
the nations.

...Fund the research...
...Talk to government...
...Help to move us along...

We can do more now than ever before,
To right the many past wrongs.

❧

Some family and good friends and
doctors keep sharing,
Scientists who research and really
are caring.
They keep the hope up for us to
hang on,
Without them, it would be hard
to belong.
So I say thank you to all those
beside me,
Can't always tell you the good that I
do see.
I'm still sure you know how much that
I care,
But for the illness, I'd always be there.

    …ME/CFS…
    …Neuro-immune disease…
    …These are hidden no more…

Some day they'll put all the pieces
in one,
And then all of us…WILL SOAR.

THE CHRONIC-CALL

Poem with Notes

PART I
SUDDEN FLU-LIKE ONSET
(My Age: 30 to 34)
1990-1994

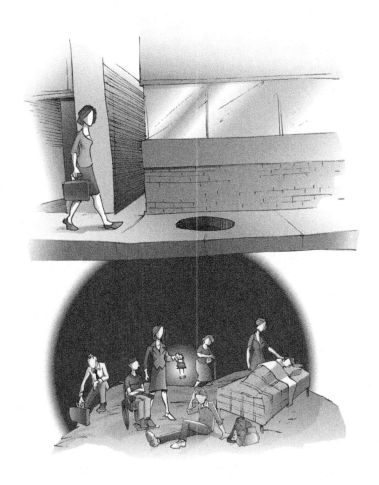

STANZAS 1-8 TOPICS

STANZA 1

Bizarre symptoms

Chinooks and low clouds and changes in pressure,
Full moons and melting and things you can't measure,
Perfumes and diesel and food allergies,
These are the things that *bring me to my knees.*

Poor memory, no focus, and wrong word retrieval,
Numbness and tingling, *Bell's palsy* – sounds evil.
Sleep deprivation and low energies,
Blood pressure drops that bring me to my knees.

…When I stand up…
…When I sit down…
…When I walk a while…

Symptoms galore visit all of my self,
Leaving me slumped in a pile.

STANZA 1 NOTES

🎐 *Chinooks and low clouds and changes in pressure* – When my story began to flow out in poem/song, these were the first words that came to mind due to how I was feeling that day.

One very notable symptom that came with my onset of CFS was sensitivity to weather, including any type of shift or change in it, and especially the barometric pressure. My parents have a decorative glass barometer with a spout that hangs in their country kitchen. It is filled with colored water that responds to external changes and pressure. You can see the water level increase and push its way out of the spout as the pressure decreases, and it lowers and settles inside the container when the pressure increases.

The body mechanism that controls and adjusts my blood volume and blood pressure seems to be broken: I tend to react like the glass barometer without a regulator in place. When the barometric pressure rises, I go down; when the pressure goes down, I come up. My symptoms worsen up to twenty-four hours before a weather change. Other patients with the illness report similar debilitating responses to weather changes.

Science has suggested these problems may be due to decreased blood volume in some ME/CFS patients,[8] as well as heart and blood pressure problems. The inability for the cells to use oxygen properly was part of some research studies in 2012.[9] Eventually I started using oxygen at two liters/minute from a tank at home to bring some relief, but this weather sensitivity is very hard on me because it is beyond my control.

🎐 *Bring me to my knees* – This is a theme throughout my story. I use the phrase both literally and as a metaphor to describe my need to surrender to severe symptoms. Sometimes it is physically true because I have trouble remaining standing due to blood pressure changes and energy depletion, so I end up close to the ground, lying or sitting. Other times, it is an emotional or spiritual metaphor. Another metaphor I use for surrender is raising an imaginary white flag. I started this early when I was still able to function and participate more in life. When the symptoms just took over and I was unable to do any more or even to quietly be with my family, I coped by retreating to the bedroom for more rest and quiet to regain some strength. It often felt like both an internal and external war was going on, and that raising that white flag allowed for it to pause.

---

8   Hurwitz, et al, "Chronic Fatigue Syndrome: Illness Severity, Sedentary Lifestyle, Blood Volume and Evidence of Diminished Cardiac Function," Clinical Science. 2009. 118, 125-135. www.ncbi.nlm.nih.gov/pubmed/19469714 (accessed July 20, 2016).

9   Light AR, et al., "Gene expression alterations at baseline and following moderate exercise in patients with chronic fatigue syndrome and fibromyalgia syndrome." J Intern Med. 2012 Jan; 271(1): 64-81. C. Johnson explores other studies on exercise at www.healthrising.org/blog/2013/04/17/are-oxygen-starved-tissues-causing-pain-and-fatigue-in-fibromyalgia-and-chronic-fatigue-syndrome-mecfs (accessed July 6, 2016).

❧ **Bell's palsy** – I had paralysis of the nerves on the left side of my face – an early symptom of my illness. My left eye drooped, my cheek hung down, and to this day, although my face appears even, the sensation in the left side of my head, face, and brain is different from the right. Viral infections, as well as Lyme disease, are some known causes of Bell's palsy. I have only heard of a few other people who have had this diagnosis along with chronic fatigue syndrome. In Chapter 1, "A Fortunate ME/CFS Patient?" Corinne mentions Bell's palsy in the early phase of her ME/CFS history.

❧ **Sleep deprivation** is common in ME/CFS because the body becomes deregulated and sleep quality is poor and not refreshing. There are many types of sleep dysfunction. Some people with ME/CFS sleep eighteen hours a day, some not at all, and others get their rhythms mixed up so they end up sleeping all day and are up all night. I remember that at one point, I simply stopped sleeping altogether. Sleep medications, natural remedies, and good sleep hygiene were the first things my CFS doctor helped me with. Although I still follow my physician's advice, mornings remain the worst part of my day because I wake up feeling horrible – like I haven't slept at all. This was the case prior to the use of sleep medication as well, except then I was awake all night with no respite.

As an example of how our contorted sleep patterns affect everyday life, I've had to take into account people's patterns and "energy envelopes" while working on this book. When I need to contact someone, I stop to think: *Oh yes, this person doesn't wake until 11:00 a.m. This one is only awake at night. I should email this one because he sleeps in the day. This one has been relapsed for a week, so do not bother her now.* And, of course, I am juggling my own strange, ever-changing schedule. It's a miracle we get anything done.

STANZA 2

Onset

Two or three weeks after *getting a flu,*
I was not any better so what should I do?
I had *symptoms of nausea, thirst, hunger, weight loss,*
Body-temp changes and blood pressure drops.

It was only the flu so just how could this be?
My anatomy books came in handy to see,
That my brain is involved – it's the master control.
When I told the docs, they gave their eyes a roll.

   …Decades later…
   …Thru the research…
   …Was confirmed the piece…

That part of the brain can be harmed in this way;
How did flu become *complex disease?*

STANZA 2 NOTES

🎕 *Getting a flu* – This "flu" started out normally enough. It was a lovely summer afternoon in mid-July. My baby daughter, almost a year old, sat in her car seat and my husband drove us on our very typical three-hour journey to my parents' home. My extended family was meeting there for the celebration of my grandmother's eighty-eighth birthday. On our way, about an hour into the trip, we made a brief stop in a small city so my husband could do some business. All of a sudden, a sweep of nausea and weakness came over me. There were very few other symptoms. By the time we traveled the remaining two hours, I felt very ill. All of my cousins, aunts and uncles, my sisters and their families, and of course my parents, were there. I sat through the outside party quietly hoping I would soon feel better. It was the day that changed my life and the lives of those around me.

🎕 *Symptoms of nausea, thirst, hunger, weight loss, body temperature changes, and blood pressure drops* – These were symptoms that started after that first day and lasted for a few months. Eventually, my sleep patterns and quality of sleep also changed. I had always been interested in the body and how it worked. I'd needed some anatomy basics to become an aerobics instructor and had continued learning more in that area. When I checked my physiology books to find out what controlled all these symptomatic areas, I learned that one possibility was the hypothalamus in the brain – one of the major control centers for the body. I did attempt to relate this to my doctor, but because there was not much understood about the illness at that time, nothing more came of my theory.

Years later, science proved that the hypothalamic-pituitary-adrenal axis is dysfunctional in some people with CFS. This complex neuro-immune communication system works in a negative feedback network to regulate the adrenal gland's hormonal activities.

"This tiny pea-shaped gland in the brain regulates a number of functions, including hormone secretion," Dr. Charles Shepherd of the U.K. explains. "Problems here could help explain symptoms as diverse as sleep disorders, low blood pressure, temperature disturbance, and heart, bowel, and bladder problems…" [10] This is only one piece of the puzzle, however. Dr. Shepherd became ill with ME in the late 'seventies after catching chickenpox from a patient with shingles. He had been well up until that time. Dr. Shepherd is the medical advisor to the ME Association in the U.K. and has spent the last two decades vigorously fighting the "all in the mind" attitude, which he says is still common among medical professionals there.

🎕 *Complex disease* – Over the years, clinicians and researchers have come up with many theories as to what is actually happening in a person with ME/CFS: Some suggest brain

---

10 "Daily Telegraph talks to Dr. Charles Shepherd." 26 Nov 2012, U.K. www.telegraph.co.uk/news/health/news/9699911/ME-isnt-all-in-the-mind-but-its-still-a-mystery.html (accessed July 10, 2016).

and nervous system involvement, while others lean towards viral and infection involvement or immune system issues. We're hopeful that researchers will soon find the root of this complex problem, which involves so many body systems, so they can finally put the many research pieces together.

STANZA 3

Career, motherhood, fatigue, and diagnosis (epidemic or endemic?)

A career of fifteen years as a court reporter,
Quick as a hummingbird – solid as mortar.
Asleep now in the car after I'd get to work,
Unable to keep up the shorthand I took.

From someone who did teach aerobics at lunch hour,
Who gardened and traveled – at hard work did not cower,
Now my baby seems heavier – muscles are weak,
Disoriented driving and it's hard to speak.

　　…Doc, what is wrong?…
　　…Something serious…
　　…My world is falling apart…

She said, *"I think you have something quite new:*
Chronic fatigue syndrome, sweetheart."

STANZA 3 NOTES

✖ *Asleep now in the car after I'd get to work* – I would never have called my experience fatigue. This is the "F-word" of CFS. Fatigue is normal tiredness or sleepiness from a long day. I was left immobilized or exhausted, like many people feel when they get the flu. The English language doesn't seem to have words that adequately convey or describe this experience. ✈

Patients have offered all kinds of descriptions of the exhaustion they feel, including "bone-crushing," and "like walking in mud up to your waist." One patient recently expressed the feeling as a collapse from prostration, which is a medical term that means "from complete physical or mental exhaustion." This comes close to how I would describe the severity of this symptom and my experience with it. Fatigue has many forms, according to L. Jason et al. in the study titled "Examining Types of Fatigue Among Individuals With ME/CFS." [11] These include:

Post-Exertional Fatigue: In this type, a person feels extremely weak, uncomfortable, or sick after minimal activity.

Wired Fatigue: In this type, a patient feels extremely low-energy, leading to a feeling of over-stimulation with a major sign of maladaptive stress.

Brain Fog Fatigue: In this type, a person experiences extreme mental fatigue, which is far more serious than physical fatigue. Mental fatigue involves confusion, disorientation, and the inability to function normally in daily activities.

Flu-like Fatigue: In this type, the patient feels weak with flu symptoms, high temperature, and sore glands.

Energy Fatigue: In this type, the patient experiences heaviness, immobilization, and depleted energy and is unable to do any activity for long periods. This is generally experienced in the first three months of illness or during a temporary relapse.

The Diagnostic Criteria Worksheet from the International Association for CFS/ME's *Primer for Clinical Practitioners* (IACFS/ME, 2014)[12] describes the fatigue of ME/CFS as "Pathological fatigue – a significant degree of new onset, unexplained, persistent or recurrent physical and/or mental fatigue that substantially reduces activity levels and which is not the result of ongoing exertion and is not relieved by rest."

---

11   Jason et al. "Examining Types of Fatigue Among Individuals With ME/CFS." Disability Studies Quarterly, Vol. 29, No 3. 2009. dsq-sds.org/article/view/938/1113 (accessed July 10, 2016).

12   IACFS/ME (International Association for Chronic Fatigue Syndrome/Myalgic Encephalomyelitis). 2014. "ME/CFS Primer for Clinical Practitioners." Chicago, IL: ME/CFS Clinical Diagnostic Criteria Worksheet. 12. http://iacfsme. org/portals/0/pdf/Primer_Post_2014_conference.pdf (accessed July 10, 2016).

🌿 *From someone who did teach aerobics at lunch hour* – As a kid, I was always in a hurry to get my chores done so that I could ride my bike, play softball, or do something with my friends. I have loved physical activity and sports all my life. I played sports in school all the way through college, and I trained as an aerobics instructor during my working years because I also loved music and dance. I worked as a court reporter in the local Queen's Bench Court House. Between courtroom assignments, my colleagues and I would quickly change into our workout clothes and hit our exercise room for forty-five minutes of aerobics. We had a great time. This is one of my fondest memories, and the inability to remain physically active due to ME/CFS is one of my deepest losses.

I still wear my runners regularly, regardless of my inability to walk very far. In the early days of my illness, I set them next to my bed, expecting to jump into them the next morning and hit the floor running. I don't remember how long it took for me to fully comprehend that this was not going to happen. Many new ME/CFS patients have told me that they too fully expect to wake up well every day. When you're young and able and you suddenly become drastically ill, it is natural to believe that the illness is temporary. For many with ME/CFS, unfortunately, it is not temporary.

🌿 *Now my baby seems heavier* – When I came down with that first flu, my daughter was almost a year old. I was physically fit and strong, lifting and carrying her with ease. Suddenly, a week or two after this flu, she felt heavy for me to lift and carry; a remarkable change. This was one important sign of new muscle weakness that I reported to the doctor.

🌿 *"I think you have something quite new."* – I realize now that chronic fatigue syndrome had only been named as an illness in 1987, and I was diagnosed in 1990. Cluster outbreaks of this unrecognized illness had occurred in various locations across North America since 1984, and the U.S. Centers for Disease Control and Prevention ended up giving it the label *chronic fatigue syndrome*.

As I look back, I can see that I was fairly fortunate to receive a quick diagnosis. My young, female family doctor, originally from South Africa, had a good grasp of this syndrome which was fairly new to North America. She diagnosed me by my sudden onset, history, and symptom presentation. My blood work was normal, which is often the case with CFS, and no other tests were recommended. In spite of the diagnosis, no treatment was available.

Currently, by most CFS diagnostic criteria, an adult has to be ill for at least six months with specific symptoms, and there needs to be a substantial reduction in activity levels before a diagnosis can be made. In children, a diagnosis can be made in three months. That is a long time to be ill, and perhaps worsening, before you know what you are dealing with. People may see ten medical professionals over a period of many years before a diagnosis is made. The International Association for CFS/ME's *Primer for Clinical Practitioners* (IACFS/ME, 2014), page 7 states: "Although considerable media attention has been given to ME/CFS, most patients with the illness have not been diagnosed." [13] [14]

Finding a biomarker for the illness has been a research goal for decades. A biomarker will enable a faster, more efficient, and more accurate diagnosis. This is the case with other diseases such as HIV/AIDS and diabetes which can now be confirmed by blood tests. These tests prove the presence of the illness without needing to exclude every other similar condition – benefiting patients and doctors alike – while lowering medical costs at the same time.

Little did I know that I was becoming part of the statistics in Canada, along with the growing numbers of people who had become ill with chronic fatigue syndrome since the early 'eighties. In 1990, I felt like I had a rare and isolated illness and did not know of others with the condition. It was very interesting for me to learn much later on that there were epidemics in different locations in North America around that same time – and for years before in other countries.

A Canadian doctor, Byron Hyde, MD, is the founder of the Nightingale Research Foundation, which is dedicated to the study and treatment of CFS and related illness, starting with myalgic encephalomyelitis (ME). Dr. Hyde has had an interest in ME and CFS since its early days in North America in 1984. Instructed by previous researchers of these epidemics, he has traveled around the world investigating ME/CFS epidemics in the United States, the United Kingdom, Australia, New Zealand, and Iceland. These epidemics are listed in his book *The Clinical and Scientific Basis of Myalgic Encephalomyelitis/ Chronic Fatigue Syndrome.* [15]

I have chosen some quotes to tie the timing together with my own illness onset in July 1990 in Canada, as well as with the onset of chronic fatigue syndrome in North America.

"1984 ... From 1984 until 1992 [at publication of this text], an endemic period occurred in which an unusually large number of clusters and epidemics of ME/CFS have been recognized in North America. After an apparent initial increase in morbidity in 1983 there seemed to have appeared in late summer of 1984 an unprecedented increase of sporadic

---

13   Jason LA, et al. "A Community-based Study of Chronic Fatigue Syndrome. Archives of Internal Medicine." 1999. Oct 11: 159 (18): 2129-37.

14   Reyes M, et al. "Prevalence and Incidence of Chronic Fatigue Syndrome in Wichita, Kansas." Archives of Internal Medicine. 2003 Jul 14; 163 (13); 1530-6.

15   Hyde B, editor. "The Clinical and Scientific Basis of Myalgic Encephalomyelitis Chronic Fatigue Syndrome." 1992. The Nightingale Research Foundation. The full list with citations can be found under, "A Bibliography of ME/CFS Epidemics." (176-186). This list begins with 1934, ends in 1990, and has 63 entries, although there have been as many as 75 epidemics of illness similar in symptoms to ME/CFS since 1934. www.nightingale.ca (accessed July 10, 2016).

and epidemic[16] cases across North America. Although certain geographical hot spots seem to have taken up much of the medical interest, this endemic[17] situation probably represents an unusual and unremitting morbidity[18] in all areas of the United States and Canada. Some of the clusters and epidemics are listed."

The next entry in Dr. Hyde's text is the fifty-fourth epidemic mentioned, which is an important one for chronic fatigue syndrome:

"1984 ... Epidemic 54. Incline Village, Lake Tahoe, Nevada Epidemic, August – September. This community epidemic, apparently started in a girls' basketball team, then involved primarily teachers in at least three high schools, and then large numbers of the community. A large number of lay and medical publications have been generated. "[19]

"Epidemic 56 ... Montreal, Quebec & Ontario, Canada – Labour Day epidemic, Montreal, S. O'Sullivan…Over 500 cases of ME/CFS documented in Ontario during the August-November 1984 period ... This endemic was active in all parts of Canada during this period and appears [to] have maintained its activity until the time of writing in 1991. "[20]

"1985... Epidemic 58. Lyndonville Epidemic – New York – This was an epidemic involving children and adults and was described by Dr. David S. Bell in his book 'The Disease With a Thousand Names'. "

These are important dates and places which were changing many lives; but most of us had no idea what was happening to us and didn't know that others were experiencing the same symptoms and serious illness. Some of the doctors in North America who became experienced in these epidemics are still involved in the illness community more than three decades later and are the pioneers and leaders in the field. (See Dr. D. Bell's story, "The Early Days" in Section 2)

---

16 A widespread occurrence of an infectious disease in a community at a particular time.

17 An endemic state for a disease is one that is in a steady state, not rising rapidly nor dying out on its own.

18 The presence of disease.

19 Buchwald D, Cheney PR, Peterson DL, et al. "A chronic illness characterized by fatigue, neurologic and immunologic disorders and active human herpes virus type 6 infection." Annals of Internal Medicine. 1992 Vol.11; 103-113.

20 Gray JA, "Some long-term sequelae of Coxsackie B virus infection." JR Coll Pract 1984; 34:3-5.

STANZA 4

Am I dying?

Bright lights and things that are too stimulating,
Things that the healthy find invigorating.
Nothing seems normal. How strange can it be?
Sensory overload ✂ – back to my knees.

Temperature changes and non-adaptation,
These are the things that bring alienation.
Humbled and quiet, I'm forced to withdraw,
Back to the place where I can feel it all.

    …Petrifying…
    …*"Am I dying?"* ✂…
    …"No, you'll stay alive"…

The doc told me this – but it's overwhelming,
And all I can do is cry.

STANZA 4 NOTES

❧ *Sensory overload* – This refers to the symptom of hypersensitivities to sensory stimuli, such as light, sound, smells, touch, and temperature. These extreme sensitivities are common to ME/CFS patients in certain phases and severities of illness. It is also known as "overload phenomena" and includes emotional overload. Many ME/CFS patients tell me they experience migraines, dizziness, and even seizures from stimulation of any type.

At certain times in my illness, I was unable to watch TV or use a computer because the visual stimulation created confusion and pain and worsened all my other symptoms. Smells such as perfumes, laundry detergents, and even aromas from certain flowers, especially Easter lilies, made me feel more ill. All sounds were overwhelming and exhausting. To this day, I am only able to take busy or chaotic environments for limited periods of time and only in my better hours. Many people with ME/CFS need to spend a lot of time in quiet, dimly lit, relaxing areas that are clear of scents and are moderate in temperature. Safe, protective, and environmentally-friendly areas are important for the ability to heal and to avoid flare-ups. The avoidance of stressful environments and people is helpful. This, of course, is not easy to do in a busy family or in our chaotic world.

❧ *"Am I dying?"* – There were times that I felt so sick that I thought I was dying. It is not uncommon for CFS-knowledgeable doctors to answer the question "Am I dying?" with "The good news is that you are not dying, and the bad news is that you are not dying."

This really sums up how extremely difficult enduring CFS is. The doctors who work with CFS patients realize how very sick their patients can be and how frightening it is. To feel that ill and not understand why you are feeling that way can be petrifying. In one breath I thought, *I hope I am not dying*, and in the next, *I wish I were*.

As you continue reading, you will learn that ME/CFS actually has no bottom to its severity or complexity. So many of us have had the belief, *Well, it can't get any worse*. Unfortunately, for many of us, it does get worse. Knowing that it can get worse is important. I know I did not understand or believe it possible at the beginning of my illness. Nor did the people around me. I might have been better prepared and sought out expert support earlier had I known.

For medical professionals, patients, and their loved ones to take this illness seriously is so important. Having updated knowledge and care can relieve so much stress and suffering. Even good care and support do not guarantee that worsening will not occur, but it may at least help alleviate the symptoms and the emotional burdens that come with the illness.

STANZA 5

Illness labels and definitions for CFS, ME, and ME/CFS

In 1990, 'twas known as C-F-S,
"Chronic fatigue syndrome," ✎ the diagnosis.
It's really not a name that tells how it is.
Until we know more, we are stuck with a myth.

Unknown at the time other countries had named this,
"My-al-gic En-ceph-a-lo-my-e-li-tis:" ✎
The swelling of spinal cord and of the brain,
Also including severe muscle pain.

> …What is the cause?…
> …We don't know yet…
> …Health destroyed; taken away…

By some mysterious force not yet understood,
That could crush life all in one day.

STANZA 5 NOTES

❧ *Chronic Fatigue Syndrome (CFS)* – The name chronic fatigue syndrome can be traced to a working group convened by the U.S. Centers for Disease Control [21] (CDC) in 1987 in response to illness outbreaks, which began in 1984 in Nevada,[22] New York State,[23] and other areas in the United States. The group looked at the "symptom complex" being called chronic Epstein-Barr virus infection or chronic mononucleosis syndrome. Other labels in use at that time included Raggedy Ann syndrome, post-viral fatigue syndrome, and the yuppie flu.[24]

The U.S. outbreaks were similar in nature and symptoms to numerous outbreaks of myalgic encephalomyelitis (ME), which had occurred in many parts of the world prior to 1984.[25] Despite this, the CDC group labeled the condition as new and published a case definition for it known as the Holmes criteria[26] which primarily focused on the symptom of chronic fatigue. The Fukuda definition that succeeded it in 1994 was also created by the CDC[27] to standardize CFS research, and it similarly focused on fatigue. As of 2016, the Fukuda definition is still widely utilized for research studies as well as for diagnosis. Many claim it is too broad, allowing those with both physical and psychiatric illness to be captured, which creates misleading outcomes for research. Other CFS definitions – i.e., those with a singular focus on fatigue – include Oxford (1991) and Reeves (also known as the Empirical definition, 2005).

Patients and advocacy organizations have been trying to change the CFS label since it was named, arguing that it is vague and trivializing. They are not alone in making this assertion.[28] It should be noted, however, that a considerable amount of fruitful biomedi-

---

21 Later to be named Centers for Disease Control and Prevention.

22 Notably Incline Village, Nevada, where Drs. Peterson and Cheney were in practice. Remarks from Dr. Peterson can be found in Section 2.

23 Notably in Lyndonville, upper New York State where Dr. Bell had his practice. More information about Dr. Bell can be found in Section 2.

24 Chronic Fatigue Immune Dysfunction Syndrome (CFIDS) is still used by some. Chronic Fatigue Immune Dysfunction Syndrome (CFIDS) is a name proposed by researcher, Dr. Seymour Grufferman, in the late 1980s to differentiate the condition from ordinary chronic fatigue. See Dr. David Bell's book, "A Doctor's Guide to Chronic Fatigue Syndrome: Understanding, Treating and Living with CFIDS," 1994 Revised edition of "A Disease of a Thousand Names."

25 See Stanza 3.

26 Holmes GP, et al. 1988. "Chronic fatigue syndrome: A working case definition." Annals of Internal Medicine 108(3): 387-389. annals.org/article.aspx?articleid=701163 (accessed July 27, 2016).

27 Fukuda K, et al. 1994. "The chronic fatigue syndrome: A comprehensive approach to its definition and study." Annals of Internal Medicine 121(12): 953-959. annals.org/article.aspx?articleid=708271 (accessed July 27, 2016).

28 The Institute of Medicine committee agreed with this, stating: "…the term "chronic fatigue syndrome" often results in stigmatization and trivialization and should no longer be used as a name of this illness." IOM (Institute of Medicine). 2015. "Beyond myalgic encephalomyelitis/chronic fatigue syndrome: Redefining an illness." The National Academies Press. Washington, DC. 60. www.nationalacademies.org/hmd/Reports/2015/ME-CFS.aspx (accessed July 27, 2016).

cal research has been ongoing under the CFS label over the years, particularly in the United States.

✿ *Myalgic Encephalomyelitis (ME)* – "Myalgic encephalomyelitis (ME) is a distinct systemic disease characterized, primarily, by a central nervous system dysfunction that impacts all body systems." [29] Benign myalgic encephalomyelitis was a term coined in an editorial in the *Lancet* in 1956 to describe patients who became ill in multiple epidemics, including one at the Royal Free Hospital in London.[30] (*my* = muscle; *algic* = pain; *encephalo* = brain; *myel* = spinal cord; *itis* = inflammation). ME had many prior names, including atypical poliomyelitis, Royal Free disease, Iceland disease, epidemic neuromyasthenia[31] and post-viral fatigue syndrome. Historical figures such as Florence Nightingale and Charles Darwin suffered from a similar illness as far back as the mid-1800s.

Even in early reports it was noted that the condition described had "the same pattern of neurological illness with myalgia, pareses, and sensory phenomenon and quite distinct from poliomyelitis…" [32] In 1969, benign ME was classified as a disease of the nervous system in the ninth revision of the World Health Organization's (WHO) *International Classification of Diseases*, the ICD-9. The word "benign" continues to be used in their current ICD-10[33] classification but has been dropped from general usage as the disease, although not usually fatal, is anything but benign.

The first comprehensive description of the multi-systemic condition ME was by Melvin Ramsay.[34] Other case definitions for myalgic encephalomyelitis (ME) include: London criteria 1994; Hyde 2007; Goudsmit 2009; and the International ME definition (Carruthers, et al. 2011).

---

29 www.ncf-net.org/faq-home.htm#4National CFIDS Foundation (accessed July 15, 2016).

30 Galpine JF, "Benign Myalgic Encephalomyelitis." The British Journal of Clinical Practice, Vol. 12, No. 3, March, 1958. me-ireland.com/ME1958.doc (accessed July 5, 2016). Acheson ED. "The Clinical Syndrome variously called Benign Myalgic Encephalomyelitis, Iceland Disease and Epidemic Neuromyasthenia." American Journal of Medicine 1959 Vol 26, Issue 4. www.meresearch.org.uk/wp-content/uploads/2012/11/Acheson_AmJMed.pdf (accessed July 25, 2016).

31 This was a term which at least one author (Acheson, 1959) noted was unfortunately close to neurasthenia (a term formerly used for a psychological disorder characterized by fatigue and weakness).

32 Galpine. 1958. op. cit.

33 The coding is for post-viral fatigue syndrome and includes both benign myalgic encephalomyelitis and chronic fatigue syndrome (a connection which was added in 1992) under the same neurological category G93.3 (other disorders of the brain). This can be revised by each country. Canada has the same categorization but the U.S. clinical modification, in force October 1, 2015, is an exception with a code for both ME and post-viral fatigue syndrome (under G93.3 neurological) and a different one for CFS (under R 53.82 malaise and fatigue – signs, symptoms and abnormal clinical and lab findings, not elsewhere classified).

34 Ramsay AM, 1986. "Myalgic Encephalomyelitis: A baffling syndrome with a tragic aftermath." ME Action U.K. terms this "the definitive description of ME." www.meactionuk.org.uk/ramsey.html (accessed July 10, 2016). Also see Dowsett EG, "Redefinitions of ME/CFS: a 20th century phenomenon." www.name-us.org/DefintionsPages/DefinitionsArticles/DefinitionsBy%20Dowsett.pdf (accessed July 5, 2016).

The case definition for ME/CFS (Carruthers, et al. 2003 known as the CCC),[35] is also widely considered an ME definition. It is the foundation of this book. See ME/CFS below.

Myalgic Encephalomyelitis/Chronic Fatigue Syndrome (ME/CFS) is an umbrella term created in 2003 by an international panel of experts. The definition, which describes a complex physical illness, is now commonly referred to as the Canadian Consensus Criteria (CCC), (Appendix A). (In the U.K., CFS/ME is also used as an umbrella term but has different criteria.)[36]

The criteria and the names of ME and CFS were combined in the CCC for a number of reasons, including dissatisfaction with the name CFS alone – which fails to communicate the seriousness of the illness – as well as research showing that the term ME is taken more seriously by medical professionals.[37] This decision also joined patients with similar experiences around the globe.

ME/CFS (or CFS/ME) are not labels that are used to code the illness in any country.

Some patients and professionals feel that ME/CFS should *not* be used as the name of the illness, preferring ME for many reasons. In addition to the concerns that the label, chronic fatigue syndrome, trivializes the illness and has a focus on fatigue, some feel that adding the name and history of CFS to ME confuses the distinct illness of ME as described by the respected ME definitions mentioned previously. As noted in Mary Dimmock and Matthew Lazell-Fairman's Background paper, "Thirty Years of Disdain": [38]

> "Finally, the CCC established the term 'ME/CFS', intending it to be a bridging term until the term 'ME' was adopted. With hindsight, many now see that this likely contributed to the definitional confusion."

---

35   See Appendix A for this definition: Carruthers BM, Jain AK, De Meirleir KL, Peterson DL, Klimas NG, Lerner AM, Bested AC, Flor-Henry P, Joshi P, Powles ACP, Sherkey JA, van de Sande MI "Myalgic Encephalomyelitis/Chronic Fatigue Syndrome: Clinical Working Case Definition, Diagnostic and Treatment Protocols." J CFS 11(1):7-115, 2003. www.mefmaction.com/images/stories/Medical/ME-CFS-Consensus-Document.pdf (accessed July 5, 2016).

36   The U.K. Report of the CFS/ME working group, "Report to the Chief Medical Officer of an Independent Working Group." January 2002 noted re: terminology on page 5, "While awaiting such a solution (a consensus on definition and terminology), the Working Group suggests that the composite term CFS/ME is used as an umbrella term and considered as one condition or a spectrum of disease for the purposes of this report." www.erythos.com/gibsonen-quiry/docs/cmoreport.pdf. (accessed July 14, 2016).

37   Jason LA, Taylor RR, Plioplys S, Stepanek Z, Shlaes J. "Evaluating attributions for an illness based upon the name: chronic fatigue syndrome, myalgic encephalopathy and Florence Nightingale disease." Am J Community Psychol, 2002 Feb; 30(1): 133-48. "Abstract:…findings indicated that the name, chronic fatigue syndrome, may be regarded less seriously than the Myalgic Encephalopathy name with respect to some important aspects of the illness. In this study, specialty of medical trainee also played a role in how the illness was perceived."

38   Dimmock M, and Lazell-Fairman M, "Thirty Years of Disdain" (Background) December 2015. p 45. http://bit.ly/The_Burial_of_ME_Background (accessed July 26, 2016).

On the other hand, some people with a CFS diagnosis are concerned about how ME has been researched and treated in the United Kingdom and do not want those associations with their illness: ME has been psychologized with cognitive behavioral therapy (CBT) and graded exercise therapy (GET) as the only treatments offered. CBT and GET have dominated the studies regarding treatment for ME in the United Kingdom.

These modalities, CBT and GET, as described in the study trials, are not curative, have some benefit for a few, and have caused harm for some. Using research dollars in the U.K. on treatments such as CBT and GET instead of biological research has wasted time, money, and lives.

I witnessed the dangers of the U.K. model of CBT and GET firsthand in Canada recently when my friend, Peggy, who has ME/CFS, was told by her disability insurance company she would need to undergo a rehabilitation program to qualify for her disability income. The therapists insisted that she ignore her symptoms and/or relapses and add more exercise, while changing her beliefs about her illness.

Over the course of months, she lost all the gains that the time off from work and resting had given her – physically, mentally and emotionally. She dropped from 60 percent functioning on the adapted CFS scale (Appendix H) to 30 percent. It was upsetting for me to observe her relapse and the trauma it created for her, while I was unable to help. Even her supportive doctor was unable to prevent this.

It was only after Peggy went to an out-of-country expert, who then got involved, that a new treatment trial was started using anti-viral medication. She has been given a limited period of time for this trial before the disability company will continue its demands.

These definitions and illness labels are evolving hand in hand with research and science. At the time of writing, we are still in transition. In 2015, there was a new proposed label and diagnostic criteria for ME/CFS suggested to the U.S. Health and Human Services (HHS) by the Institute of Medicine (IOM) which had been contracted by HHS for this purpose.[39] The name suggested is "systemic exercise intolerance disease" (SEID). The IOM report claims that these new evidence-based criteria are very similar to the CCC.[40]

This currently proposed clinical diagnostic criteria for ME/CFS (SEID)[41] can be found in the Institute of Medicine's (IOM) report.

---

39   The full report "Beyond Myalgic Encephalomyelitis/Chronic Fatigue Syndrome: Redefining an Illness" is available at www.nationalacademies.org/hmd/Reports/2015/ME-CFS.aspx (accessed July 10, 2016). The report contains a very good discussion of the history of ME and of CFS as well as an analysis of a number of the criteria used to define them.

40   "Beyond Myalgic Encephalomyelitis/Chronic Fatigue Syndrome: Redefining an Illness." 212.

41   "Beyond Myalgic Encephalomyelitis/Chronic Fatigue Syndrome: Redefining an Illness" Box S-1,6.

We do not know what HHS or others will do with these 2015 recommendations. We do know that there is considerable controversy in many areas of this newly proposed name and diagnostic criteria.

Everyone afflicted and affected by the illness hopes for the universal determination of one appropriate name, one diagnostic definition to describe the illness, and a biomarker clarifying subsets of patients. This will change the quality of life for people who suffer from these illnesses in so many ways (Appendix D). I trust we will get through this transition of multiple names and definitions by means of a scientific process… eventually.

Over time, experienced doctors have diagnosed me with CFS, ME, and ME/CFS, using the distinct, respected criteria I have mentioned. When I wake up in the morning, I still feel as ill, regardless of what it is called. I believe that each term refers to the same illness in my case. As a reminder, I use the labels CFS, ME, or ME/CFS interchangeably. I am always referring to the criteria set out in the Canadian Consensus document (Appendix A) when I use these terms as a foundational framework.

Comparisons between the many definitions are laid out in an easy-to-read table in "Thirty Years of Disdain," Dimmock M, and Lazell-Fairman M.[42] (Appendix E).

---

42   Dimmock M, and Lazell-Fairman M, "Thirty Years of Disdain" (Background) December 2015. Appendix 1. http://bit.ly/The_Burial_of_ME_Background (accessed July 26, 2016). The Summary is at http://bit.ly/The_Burial_of_ME_Summary (accessed July 26, 2016).

STANZA 6

Pre-illness health, loving life, expecting to heal, and prognosis

As someone who biked and who camped in the woods,
And *loved all of life, trying all that she could,* ❧
"My body will heal. I'll just wait for that day, ❧
I know I'll be back my original way."

Over time I'm improving, although not the same,
It will be okay and there's no one to blame.
I'm sure I can fight this. I know that I'm strong,
I've never been sick when it has lasted long.

...How could I know...
...It would get worse?...
...This was only the start...

Nothing prepared me for what was to come ...
Chronic illness that would break my heart!

STANZA 6 NOTES

☙ *Loved all of life, trying all that she could* – I am so grateful for all the things I was able to do until my health became shaky. My husband is an adventurous soul, with few limitations to his abilities or creativity. His influence definitely encouraged an interesting life, as well as a hard-working one. We traveled quite extensively and purchased an acreage where we boarded a couple of horses and some rabbits. He created a specialty vehicle restoration business on our acreage, which grew and transformed into other businesses over the years.

When our daughter was born, we still spent lots of time traveling and playing. Although I was working, it was really enjoyable. I loved to garden, and I clearly recall setting my ten-month-old in the wheelbarrow with the needed tools and singing as I went to prepare the land for spring planting. My husband and I both have large families who live a few hours from our home, and we were always active with them. There was often a wedding, birthday, shower, or christening for a new baby. I loved it all.

On many days, I realize how important and fortunate it was that I had a full life before becoming ill. At least, I had experiences to draw on, like driving, working, and earning a living. Often, I think those experiences are the reason I have done as well as I have in maintaining some normalcy.

At thirty-five, I became so ill that I was unable to learn new things easily or to adapt to our fast-paced culture. For the first years, I tried to keep up and push through it, but eventually life moved ahead without me, and I could not even hope to catch up.

I often think this is another reason to focus on the youth who encounter ME/CFS. Yes, they may recover on their own with some support and good medical decisions, but too often they do not, leaving them to face a very long life without the ability to take part in these important life experiences.

☙ *My body will heal. I'll just wait for that day* – For most of my ME/CFS experience, I believed I would find a way to achieve great improvement or full recovery. It wasn't until many years later – when I learned the facts about prognosis and hadn't improved or recovered despite my great efforts – that I understood more about my realistic chances for total recovery. Improvement levels are more likely than complete recoveries, especially in the earlier years, but there are no guarantees.

Complete, sustained recovery back to pre-illness health is rare for people with ME/CFS, according to the International Association for CFS/ME's *Primer for Clinical Practitioners* (IACFS/ME, 2014). Recovery rates and improvement rates vary in different studies, but the CCC *Overview* 2005[43] claims that in most of the studies they referenced, the recovery rate for adults who return to their pre-illness levels of functioning is ***less than seven percent, leaving ninety-three percent waiting for effective treatment to restore their lives***. It also describes the prognosis for children and youth as much better, claims symptom severity as the best indicator of outcome, and explains that an accurate prognosis cannot be predicted with certainty for any individual. Even when a patient has improved or attained wellness, relapses can occur several years after remission – a difficult fact to live with.

Out of the few people I have personally met who have completely recovered, or who improved and sustained more normal levels of functioning, most have been young males who took an average of four to seven years to do so. Losses and repercussions occur in many areas of life as a result of such a degree and duration of illness. We need more research and effective treatments to change these statistics, improve recovery rates, and make them much more timely.[44]

There are people who have improved greatly or who have recovered to excellent health. Some write about their healing experiences which are very inspirational. They include those in Chapter 8: Recovery, Improvement and Hope, as well as: Gretchen Brooks Nassar's *CFS is a Call for Soulwork* (www.amazon.com), Alexandra Barton's *Recovery from CFS: 50 Personal Stories,*[45] *and* Dan Neuffer's *CFS Unravelled.*[46] I personally love reading recovery and improvement stories as well as listening to D. Neuffer's interviews of people who have found ways to improve and restore their health and their lives. D. Neuffer has also launched the *ANS Rewire* program in 2016 to aid people on their recovery journeys. It is important for me to keep these possibilities in mind as I move forward in my own experience. An increase in research as to why some people do recover over time, and others do not, would be interesting.

---

43   Carruthers B, and van de Sande M, "Myalgic Encephalomyelitis/Chronic Fatigue Syndrome: A Clinical Case Definition and Guidelines for Medical Practitioners: An Overview of the Canadian Consensus Document." 2005. www.mefmaction.com/images/stories/Overviews/ME-Overview.pdf (accessed July 25, 2016).

44   For more on improvement and recovery insights, see the following study: Bell DS, Jordan K, and Robinson M. "Thirteen-year follow up of children and adolescents with Chronic Fatigue Syndrome." Pediatrics Vol 197 No. 5, May 1, 2001. 994-998 doi: 10.1542/peds.107.5.994.

45   www.amazon.ca/Recovery-CFS-50-Personal-Stories/dp/1434363589 – May 30, 2008. (accessed July 10, 2016).

46   cfsunravelled.com/books (accessed July 10, 2016).

STANZA 7

Growing stronger and carrying on

As a kid I ran behind the lawn mower,
Then jogged behind baby while pushing the stroller,
So I thought it would help adding exercise in;
But *muscles were burning* ❧ – slowed my regimen.

Although I was able to keep up part-time, ❧
Physical effort is for me the worst kind.
Sitting and thinking – though different – could do,
But walking or gardening, my symptoms renew.

…We did not know…
…This could harm me…
…No one said a thing…

In the early '90s, no one really knew,
No knowledge could anyone bring.

STANZA 7 NOTES

❦ *Muscles were burning* – This was another of those early signs that something had changed in my body after the initial flu-like onset. When I danced or did aerobics, my thigh muscles would burn and recovery began to take longer and longer. I did not know, nor did anyone else, that continued exercise was probably worsening my condition. We are generally trained to think that activity is good. Unfortunately, back in the 1990s – and even in 2016 – people with ME/CFS may be advised by their doctors to exercise and push through the symptoms. It is very important for those considering ME or CFS as their diagnosis to stop all activity, or at least decrease it, until they know for sure. Early diagnosis, aggressive rest, and good care, including medication, diet, and supplementation, may lead to better outcomes than many of us have experienced.

Some research is focused on potential abnormalities in the muscles of ME patients, with evidence that some sufferers produce excess acid when they exercise. One study at Liverpool University in the U.K. is also examining potential structural abnormalities in the mitochondria – cell components that produce energy in a usable form – in skeletal muscle, as reported by Dr. Charles Shepherd in the November 26, 2012 issue of *The Daily Telegraph*.[47] More current studies in this area are in footnote 47.

❦ *Although I was able to keep up part-time* – I had switched from working full-time to working part-time at the courthouse when I was pregnant which was prior to my illness. It was just after my nine-month maternity leave in 1990 that I first became ill after the flu-like onset. From 1990 through 1994, I was still able to work part-time and slowly regained approximately seventy percent of my pre-illness function. I knew that something was different in my body, but life goes on, and we did not know much about CFS or how to manage it. I did what I always did – tried to eat well, exercised when I could, and cared for my family. As I slowly regained some strength, I began to make more life changes.

---

47   www.telegraph.co.uk/news/health/news/9699911/ME-isnt-all-in-the-mind-but-its-still-a-mystery.html.
(accessed July 10, 2016). Excess acid study: Jones DEJ, Hollingsworth KG, Jakovljevic DG, Fattakhova G, Pairman J, Blamire AM, Trenell MI, and Newton JL, "Loss of capacity to recover from acidosis on repeat exercise in chronic fatigue syndrome: a case-control study." European Journal of Clinical Investigation, 2012, 42: 186-194. Doi: 10.1111/j.1365-2362.2011.02567.x.

   Mitochondria studies: As recently as March 2016, the ME Association announced that it continues to fund studies related to mitochondria in ME/CFS. www.meassociation.org.uk/2016/03/me-association-to-fund-fourth-study-into-the-role-of-the-mitochondria-in-mecfs-10-march-2016. Preliminary results from the study Dr. Shepherd spoke about to the Daily Telegraph were published in 2015. The study can be found at Earl K et al. "The Role Of Cytokines in Muscle Fatigue in Patients with Chronic Fatigue Syndrome (CFS)." The FASEB journal, 2015, vol. 29, no. 1 Supplement, 1055.34. A write-up about this study can be found at www.meassociation.org.uk/2015/04/mitochondrial-dysfunction-and-the-role-of-cytokines-in-mecfs-preliminary-results-from-research-being-funded-by-the-mea-ramsay-research-fund-and-the-medical-research-council-2-april-2015 (accessed July 25, 2016). Dr. Sarah Myhill is also doing mitochondrial related work. More about her and her work can be found in the notes at Stanza 16.

STANZA 8

Education and cognitive symptoms

I thought a job change would be what to do,
So *I added to my plate a natural health school.* 🌿
I studied for three years to make myself well,
But couldn't complete – down the hallways I fell.

Now *cognitive troubles,* 🌿 with numbers a problem,
To read or multitask – not even an option.
To balance a checkbook would make my brain freeze,
I needed to know: *"Who's watching over me?"* 🌿

　　…It's Alzheimer's…
　　…Or depression…
　　…Or MS I fear…

These are the things that ran through my poor mind,
Not CFS symptoms – severe.

STANZA 8 NOTES

🕊 *I added to my plate a natural health school* – As I slowly and partially recovered, I decided to go back to school part-time for my Natural Health Practitioner Diploma in order to eventually switch careers into something more health conscious. This made for a very full schedule: work, school, parenting, and duties around home. Although I was not physically as strong and energetic as I had been prior to illness, I was able to do all of this fairly comfortably for a while – until it all came crashing down. While taking some courses, I began to have trouble standing up without crumpling down to sit on the floor. One day, we were in a lab studying the body for an anatomy class, and the professor was speaking to us in a group while we stood around him. I found myself feeling faint and quickly found a wall, which I literally pushed against and slid down to the ground. I was later lucky enough to get the final exam done with successful marks before I had to drop all hopes of continuing my studies.

🕊 *Cognitive troubles* are part of ME/CFS. Some people call this "brain fog." I neither refer to it nor experience it that way. I learned through personal experience and research that many cognitive symptoms are common, including disorientation, confusion, slowed information processing, slowed reaction time, difficulty in word retrieval or speaking, trouble concentrating and paying attention, and short-term memory problems. Along with some of these symptoms, multitasking became impossible for me and remains so.

My ability to work with numbers has been permanently affected, though I was good at math and enjoyed it prior to illness. In fact, when I worked at the courthouse with more than twenty other stenographers, I was part of the Finance Committee, which was responsible for managing the $500,000 per year income earned by the group. My responsibilities included dividing the money equally amongst the partners and setting per-page transcription rates for clients including lawyers and judges. However, since my illness, I have never even been able to play a good game of cribbage and have had difficulty mastering the simplest math skills.

I was a court reporter for more than ten years, comfortable taking machine shorthand in stressful courtrooms for more than two hours at a time, twice a day. Sometimes multiple people would speak at once, many of them speaking up to 220 words per minute. There were times when the judge or lawyer required instant read-backs from me, and I would read my shorthand notes back to them, confirming what had just been said. Then I was responsible for producing a perfect, verbatim transcript of the proceedings, which required the use of fairly elaborate computer software and a great deal of time and detail going into each transcript's preparation. All of this was pre-illness.

As my illness worsened, I could no longer read or write English at times, never mind use the shorthand machine that had become second nature. I would get confused or exhausted from a normal conversation with a friend, or get lost in a familiar neighbor-hood. It was all so petrifying.

Concentration and memory impairments are cited as some of the most disruptive and functionally disabling symptoms of ME/CFS. Reactive or secondary depression and anxiety also can occur from the illness, just as from most other serious illnesses. However, ME/CFS should not be confused with primary depression. A lot of research has been done to distinguish ME/CFS from primary depression. I've included a chart[48] (Appendix F) outlining these differences as described by Dr. E. Stein.[49] Emotional lability – which is unstable or disproportionate emotional reactions such as involuntary or uncontrollable crying – can occur. This is also true for other conditions such as M.S., stroke and trau-matic brain injury. These symptoms vary over time and from person to person. I do not know how we can go through such severe physical changes, affecting both the body and mind, without experiencing some of these fears and reactions.

There are studies that explore the brain changes in ME/CFS, as explained by Gudrun Lange, neuropsychologist, in a May 2012 presentation for the CFIDS Association of America.[50] In her slide presentation, Lange relates: "On neuropsychological exam, patients are likely to show subtle and relative deficits in: efficient information processing with decreased thinking speed, ability to keep information 'online' with decreased amount of information for use available, and sequencing pieces of information and prioritizing their use (decreased ability to make quick decisions)."

I can relate to all of these. The only happy thought after all this heavy knowledge (*my poor brain*, I am thinking right now) is Lange's comment that "there is generally NO decrease in overall intellectual function." Whew! There is some hope, isn't there?

✎ *"Who's watching over me?"* was an ongoing concern I had due to the increasing sever-ity of my symptoms. Because ME/CFS affects thinking processes, emotions, and body systems, it is very frightening. With little information and no treatment available, there was nowhere to turn for knowledgeable or effective help at times, so the fear was perpetuated.

The hospital wasn't even an option, though at times I felt like I was dying. Because very few medical professionals understood the illness early on, they could do very little for me there. Unfortunately, much of this still remains the reality for people with ME/CFS in 2016.

---

48   Stein E, MD FRCP(C) Presented at the AHMF 3rd International Meeting on CFS, Manly, Australia, Dec 2001.

49   Stein E, MD FRCP(C) "Let Your Light Shine Through – Strategies for Living with Myalgic Encephalomyelitis/ Chronic Fatigue Syndrome, Fibromyalgia and Multiple Chemical Sensitivity." 2012. Session 8 – Depression and Anxiety p.8 - 13.

50   www.youtube.com/watch?v=ErcJCI-sm_A (accessed August 6, 2016). The CFIDS Association was renamed Solve ME/CFS Initiative in 2014.

PART II
MY RE-FLU AND SEVERE CHRONIC ILLNESS
(My Age: 35 to 39)
1995-1999

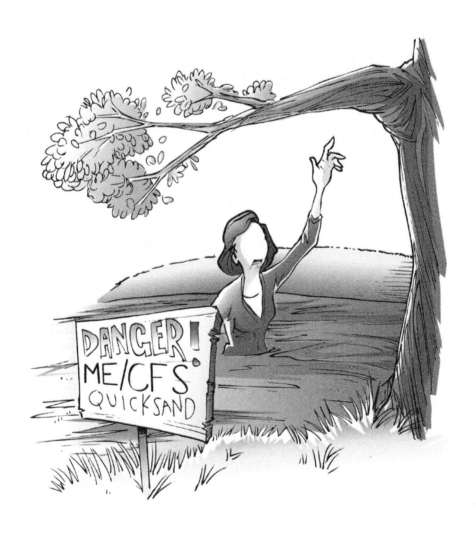

STANZAS 9-21 TOPICS

STANZA 9

Re-flu, relapse, and energy scales

Zero to one hundred percent on *the scale,*
To measure functioning, stronger or frail.
An easy 100 when I was still well,
But on this *re-flu,* to 10 percent I fell.

People with CFS, they know "the lingo,"
Healthy folk can't contemplate all this jingle.
I hope that they know just how lucky that is,
To not understand "it" means they don't have THIS.

...20 percent...
...Maybe 30...
...Oops, *"flatlining"* again...

This little engine that thought that she could,
Her DRIVE and WILL could not defend.

STANZA 9 NOTES

❧ *The scale* – I use the Karnofsky Scale Adapted for ME/CFS.[51] It is one of the most widely-used scales available for charting energy and function, and it can be used to monitor severity status. The Karnofsky scale outlines levels of energy and functionality from 10 percent to 100 percent. One hundred percent on this scale is described as "Totally well; no concerns about fatigue. You can think clearly and do several things at once. You can exercise to your maximum potential without any problems." At 10 percent: "You are in bed for most of the day and you have zero tolerance for anything extra. You are frequently too exhausted to even eat."

I have spent most of my ill years between 10 and 50 percent on this scale, which puts me on the spectrum of severity ranging from extreme to moderate ME/CFS.

Another widely-used scale is that of Dr. Alison Bested.[52] I have included it in Appendix H along with the Karnofsky scale. It is outlined in Dr. Bested's book along with other patient resources.

The levels of severity are described by Canadian psychiatrist Eleanor Stein, MD FRCP (C) in her treatment guidelines paper:[53]

"Mild – still able to work/study full time though with effort, and rest on weekends.

Moderate – able to work or study part time with effort.

Severe – unable to work/study and requires assistance to live independently.

Extreme – unable to live independently, virtually house and sometimes bedbound."

(More information on severity is contained in the Stanza 15 Notes.)

Most people think of the percentages as the percentage of functioning compared to being healthy. However, as the late Emily Collingridge from the U.K. commented in her book *Severe ME/CFS: A Guide to Living*: "Clinicians and carers should not view 50 percent ability as meaning, for example, that a patient is able to walk half the distance of a healthy person." The Karnofsky scale describes the 50 percent range as: "Your energy only allows you to do about three tasks per day (2-3 hours of activity). Your energy is easily

---

51 Karnofsky Scale adapted for ME/CFS, Appendix H.

52 Bested AC, Logan AC and Howe R, "Hope and Help for Chronic Fatigue Syndrome and Fibromyalgia." Cumberland House. 2008. 2nd ed. Print.

53 Stein E, MD FRCP(C) "Assessment and Treatment of Patients with ME/CFS: Treatment Guidelines for Psychiatrists." This paper was posted on the Internet in December 2006 and has been translated into three languages (Norwegian, German and Italian) in addition to its original English. www.eleanorsteinmd.ca/publications (accessed July 26, 2016).

drained. Thought processes are difficult. Your exercise tolerance is poor; walking up stairs is difficult."

If I rate my energy and functioning at 30 percent, I do not function at 30 percent of the 100 percent I was in good health. It is more like some small fraction of that. For example, I am able to do 30 percent of the easiest things that I could previously do, for 30 percent of the day, while feeling 30 percent – in other words, I am not feeling like a well person doing even 30 percent of my former activities. I feel multiple symptoms most of the time while doing tasks, and I never feel well, even at rest. I do all tasks differently from when I was healthy, such as while sitting or lying down rather than standing. It can help to switch tasks around regularly, so I only focus for brief time periods on one thing and then do something else. For example, I do a few dishes, then spend a while using my mind on the computer, then rest. I often default to television or quiet rest when all else fails.

Along with that, I cannot do as good a job as I would have in wellness. I run out of stamina, have trouble standing long enough to finish tasks properly, or lose focus. So I have to leave things partially undone. Then for the rest of the day, I simply do not have the energy and feel too unwell to do anything else. That means it might be three days before one load of laundry gets put away or that the dishes are washed poorly and left to air-dry, not getting them into the cupboard until the next day. This goes against my nature as a highly efficient and fast-moving person and is not how I worked when healthy.

It is easy for this to become a point of contention with those around me, because often their expectations are higher than I can meet. It is very hard for loved ones to understand when looking at the situation from the outside. It can appear as laziness, selfishness, selective illness, or even as not caring or craziness when I can do one job and then not another. I choose one task like folding laundry because I can sit down, but then not touch the vacuum cleaner because I have to remain standing.

Another perplexing piece of this is that a person could be 70 percent on their cognitive function and 30 percent on their physical function, while 90 percent on emotional stability. We are always changing, and this can also be confusing for everyone. It is so abnormal that I can't fully express it.

Education and communication are key, and I hope that doctors call in patients' supporters to teach them what and why this may become a problem between family members, especially as improvement begins and one is no longer bedbound.

I personally find pressures, both from myself and others, to be the worst when I have adapted to a 40-50 percent contained lifestyle because I appear to be more able-bodied than I actually am. That level of well-being is only due to the choices that I am making which I call "Adapting and Adjusting" in my personal scale lingo. Unfortunately, it is not only the sick person who has to adapt. It is everyone around him or her. Adaptation and adjustment to my lifestyle, caging to a tighter and tighter boundary, is not the same as recovery!

For the **extreme and severely ill** levels, although it is not measurable on any chart, I feel there is a much lower level of energy and well-being than 10 percent on the Karnofsky scale. I call it "**the negative zone**" where I feel I am not even at 10 percent. During this relapse in 1995, when I became bedbound and unable to do anything, I thought feeling worse should stop there. But I felt so extraordinarily ill that I was sure the scale should comprise numbers below zero and that it should go down to negative 100. During the worst times of my illness, it was possible to feel more and more sick with energy going lower and symptoms increasing, even when bedbound and staying still.

Many ME/CFS patients would say they feel and exist at negative 100 in their bedbound life with bodies and brains in torment 24/7. Page 27 of the International Association for CFS/ME's *Primer for Clinical Practitioners* (IACFS/ME, 2014) lists some symptoms that the most severely ill patients may experience – symptoms that I have not spoken of in my story. These include severe nausea and inability to feed oneself, which may necessitate tube feeding; inability to walk to or use the toilet, possibly requiring use of a bedpan, diapers, or catheter; inability to turn over in bed; atypical seizures; and difficulty communicating needs to a caregiver due to speech difficulties or exhaustion. This is a short list of many more possible symptoms. Chapter 3: Severity, and Chapter 4: Those Who Have Died, illustrate many of the severe and extreme experiences of ME/CFS patients and their caregivers.

Over the years and looking back from 2016, I have determined that the use of the severity or functioning scale is valuable because it creates a common language for those with the illness to communicate with each other or with their doctors and loved ones. This can create a better possibility of self-care and care by others. However, in the end, it is an individual journey, which really cannot be compared to another person's experience because of all the differences in symptoms and stages of illness.

✎ *Re-flu* (my second-time stomach flu that caused relapse) – Between 1990 and 1995, I had regained my functioning and energy back to 70 percent on the Karnofsky scale. I still needed to be very careful with managing my energy and activities, but if I took precautions, I was able to do a fair bit, including part-time work and study. It was not my pre-illness health level, but as I mentioned in Part I, I'd begun classes to become a natural health consultant in hopes of regaining my good health.

In the winter of 1995, in the midst of writing a physiology exam at the university, a wave of flu-like feelings began, which I recognized immediately from the ME/CFS onset five years prior. I knew I would need rest and that it would be a slow recovery. I was prepared for that, but not for how things turned out following what I call my "re-flu." My life changed completely. I had to face that I was living with a very severe chronic illness.

 Flatlining is a term I use to describe those bedbound times in the negative zone mentioned above: when my symptoms are so severe and my energy so low that I feel that consciously breathing is the only thing keeping me alive. I fear that if I don't pay attention to my breathing, this thin thread attaching me to life will be gone, and so will I. On my personal functioning scale, I refer to it as the "Blink and Breathe" state, because that is all I can do during those times. I am glad to report that this state is not happening as often as it did during the early years, but if I wander out of my safe energy zone for long, this can still happen.

STANZA 10

Sudden worsening with increasing symptoms

My brain is now tired, my stamina gone. ✀
Everything's slower, my thoughts take too long.
Energy's draining right out from my feet,
What odd sensations starting to repeat.

This herb – no, that med – oh, yes, it is this one.
Oops, maybe not – I am worse now! So not fun.
Time to pray harder and witness it healed,
"They" say this is done in the large *Quantum Field.* ✀

> …When I exert…
> …When I think hard…
> …When I talk too long…

That's when I end up in bed *"paying back,"* ✀
Just wondering what went wrong.

STANZA 10 NOTES

❧ *My brain is now tired, my stamina gone* – In 1995, I had a major relapse that was life-altering for me and for my family. My brain was tired and I had a complete lack of stamina along with the feeling of energy draining out from my feet. In addition, I had trouble eating, became more sensitive to foods, and had pain on the right side of my abdomen. My muscles continued to burn when used and would fatigue easily.

❧ *Quantum field* – This is a concept or theory put forth by people like Deepak Chopra. My interpretation is: Universal law states that "energy comes before matter," and we can use our intentions, thoughts, and actions to exert some influence over what happens in our lives. Science has proven that underlying everything is energy, the very essence of all that is, including us. Each culture seems to have its own name for this energy. In the West, we call it the soul or spirit. Some Eastern cultures refer to prana or qi.

With that concept in mind, the practices of hypnotherapy, prayer, visualization, energy and emotional work, in addition to other modalities, have kept me occupied, and I found them very helpful in keeping my spirits up.

❧ *Paying back* is another way to express the common symptom of post-exertional malaise (PEM), post-exertion relapse, and, as some patients call it, post-exertional collapse or simply "crash." This is the impact from the overuse of our reduced energy. This reaction can be immediate or delayed for more than twenty-four hours after the overexertion. It exacerbates existing symptoms and/or creates new ones that can last days, weeks, or months. Many experts regard PEM as a key feature, or a cardinal symptom, which distinguishes ME/CFS from many other conditions.

Payback can occur even from minimal physical or mental activity, such as a brief walk down the hallway, sitting or standing too long, having a shower, or reading for just five minutes. Think of it like spending more money than you have: Doing so has many repercussions, but you may not feel them until later. So my first CFS doctor advised me to put my bed on the main floor so I would not have to walk the six steps to my bedroom!

Each patient's "energy bank" or "energy envelope" is different and can change frequently and rapidly. As examples, one person with ME/CFS may be unable to roll over in bed without feeling more ill because he is immobilized and bedbound. Another may function at a higher level, which may mean she can work at a quiet desk job three days a week, four hours per day. However, in order to keep that up, she must rest a lot in between work days and cannot do much socializing or many chores without worsening and becoming unable to work at all. Others may be able to walk in the house a bit but cannot walk up the stairs without worsening. A more fully recovered person may function fine for months with intermittent relapses that take him or her out of commission.

STANZA 11

Needing disability insurance

Too sick to work after *second flu onset,*
Insurance for illness, a long fight to get it.
Too ill to sort out all this crazy stuff,
With a union and doctor, it still felt quite rough.

Never dreaming I'd need disability pay,
At age thirty-five; and still get to this day,
For an illness I never had heard of before.
On work and on play, it had closed all the doors.

 …I am lucky…
 …To have had help…
 …And some financial aid…

And though one could never live on that amount,
It has helped me along the way.

STANZA 11 NOTES

❧ *Second flu onset* – Eventually, I learned that a flu-like onset was quite typical for CFS and for ME. The International Association for CFS/ME's *Primer for Clinical Practitioners* (IACFS/ME, 2014) on page 8 says: "ME/CFS may be preceded by: an acute infection (viral, bacterial or parasitic); exposure to environmental toxins (e.g., organophosphate pesticides); a recent vaccination; or a significant physical or emotional trauma.… A high percentage of patients date the onset of their ME/CFS to a flu-like illness."

Although there have been cluster outbreaks of both CFS and ME throughout history, most cases of these illnesses occur, like my own, as isolated or sporadic incidents. A common story is that a group of people contract the "flu" – something going around the office. Most recover, but one doesn't. Why this happens is one of the mysteries of the illness. These single occurrences add up to millions of people worldwide.

❧ *Insurance for illness* – It was after this relapse at age thirty-five that I applied for long-term disability payments, and I have been reviewed every year since then. My long-term disability is for a primary diagnosis of chronic fatigue syndrome. It also now covers celiac disease and orthostatic intolerance – but this did not happen without a lot of time and wear and tear. Unless we find solutions for this illness, I expect to qualify for disability income for the rest of my life. Personally, I'd rather have a cure than the disability payments.

Applying for long-term disability was the last thing I wanted or expected to do. Not only did I not want to acknowledge the long-term nature of my illness, but I found it difficult to go through the necessary steps when I was so ill – cognitively, as well as physically. I was very fortunate to have disability coverage through my work, a union to represent me, and a CFS doctor to provide accurate and relevant information to my insurance company. Without a good union representative, I am sure I would have failed. Without a doctor who was knowledgeable about CFS, I do not think I would have continued receiving the payments for all these years.

Despite their support, it took one year to complete the complicated process, including meetings with the insurance company in a city three hours from my home, a review by independent psychiatric and internal specialists, and much later, a physiotherapy assessment.

Although my ME/CFS onset was sudden, and I was diagnosed quite quickly, my insurance required me to make a trip to an independent psychiatrist to rule out primary psychiatric disease (eg. Major depression). The requirement for an independent psychiatric examination in cases of ME/CFS, regardless of the type of onset, is common. Some disability insurance companies (dependent on the country) deal with depression differently than they do an illness like ME/CFS. For example, depending on the disability company and the diagnosis, there may be different time limitations for how long a person can receive payments.

It was very difficult not to be frightened by the many experiences this illness brought into my life.

During the time I was qualifying for coverage, the insurance people followed me and watched my home life. I've learned this is standard in these types of cases, but it was disconcerting. Because I live on an acreage, it was easy to spot them in their vehicle outside the driveway – morning, noon, or night. I remember thinking: *What if they see me drive my daughter to the bus?* I found myself questioning my own level of illness because I really had no idea just how bad it was myself.

In a few years' time, I was asked to have an independent physiotherapist review. It took place over two days and was composed of meetings and physical exercises, following which a report was sent to the insurance company. I showed up as requested, met the assessor, and did my best to answer her questions and follow her instructions. But I never lasted more than half the day even with the light physical demands. So after the assessor monitored my heart rate and recorded all her observations, we spent the rest of the day reviewing the Canadian Consensus Criteria Overview for ME/CFS that I brought. She expressed sincere interest in the facts and in learning more about the syndrome. Her report ended up in my favor, with a recommendation to continue the insurance payments.

Other patients can have a more difficult time. Some are denied coverage and have to defend their diagnoses in court. Sometimes insurers ask patients to go through rehabilitation protocols in order to continue receiving payments: for example, graded exercise therapy (GET), which can worsen the person's health to a more serious state. These situations put extra stresses on a person with a serious illness, so you can only imagine the toll it can have on our health. Insurance "fights" are a very difficult aspect of any illness, but ME/CFS, with its uncertain standing within the medical community, is particularly vulnerable to unfair and inequitable treatment. In Part I, Stanza 5 Notes, Peggy's example of disability insurance challenges does drive home this important issue.

I am grateful for my disability income, but it is far from an amount on which an individual – or family – could live, and I am lucky that my husband has financially provided for our family. Many people do not have disability coverage through their jobs, have no medical support, and are left uncared for. They can quickly become financially destitute unless family members or others step in to help them.

STANZA 12

Grieving and losses, the best job of family and motherhood

Leaving professions and schooling behind,
Leaving my social life – could I rewind?
Leaving the dreams and the goals that I made,
These were the hardest of all to have fade.

Some jobs were left for me so I was grateful,
Still a mother and wife, though my health had a big fall.
Parts of my life remained – they were still there.
Thank God 'cause it helps with the losses I bear.

…Loving family…
…A home and friends…
…A CFS doctor, too…

These were the important things that were left,
That always kept me moving through.

STANZA 12 NOTES

✒ *Leaving professions and schooling behind* – I was too ill by the time I left my job to realize the full impact of what was happening. It wasn't until many years later that the impact and losses became clear. Even at the time, I recall being staggered that I had to give up my career of fifteen years. I tried to return to work twice, but collapsed both times after just one day. I also remember how upsetting it was to pull out of the courses I was taking in hopes of making the career switch I was working towards. Although it hasn't worked out that way, for a long time I believed it would be temporary – that I would be able to return to work or school.

This is an all-too-common reality for ME/CFSers of all ages. Children and adolescents can also become ill with ME/CFS, creating special needs for their education and training, and sometimes it is not possible for them at all.

✒ *Parts of my life* – As difficult as my illness has been, I have been fortunate to have a supportive family. Even though I lost my career, social life, my favorite hobbies, and many close friends and colleagues, I was still able to care for my daughter and husband in some ways. I call it "the best job." They cared for me in ways we never expected that they would have to. I also stayed connected to my parents, siblings and their families as best as I could.

Most of the time, I could be a loving and attentive mother, even though I was often lying down, feeling ill, and unable to do many of the things other mothers could do. My daughter and I have developed a quirky sense of humor as a coping skill, and we maintain a very close relationship. When I felt able, I was happy to plan a birthday party or a Halloween party, drive the kids somewhere, or have other children at our home. As my daughter grew up, my husband and I were able to help Jenna plan her University education and to follow through with an opportunity to go to South Africa to do some modeling. We supported her in every way possible, and continue to do so today. Conversely, there are no words for the gratitude I feel toward her for all the help and support she has given me this whole time both physically and emotionally. Even as a child, she was helping by giving me purpose and motivation to not give up.

My husband has been a very hands-on father, and he and my daughter did many of the activities that my daughter and I could not do together, such as bike riding, skiing, and skating. The ability to focus on my health and to be a good mom was largely possible because of my hard-working, independent husband, relatives and friends who lived close by, as well as a loving extended family (unfortunately three hours away).

STANZA 13

Stopping exercise and learning pacing

Have to *stop all exercise that I love now,* &
No physical working – *spread two tasks out* & somehow.
No dancing, no yard work, no biking, no fun.
Walking is hard – never mind a good run.

Stay connected to others, and share their life stories,
Hear their celebrations, their bad times, and glories.
Living vicariously I don't always mind,
But I hear my heart break when I must stay behind.

   …When the pain strikes…
   …When my brain hurts…
   …With my muscles weak…

Leaving a mere shell of myself behind,
I have to continue to seek.

STANZA 13 NOTES

❧ ***Stop all exercise that I love now*** – By 1995, even walking was becoming more and more difficult. I remember going to my hometown with my husband and daughter to stay at my mom and dad's. There was a dance at the local community hall that evening, and we had always liked to go together. That night, I had to tell my dad that I would not be able to dance. For the first time in my life, we would not be able to twirl around the dance floor in a polka – like two kids set free. I don't think he really comprehended the permanence of my situation at the time, nor did I. I have not danced since; just listening to good music for any length of time is exhausting, although I still love it. For me, it has been an ongoing struggle to accept that I can't use my body for very much. It seems such a waste and such a loss.

I have observed that many people I know with ME/CFS had very active lifestyles before falling ill and that athletics or a love of physical recreation and exercise is part of their nature. I am sure that one day we will understand this connection that we had.

❧ ***Spread two tasks out*** – This refers to one of the strategies for coping with ME/CFS and is part of pacing oneself. Depending on one's illness severity, modifications may involve the following: sitting or lying down instead of standing while doing a task; taking breaks every few minutes while on task; and spreading tasks out over the day with quiet, lying-down rests in between. These are ways of self-management to reduce suffering and increase functioning. At times, for me, this has meant eating and taking a bath as my tasks for the whole day – though feeling very ill doing even those.

Just because people with ME/CFS do tasks or go on outings does not mean they feel well. They may be forcing themselves because they don't have an option, or it is a choice they have made not to miss out on an important event. At times, I had to decide whether to run an errand in town OR make supper; to work on the computer OR do the dishes. My friend Randy says that some days he must decide whether to shave OR empty the litter box – and that is it for the whole day. Most days, I think the cats win.

For those in very severe states of ME/CFS, there are no choices at all. The only option is to remain bedbound and rely completely on caregivers. At times, I have phoned other patients to do research for this book, and they might speak with only the hint of a whisper and talk for less than a minute before total exhaustion takes over. Many cannot speak on the phone at all, due to the toll it takes. It affects me deeply to see and hear others suffer like this, and to remember my own similar stages of illness.

STANZA 14

Lab tests and charting

Lab tests and blood work and alternate care,
Resting and *charting* — Don't worsen a flare!
Going against all that's natural for me,
How am I able to set myself free?

Denying, justifying, and rationalization,
Everything needing valid explanation.
Or how will the others know just what I need?
Even with that, I don't always succeed.

    … Can I sit down?…
    … Can't stay too long…
    … Can we do it by phone?…

Needing to always excuse or defend,
I seek respite in my space at home.

STANZA 14 NOTES

❧ *Charting* is a self-observation tool for managing ME/CFS by documenting one's activities for the day, as well as keeping track of symptom severity and functioning ability. I have already introduced the Karnofsky scale as part of this system. The other part is a chart with a graph to document sleep, activities, and percentages of overall functioning, as well as medications, supplements, and diet. The idea is that this information is then used to make modifications to activity levels and sleep, as well as food and medicines, in order to prevent worsening and push-crash cycles.

The push-crash cycle is very straightforward: The more a patient pushes, the more he or she crashes or worsens symptoms. I have not mastered the art of pacing despite my best efforts. There are many outside variables and unpredictable influences that affect me, such as the weather. Charting also takes time and energy, and I can't even chart when the illness is too severe.

I have found that overriding my personal energy safety boundaries is probable when parenting – chart or no chart. At the onset of my illness, I was the mother of a one-year-old and at the time of the relapse in 1995, she was five. As all mothers know, it is natural and necessary to put a child's needs first as long as there is a choice, especially when they are infants or very young children. So unless there is help in the home during those times, a mother will mother as best she can.

One really great example of the benefits of charting and tracking one's progress, even when parenting young children, is one I read in the book *Defeat Chronic Fatigue Syndrome: You Don't Have to Live with It.*[54] Martha Kilkoyne, the author, had CFS and did recover. In fact, she climbed Mount Kilamanjaro with her husband just to make sure she really had healed completely. What was so astonishing to me about her CFS journey was that she had a new baby and a toddler at the time of her illness onset. She, along with her husband and doctor, formulated a plan to conserve her energy and to keep track of her activity and medications. This charting was helpful for them to understand her limitations. Her husband and advocate, John, became affectionately called "The Jailor" by Martha because he restrained her from doing more than she should. This meant he had to do a lot of the parenting and working, both financially and at home. She did not lift or carry her children for a very long time.

❧ *Going against all that's natural for me* – It took many years for me to understand why I was so poor at knowing my new energy limits and why my symptoms kept worsening. First of all, they were always changing, and I could not intuitively sense when I was overdoing it. Eventually, I came to understand that ME/CFS is a *counterintuitive*

---

54   www.defeatcfs.net (accessed July 29, 2016).

condition, and that is why charting became so important. This is because it took so little to exhaust me, like walking a few extra steps, standing five minutes too long, or mashing the potatoes. The common sense I had used to listen to my body while I was in health was no longer working to manage this illness.

Another part of the problem is that post-exertional malaise (PEM or payback, as I have called it before) can be delayed for more than 24 hours, and recovery can take days, weeks, or months. I generally do not start my payback until 24 hours after too much activity. Then all symptoms flare including pain, weakness, cognitive difficulties, fevers, and the inability to stand or sit long. It worsens for up to two more days, unwinding me to 20 percent. I eventually and slowly head back up the scale to my usual 30 to 50 percent.

Remaining in the "safe zone" can be so limiting and unpredictable that even the tasks of personal care or preparing a meal can mean overdoing it. Thankfully, there are tools that can give outside signs when overexerting and crossing the line into the danger zone. These tools include things such as pedometers to track steps taken per day, heart rate monitors that beep when the heart rate is too high, and blood pressure machines to track the drops and spikes that occur when one is overdoing without realizing it. These tools can help patients stay within their safe energy zone, or "energy envelope" as some call it.

These tools record the impact of *physical* effort but not of *mental* or *emotional* effort. So without charting and tracking, there is no way of knowing how much of those we can tolerate without worsening.

The blood pressure monitor was a very helpful tool for me: It provided an objective indication of my ill health – something that is often difficult for people with ME/CFS to find. When I first relapsed, sometimes my blood pressure wouldn't even register or was dropping to numbers like 80/50 (120/80 being normal). Nobody can stand up with blood pressure like that! It brings you to your knees pretty quickly, as I express in my poem. Even now, my blood pressure is about 100/60 and can drop suddenly with any movement.

I did try the heart rate monitor over a two-month period while my daughter was in junior high school and my husband was very busy with a new business. When I was healthy, my resting heart rate was below 70 beats per minute, but is now often over 90. I set the monitor to beep at a maximum heart rate of about 110 beats per minute based on the formula for a CFS patient my age. It was almost comical because I could not get off the couch without the monitor's incessant beeping which let me know that I was in trouble. This is perhaps the only device that can also demonstrate to the people around us that something is not normal and how severe it can be. I found there were things I needed to do regardless – like making meals, and caring for my family and myself – so I could not always heed its warnings. Eventually I gave up on using these tools.

STANZA 15

Erasing my life – severity and battle fatigue

Fighting a war inside twenty-four/seven,
Hope it's relieving when I get to Heaven,
'Cause the "Chronic" in CFS means 'til I die.
Try to keep suffering low; functioning high.

This is exhausting for all, you can see,
Including caregivers and my family. ✒
I'm sorry to put them through all of this stuff,
It has not been my choice – we've all had enough.

   …Not a fair fight…
   …Erasing my life… ✒
   …With what, we only guess…

But let it be hoped that the enemy dissolves,
And that God can clean up the rest.

STANZA 15 NOTES

❧ *Including caregivers and my family* – An illness like ME/CFS affects everyone: family, friends, employers, doctors, and society as a whole. Each person has a different "total illness burden," (a burden that is dependent on the severity of his/her illness coupled with his/her family/social/financial circumstances). I heard the term "battle fatigue" recently applied to chronic illness. Because the illness itself is an internal war, which can be ongoing 24/7 and for years, this individual battle is often difficult enough. However, when external circumstances occur on top of that, each becomes an additional battle. This includes things such as relationship issues, finances, and/or medical estrangement. These can add up over time, leaving people in dire straits with risks of suicide or other desperate measures. Chapter 4, "Missing Lisa" by V. Free, describes how internal and external circumstances sometimes add up to a devastating ending.

As with many other serious illnesses, significant support is required, and it is difficult for immediate families to bear the entire burden. Caregiving and other help from outside the immediate family circle are often needed.

During the worst times of my illness, my mom and dad would come, food in hand, to care for us. What a relief that was! They were always sad to leave us, knowing it was so difficult. I also considered moving back to their place with my young daughter who had just started school. However, I would not have had access to the helpful medical or alternative care that I had at the time, my daughter would have had to change her school, and my husband had his business to tend to, so I chose not to move.

As opposed to false hope or no hope, maintaining realistic hope for improvement is important – but not that easy to keep up – when dealing with cognitive, emotional, and physical disability. With ME/CFS, the medical care and treatment are so lacking that hope can be swept away. Some families do not stay together, and many patients end up on their own, in situations that range from challenging to impossible. And because so few resources are available to those with ME/CFS, we very often fall through the cracks.

❧ *Erasing my life* – The severity and intensity of my relapse of 1995 was shocking. In the section on Presentation and Course of Illness, the International Association for CFS/ME's *Primer for Clinical Practitioners* (IACFS/ME, 2014) states on page 7:

> The illness can vary from mild to severe, with symptoms that may fluctuate significantly from hour to hour and day to day. A substantial number of patients with ME/CFS are bedridden, housebound, or wheelchair dependent. Many of these patients are too impaired to travel to office visits. Others, if not housebound, may be unable to hold a job. Those least affected may work part-time or even full-time if their occupations

are not too exhausting or if suitable accommodations are made. Some may need to find less demanding employment in order to continue working. Yet these higher functioning patients are often so exhausted from working that they spend many of their non-working hours resting.

I'm not the only one I know with this illness who has trouble grasping its realities. For instance, my friend Linda can't handle normal tasks of daily living due to her illness. She tells me that she is shattered from an outing to get groceries, but then wistfully utters, "Maybe I could work a little." Living with this illness and its fluctuating challenges is so confusing for those who have it and those around them, including the medical professionals. This may be what CFS should stand for: **Con-Fu-Sing.**

STANZA 16

Hallmark symptoms: energy problems

The body works well with two energy systems,
Aerobic ✒ is one, using oxygen pistons.
It's used for sustaining long-term energy,
But now it's not working – brings me to my knees.

The other is called the *Anaerobic* ✒ system,
Not needing oxygen; short, sharp emission.
Like weights or the one-hundred yard relay sprint,
Research reveals only this one is "mint." ✒

    …Stairs a mountain…
    …Resting between…
    …Do things differently…

To have a *relay for life's work and demands,* ✒
I'd need 50 of me with ME.

STANZA 16 NOTES

❧ *Aerobic* means "needing oxygen" and is the energy system we rely on for long-term activity when healthy. This energy system has been proven dysfunctional in ME/CFS, so sustained activity of mind or body is a challenge. This is one reason that exercise, as I knew it in health, is not even remotely possible. Even walking challenges the aerobic system for me, and if this system is pushed beyond capacity, worsening and/or permanent damage can occur. There are measureable physical differences in response to exertion between healthy people and those who have ME/CFS, including resting heart rate, cardiac output, and cerebral blood flow. For more details on these differences, see Appendix G.

❧ *Anaerobic* means "not needing oxygen" and is the energy system that is more intact in ME/CFS. So short, small movements are sometimes more manageable. In the healthy, a short, quick sprint primarily uses the anaerobic system, and we all know what the soreness feels like from the lactic acid produced from it. I can carry a large water bottle a few yards to the dispenser without much problem, as long as that's all I do. But walking 100 yards, which utilizes the aerobic system, is very difficult; and payback is imminent if I do it too often. That is because my body shifts to the anaerobic system for fuel too early, creating pain and relapse. The ratio we are taught for energy management is 1:3, 1 part effort to 3 parts rest, as in the next stanza. Alternately, there's the 90-second rule: 90 seconds of activity, and then rest.

Unfortunately, due to lack of accurate knowledge and understanding about ME/CFS by health professionals, exercise may be recommended as a form of treatment, or at least encouraged. In countries such as the United Kingdom, graded exercise therapy (GET) is a standard part of their recommended treatment protocol. However, without proper guidance and monitoring, this can be dangerous and counterproductive.

The anaerobic threshold is what we can use to measure the limit that is safe for physical activity for those with ME/CFS at certain stages. The threshold can be calculated through cardiopulmonary testing by clinicians who, ideally, are experienced in reading the results for ME/CFS patients. This is where the use of a heart rate monitor comes in, which can help gauge when our energy crosses over from the aerobic system to the anaerobic zone. See Chapter 10, "Adapting" by J. Spotila for an example of how using a heart rate monitor alters doing an activity.

Another area of research in ME/CFS is the production of energy, or lack thereof, called mitochondrial dysfunction. The mitochondrium are found in most cells and produce the enzymes for the metabolic conversion resulting in energy. Dr. S. Myhill has completed three studies in this area which are found on her website.[55]

---

55   drmyhill.co.uk/wiki/Main_Page (accessed July 25, 2016).

❦ ***Research reveals only this one is mint*** – There is validating science to shed light on the serious symptom of post-exertional malaise or relapse which illustrates why so many ME/CFS patients have such resistance to the word "exercise." [56] Mark VanNess and fellow researchers monitored ME/CFS patients during an exercise challenge on two consecutive days, 24 hours apart. First, the patients' respiratory gases and cardiovascular, pulmonary, and metabolic responses during exercise on the treadmill were measured, and then measured again, at rest. This is called cardiopulmonary exercise testing or CPET. (The more usual purpose for CPET is to measure the performance of athletes).

Researchers noticed both abnormal symptoms and biological measurements following exercise in ME/CFS patients that are fairly unique to the illness.[57]

The researchers then charted how long these abnormal reactions and symptoms lasted after the challenge. Believe it or not, some of the increased symptoms that the CFSers experienced after this exercise challenge – including fatigue, light-headedness/vertigo, muscular/joint pain, cognitive dysfunction, headache, nausea, weakness/instability, trembling, insomnia, and sore throat/swollen glands – were reported as increased for up to 15 days.

Mark VanNess and this research group found that the recovery time from the two-day challenge was, on average, 4.5 days for CFS patients and 24 hours for healthy control subjects. So post-exertional relapse is now provable and measureable. This is very important for me and many patients in understanding our experience better – and in encouraging us to be kinder to ourselves as a result.

These results are not the same as those for deconditioned healthy people or those who are unfit. However, the consequence of deconditioning from long-term reduced movement in ME/CFS patients can worsen these readings. The good news is that trained professionals can create programs for the ME/CFS patients to help them remain more mobile and strong and to make the tasks of daily living a little easier. That might mean five minutes of certain exercises on the floor or a slow-paced, five-minute walk once a week, working up in time or intensity if and when possible. This is done with the heart rate monitor and lots of charting.

Two other examples of well-informed and respected professionals/researchers in this field are Staci Stevens, MA and Betsy Keller, PhD. Staci Stevens is with the Workwell Foundation in California and is the originator of the two-day CPET testing, known

---

56   VanNess JM, Snell C, and Stevens S, "Diminished Cardiopulmonary Capacity During Post-Exertional Malaise" Journal of Chronic Fatigue Syndrome. 01/2008;14(2): 77-85.

57   VanNess et al. found a mean decline of 22 percent in VO2 max. This revealed increased oxidative stress. VO2 max indicates peak oxygen consumption, which is measured by liters of oxygen consumed per minute.

as the Stevens protocol, which is useful to objectively demonstrate dysfunction in ME/CFS patients.

I had the good fortune to learn from a phone consultation with Ms. Stevens about the type of energy dysfunction that ME/CFS brings to my life. She helped me understand my energy limitations and orthostatic intolerance[58] better and said that small movements, while lying on the floor, could help me maintain some strength and flexibility. She also taught me how to better protect myself from overdoing. It was hard to hear that the 1:3 effort/rest ratio was the way I needed to live, but understanding it was better than the consistent crash/burn cycle I was used to. I go into more detail about this in the next stanza.

Betsy Keller is a professor in the Department of Exercise and Sports Science at Ithaca College, New York. She has published a paper supporting metabolic dysfunction in ME/CFS patients.[59] [60]

One day, maybe one or more of these tests will make up the biological markers for diagnosis – either on their own or in combination with other testing. However, for the severe and extremely affected, these tests will not be accessible or doable. I personally have not done the CPET 2-day challenge because I know the severity of the relapse that would occur from the travel and testing.

ᔦ *Relay for life's work and demands* – I look at my daily routine as a relay and am glad I have partners to help. I make the grocery list; my husband works to pay for the groceries; my daughter gets the groceries; I unload the groceries; my daughter makes dinner; I do the dishes, and on it goes. The worse my health becomes, the more partners I need to tend to life or to keep up any quality of life. I really would need 50 of me with ME to keep up with a full and productive life.

Of course I realize that as time goes by, life changes, as do the people around me, and that my relay partners may not always be there or be the same.

I know that some who are on their own may not have anyone for support which must add significantly to the already significant burden of ME/CFS.

---

58 Orthostatic intolerance (OI) is the development of symptoms while standing upright, which are relieved when lying down. See Stanza 19 for more information.

59 Keller BA, Pryor JL, Giloteaux L, "Inability of myalgic encephalomyelitis/chronic fatigue syndrome patients to reproduce VO2 peak indicates functional impairment." J Transl Med. 2014 Apr 23;12:104. doi: 10.1186/1479-5876-12-104.

60 Other important and ground-breaking studies that also used exercise challenges were those demonstrating increased inflammation. White et al. 2009. www.ncbi.nlm.nih.gov/pmc/articles/PMC4378647 (accessed July 7, 2016) and "Increased expression for sensory, adrenergic, and immune genes in CFS patients." Light et al. 2009. www.ncbi.nlm. nih.gov/pmc/articles/PMC2757484 (accessed July 25, 2016).

STANZA 17

Living in quicksand:
One-part effort to three-parts rest

Living in quicksand, I find quite descriptive:
Try to crawl out and the symptoms get vivid.
Stay in the zone where your energy's best,
One small part of effort to three parts of rest.

It sounds do-able, until one has to try it.
After one day, I'm sure you would despise it.
Like quicksand it feels – doomed, if still or in fits,
The harder one fights it, the deeper it gets.

   …Limitations…
   …And restrictions…
   …Special needs galore …

How I wish I could feel solid ground 'neath my feet,
Which I took for granted before.

STANZA 17 NOTES

❧ *One small part of effort to three parts of rest* – This is something worth repeating. In health, can you imagine someone telling you that for every minute of effort, you need to rest three times as much in order to proceed (and only if you do not exceed your heart rate limit as calculated by your anaerobic threshold)? Living with this 1:3 ratio, as well as pacing and determining my changing energy envelope, is a full-time job and is so unnatural to do.

I have learned that it is important to be able to take care of essential activities of daily life first: self-care, eating, and paying basic bills. Then, if and as I improve, I add other activities. If someone improves to 60 to 80 percent, this might enable them to stay awake all day without rests, work at a job part-time, and slowly add aerobic exercise into their lives. Most doctors require people to be very functional before adding aerobic exercise because if we worsen, it can become harder and harder to pull us out of the ME/CFS quicksand.

❧ *Special needs galore* – Who would ever think from its name that an illness called "chronic fatigue syndrome" would have special needs or require accommodations beyond extra sleep? Unfortunately, most people, myself included, develop many additional considerations such as dietary exclusions, mobility concerns, medication and supplement requirements, oxygen use, energy-conservation accommodations, climate challenges, pain considerations, and always needing a place to rest. And on the sleep front, good deep sleep is elusive for most people with ME/CFS, just adding to the list of their unique needs: darkened room, earplugs, eye covers, no TV/computer in the bedroom, a good bed to reduce pain, and on and on. The list of special needs is shorter for some, while it grows longer for others.

STANZA 18

Post-exertional malaise

The *payback is named "post-exertional malaise."* ⮞
It aggravates illness for months, weeks, or for days.
It means ... after one exerts any way, shape, or form,
New symptoms show up – old ones worsen with scorn.

So instead of exertion that's making us "stronger,"
The system is goofy – It's making us "wronger."
Post-exertion relapse is one *diagnostic key,* ⮞
And this type of relapse brings me to my knees.

   …Doomed if I do…
   …Doomed if I don't…
   …*Doing this tightrope dance* ⮞ …

I try to stay grateful to struggle each day,
Some illnesses don't get a chance.

STANZA 18 NOTES

✍ *Payback is named "post-exertional malaise"* (PEM) – You have already been intro-duced to this unique symptom, and PEM is, without a doubt, one of the banes of ME/CFS. In the 2011 ME ICC definition,[61] post-exertional malaise is called post-exertional neuroimmune exhaustion (PENE). The terms differ, but the experience is the same. Although in medicine the term is correct, many patients do not like the term "malaise." Some people interpret it to mean being lazy, complacent, or insignificant, and one of its dictionary meanings is a general feeling of illness or sickness of no diagnostic significance. This does not describe our experience. That is why patients often choose to call it post-exertion relapse or collapse. So much depends on the language used and the perception it creates.

✍ *Diagnostic key* – PEM is only one diagnostic key, and other symptoms, especially when found together, are very unique to ME/CFS. One example of this constellation of symptoms includes illness-type fatigue, PEM, pain, and cognitive and neurological difficulties. Their appearance together is a significant indication that ME/CFS may be the correct diagnosis; but other conditions still have to be ruled out.

✍ *Doing this tightrope dance* – (Illustration at Section 2: Chapter 9) In so many ways, managing this illness is like walking a tightrope high off the ground, with clown shoes on, while snapping alligators wait below for the fall. It is difficult to balance a safe and comfortable activity level while accomplishing necessary activities of daily living. At the lower to mid-end of functioning, it is only possible to do light tasks two or three times a day, have some computer and TV time, and maybe go out twice a week for drive-through errands.

I sometimes feel that each choice is a risk: I lose if I try hard and lose if I don't. If I do too much, my symptoms increase – pain, poor concentration, and orthostatic intolerance for example. If I don't do enough, tasks remain undone, my self-esteem is affected, and others in my family have to pick up the slack or we have to pay someone to do them. And I am just talking about daily tasks here, not including physical work or a social life, except for some phone and Internet.

---

61   ME ICC definition – Carruthers BM, van de Sande MI, De Meirleir KL, et al. "Mylagic encephalomyelitis: International Consensus Criteria." J Inter Med. 2011. 270(4):327-338.
http://onlinelibrary.wiley.com/doi/10.1111/j.1365-2796.2011.02428.x/abstract (accessed July 25, 2016).
ME ICC Primer – Carruthers BM and van de Sande MI (eds). "Myalgic Encephalomyelitis – Adult & Paediatric: International Consensus Primer for Medical Practitioners." International Consensus Panel. 2012. Carruthers & van de Sande publishers. www.investinme.org/Documents/Guidelines/Myalgic%20Encephalomyelitis%20International%20Consensus%20Primer%20-2012-11-26.pdf (accessed July 25, 2016).

It is challenging to find an activity that keeps me from becoming deconditioned without worsening my situation. I have tried to stand for ten minutes in a warm pool, moving slowly: That relapse lasted four days. I have tried yoga on the floor, mostly stretching: That relapse started within twenty-four hours and lasted a couple days. I have tried ten minutes of light housecleaning with a vacuum: That did me in for two days. A visit to an aggressive chiropractor who did not take into account my fragile system ended in a five-day relapse.

STANZA 19

Orthostatic intolerance

Orthostatic intolerance 🌿 is a big symptom,
It means all "signs" worsen in upright positions.
The more I sit or stand, the more ill I feel,
If pushing it, fainting or dizziness reel.

Neurological problems I cannot control,
Blood pressure, blood volume down, heart rate that soars.
When upright my mind needs more blood than supplied,
One symptom, hard – never mind the whole pie.

…Keep your legs up…
…Keep your head down…
…Try some salt and meds…

How can I live life the way I was meant,
When lying on the floor instead? 🌿

STANZA 19 NOTES

❧ *Orthostatic intolerance (OI)* – My need to stay sitting or lying down is partly due to orthostatic intolerance. It is common in ME/CFS and is difficult to manage. There are different kinds of OI – postural orthostatic tachycardia syndrome (POTS) is the one I have. Orthostatic intolerance is a separate diagnosis, but many of its symptoms overlap with ME/CFS. The term means "intolerant to being upright." Symptoms include dizziness, fainting, fatigue, nausea, lightheadedness, heart palpitations, sweating, and sometimes fainting. Abnormal heart rates and blood pressures are measurable when changing positions from lying to standing, or vice versa. Dr. D. Bell states: "OI is the presence of symptoms due to inadequate cerebral perfusion (blood flow to the brain) on assuming the upright posture. Many persons with medically proven OI have been assumed to have emotional problems when they don't." [62]

Another contribution to OI symptoms is low blood volume. It has been shown that some persons with ME/CFS do have low blood volume – a liter or so short![63] You know what happens when a vehicle is low on oil, right? Well, just as a car cannot run efficiently once the oil level is too low, so a body can't function without adequate blood volume and flow. This is definitely one of my most consistent and challenging symptoms! OI makes certain things difficult to impossible, like standing up while putting on my makeup, standing in a shower, or standing in a line at an event.

Treatments such as salt loading, compression socks and garments, and certain medications can be helpful. I did try saline solution intravenous therapy during a recent winter and the nurse came to my home to run it through my arm, which took a few hours from start to finish. But I did not find it helpful long-term. Some people do have good results, but the treatment must be ongoing, and IVs always have some risk of infection.

❧ *When lying on the floor instead* – During relapses and times when my symptoms are worse, I find that lying on the floor with my feet resting up against the wall is the most comfortable place for me. It is where I feel less symptomatic, as my body can rest without the tensions and energy demands of being upright. This is partly due to orthostatic intolerance.

---

62   May 2000, Lyndonville Journal. www.oiresource.com/tresults.htm (accessed July 26, 2016).

63   Hurwitz BE et. al. "Chronic Fatigue Syndrome: Illness Severity, Sedentary Lifestyle, Blood Volume and Evidence of Diminished Cardiac Function." Clin Sci (Lond) 2009 118:125-135. doi: 10.1042/CS20090055. www.ncbi.nlm.nih.gov/pubmed/19469714 (accessed July 26, 2016).

STANZA 20

Pain

Another loud symptom is that of pain,
In *Fibro* ✦ 'n CFS, it makes many lame.
All kinds of pain are prominently there,
I have spine pain and bone pain and at times my hair!

The treatment for pain is to give things a test,
Small doses of this or that – try to get rest.
Some need to use the most powerful drugs,
Even morphine hardly gives theirs a tug.

...We can't bear it...
...Always hurting...
...Why the chronic pain?...

Sometimes the chaos inside of ME,
Could drive a sound person insane.

STANZA 20 NOTES

❧ *Fibro* is short for fibromyalgia syndrome (FMS), also simply known as fibromyalgia. It is another complex condition that is separate from, but can overlap with, CFS. Severe chronic pain can be a symptom of both ME/CFS and of FMS.[64]

This has led me to wonder about the meaning of the term "syndrome" in many illness labels: chronic fatigue *syndrome*, acquired immune deficiency *syndrome* (AIDS); fibromyalgia *syndrome*. In this book, I refer to these as "illnesses."

- The dictionary defines a **syndrome** as: *n.* a set of symptoms occurring together; the sum of signs of any morbid state; a symptom complex.

- **Illness** is defined as: *n.* 1. Poor health resulting from disease of body or mind; sickness. 2. A disease.

- A **disease** is defined as: *n.* an abnormal condition affecting the body of an organism. It is often construed to be a medical condition associated with specific symptoms and signs.

There is medical argument that these are not diseases but are syndromes because of the unknown pathology or marker. As a person who has an illness labeled as a syndrome, I don't find these labels make much difference to the experience. However, I have found that people often do not think of a syndrome as being as serious as a disease. Interestingly, in the 2015 IOM report, the new label suggested to the U.S. Department of Health and Human Services was "systemic exertion intolerance DISEASE." (emphasis by the author)

---

64   An important document of reference for fibromyalgia syndrome is "Fibromyalgia Syndrome: A Clinical Case Definition and Guidelines for Medical Practitioners – An Overview of the Canadian Consensus Document." Carruthers et al. 2005. www.mefmaction.com/images/stories/Overviews/FMSOverview08.pdf (accessed July 26, 2016).

STANZA 21

No cure, taking up yoga and symptom management

No cure, 🙞 *no treatment that's standard for care yet,* 🙞
Coping and pacing and symptom management.
Finding new ways to conserve energy, 🙞
New choices in lifestyle – no "style" do I see.

Things that I learned were unhealthy to do,
Now all have changed – *the CFS doc knew:* 🙞
Eat lots of salt, lots of protein from meat,
Stop moving your body, and stay off your feet.

   …I'll just lie here…
   …Resting my brain…
   …Trying to heal this "mess"…

But even *imagining a bird in flight,* 🙞
Is putting me to the test.

STANZA 21 NOTES

❧ *No cure* – At the time of my initial diagnosis in 1990, I was told there was no cure or treatment for CFS. After the severe relapse of 1995, I was told the same thing. In 2016, it is not much better. Mainstream medicine and treatment for the root of the illness has made very little progress. Treatment trials are available with specific doctors in different parts of the world and may offer a better quality of life for some. However, there are no guarantees and there is no universally effective treatment. Accessibility to these special options is an obstacle for most of us due to location and cost.

The two options that we have, if we're well enough to try them, are self-management techniques and symptom management options. In 2012, my ME/CFS doctor, Ellie Stein MD FRCP(C), created a manual to guide patients, families, and medical professionals through these strategies.[65] The goal is for people to improve and feel as well as possible with the strategies and symptomatic treatments currently available. The manual provides guidance and motivation to try to stay as healthy as possible until better options are known.

❧ *No treatment that's standard for care yet* – Until recently, I'd never thought about what it must have been like for those with other serious conditions before treatments were developed.

We know that HIV/AIDS was a death sentence when it first arrived in North America before treatments were available. The same goes for diabetes before insulin and certain cancers before chemotherapy. Those of us living with ME/CFS are in a similar position to people who lived with those conditions before they had treatment options, and although these mentioned do not have cures, they are now more manageable chronic illnesses. We ME/CFSers are still waiting for the same progress, unfortunately.

❧ *Finding new ways to conserve energy* – During the relapse of 1995, I found that one of the most efficient ways to conserve energy was by learning and practicing restorative yoga techniques. These include meditation, breathing, and restorative poses, all of which also help one to remain relaxed and strengthened. I made my home life "ashram-like." (An ashram is a retreat for spiritual and yoga practices.) I took classes in a local community center, developing friendships with some of the students who went on to become yoga instructors. They shared their knowledge with me. Then in 1999, I shared these techniques with neighbors and friends in my home, until I worsened after a disastrous treatment failure in 2000.[66]

---

65 Dr. Ellie Stein, "Let Your Light Shine Through – Strategies for Living with Myalgic Encephalomyelitis/Chronic Fatigue Syndrome, Fibromyalgia and Multiple Chemical Sensitivity." 2012. www.eleanorsteinmd.ca/manual-2 (accessed July 25, 2016).

66 See Part III.

❧ **The CFS doc knew** – When we are lucky enough to find compassionate and helpful medical help in any modality, it is often accompanied by the fear of losing the practitioner. This happens in both the alternative and Western medicine fields. Some of the doctors who know about ME/CFS have been dedicated to the illness since its onset in North America, almost thirty years ago – and many will retire soon.

During my most fragile and vulnerable phases of illness, it was not uncommon for me to feel anxious or afraid at the announcement from a trusted health care provider that he/she was taking a two-month leave or moving to another country. Many times, I felt my life was resting in his/her hands, so this has been an inevitable but added stress on my long journey. There have been three alternative practitioners who passed away from various causes while I was under their care. This was also alarming as they were quite young and their deaths happened suddenly.

After the relapse in 1995, I had the good fortune of finding a doctor in my city with a special interest in CFS, fibromyalgia, and post-polio syndrome. She was the first of two female ME/CFS experts whom I would see for my condition. Both of these doctors are around my age and also have ME/CFS, with onset dates close to mine. They have had to adapt their lives and practices to the restrictions and limitations that the illness places on everyone, but they have done such a great service for those of us who need their guidance and practical help.

Even in the absence of curative treatment, knowledgeable doctors can assist their patients by providing medications for symptom management, research updates, and self-management strategies, as well as disability reports and handicap parking passes. However, the severely affected may never be able to even show up for an appointment.

❧ **Imagining a bird in flight** – When I was able, I sought all sorts of help, including spiritual ideas. One of my spiritual healers suggested I imagine a flying bird as a way to keep my spirits up when I was unable to move off the couch or bed. I could not do it. The complete brain and body immobilization that I experienced during the worst periods of this illness meant that simply trying to visualize took more energy and focus than I could muster.

I also lost the ability to read, form a complete thought, or speak fluidly. I could no longer read music, although I had learned piano and guitar during childhood. I couldn't coordinate my mind and hands to use my stenograph machine even though I mastered it as a court reporter for fifteen years. I couldn't even remember simple directions in a familiar neighborhood.

During severe phases of worsening, sitting up at the table, as well as chewing my food, were laborious tasks; and I would have to rest for long periods between bites, storing the food in my cheeks like a little gopher, until I was able to continue. Sometimes I would just give up, spit it out, and go back to lie down.

On my personal scale, I call this the "Wishing Death or Wellness" state, because I would pray for God to either let me die or make me well. I did not want to be left somewhere in between good health and death, in a limbo land that I could not recognize or navigate. But that is exactly where many of us are living: "**the middle zone – a near-death, near-life experience.**"

Wishing to die to stop the suffering, I now recognize, is an aspect of my constellation of symptoms. It comes and goes with the severity, but is predictable when I become extremely ill for long periods of time or have feelings of hopelessness due to lack of improvement. Others report similar feelings. However, it isn't always during the worst times. Sometimes, when people start feeling better, the hopelessness grows because they have enough energy to see the whole picture and the impact the illness has had on their lives and on those of their loved ones.

It is important to identify these thoughts as part of the physical, mental, and emotional symptoms that come and go along with the changing circumstances. Having knowledge-able people to talk to who can provide perspective, compassion, and reassurance has been crucial in motivating me to keep on going.

Some of the other themes on my personal scale of symptoms, many of which started in the worst five years are: "nausea and numbness," "fever and freezing," "crumpled and crying," "sleepless and sore," "weak and wonky," and "scared and shaky." As things slowly lessened from this acute state, the themes began to shift to "stand and sit," "walk and wait," "mourn and meditate," and "push and crash," while always trying to "adapt and adjust" as best as I could.

PART III
TREATMENT, SETBACKS, POLITICS, AND FAMILY
(My Age: 40 to 44)
2000-2004

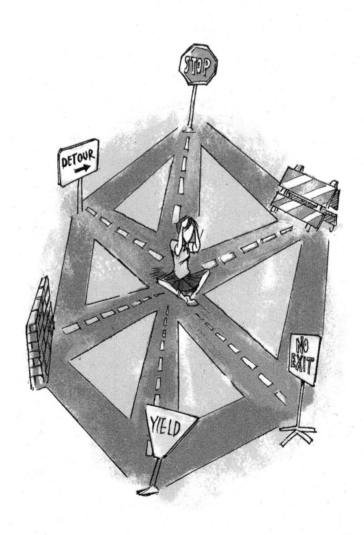

STANZAS 22-30 TOPICS

STANZA 22

Neuro-endocrine-immune disease

My immune system's different, not working the same,
No more colds for me, no more flus to tame. ✣
Even when others around me get sick,
These are the things that I no longer get.

Instead symptoms worsen, like weakness and pain,
I have learned my body and brain can inflame.
In our sick immune systems, markers they find,
One more bit of proof that it's not in our minds.

   …Where is the switch?…
   …Back to balance…
   …To work as it did before…

It's one *neuro-endocrine-immune disease,* ✣
Or N.E.I.D. for short.

STANZA 22 NOTES

✎ *No more colds for me, no more flus to tame* – When I became ill with ME/CFS, I no longer caught normal colds or flu as often as I did when I was well. I have had two brief colds in fifteen years and no flu. Interestingly, I actually felt better when I had these two short colds. Somehow everything felt more normal, and I had more energy. Some other ME/CFS patients I know report a similar phenomenon, while others catch everything they come into contact with. Now when I'm exposed to people with a cold or flu, I end up with an increase of my CFS symptoms lasting for days or weeks.

An interesting connection to this immune dysregulation is that experts recommend that "patients with ME/CFS should consider avoiding all but essential immunizations particularly with live vaccines, as post-vaccination relapse has been known to occur." (IACFS/ME Primer, 2014, 6:5) Others suggest immunizations, such as the flu shot, be given in smaller, repeated doses, if given at all, because they may worsen symptoms. Vaccinations are cited as one of the possible triggering events for ME/CFS, and I have met a few young people who have become ill after receiving multiple vaccinations in order to travel to foreign countries, as well as middle-aged people who became ill after standard immunizations required for their job. Another special concern is that of donating blood. I donated blood when I was well but as soon as I became ill with CFS, I did not think this would be wise, even during times of feeling a bit better. Over the years, there have been different views on this. But as the IACFS/ME Primer, 2014, states at 6:6:

> Blood and Tissue Donation: The American Red Cross requires that blood donors 'be healthy', i.e., feel well and be able to perform normal activities. Since people with ME/CFS are not healthy by this definition, they should not donate blood. Furthermore, given the possibility of infectious disease transmission in patients with ME/CFS, many countries have deferred or prohibited blood and tissue donation from patients who have ever suffered from ME/CFS.

✎ *Neuro-endocrine-immune disease* (or neuro-immune disease) is a term referring to illnesses that are the result of acquired dysregulation of the immune, endocrine (hormonal), and nervous systems. These illnesses share many features, including the possibility of lifelong disease and disability. Some of the illnesses included under the neuro-immune umbrella are fibromyalgia syndrome, ME/CFS, Gulf War illness, and chronic Lyme disease. They are all complex chronic illnesses affecting multiple body systems. The Institute for Neuro-Immune Medicine at Nova Southeastern University in Florida[67] is one place where these illnesses are being studied.

---

67 www.nova.edu/nim (accessed July 26, 2016).

STANZA 23

Looking okay, feeling sick

No bleeding, no bandages,  no broken bones,
Looking quite normal when out of our homes.
A strange thing for all, invisible disease,
'Cause people can't believe how sick we can be.

One patient wrote a book; the title she picked,
I Have CFS But I Don't Look Sick,
Which shows how this frustrates the patients galore,
For people to believe appearances more.

…Looking okay…
…Is a nice thing…
…But does not mean we're well…

For all kinds of disease that this applies to,
What's inside is hard to tell.

STANZA 23 NOTES

❧ *No bleeding, no bandages* – Since invisible illnesses can't be seen from the outside, it is often difficult for other people to understand there might be something amiss. When I'm in Arizona with my family at our vacation home, I use my scooter to get around. One time, I hurt my leg and had to wear a large bandage. People asked, "What happened?" It was apparent they understood why I, a young-looking middle-aged woman, needed a scooter. This is very different from my usual experience – without the bandage – when I feel people's questioning glances. Some go even further asking, "Why are you riding a scooter at your age?" This does give me the opportunity to tell people about CFS if I have the energy to do so, and maybe that is a good thing. But it is tiring, always explaining or feeling the need to explain. I've had the same experience using my wheelchair. When I stand up from it in a clothing store, reach for clothes to try on and walk a short way, and then sit back down with my daughter pushing the wheelchair, it creates confusion. Not many people know about energy illnesses. It can be hard for them to understand.

❧ *I Have CFS But I Don't Look Sick* – This is a very touchy subject for people with ME/CFS. It relates to the invisibility of the illness, how little is known about it in the general population, and how far we are from curative treatments.

I Have CFS But I Don't Look Sick is the title of a 2011 book by Pam Kidd. Pam and her two children became ill with CFS, and this book relates their experiences. At first, I was perplexed that she titled her book so specifically to one issue when there are so many, but I know first-hand that this is a frustrating aspect of this illness. After I first got ill, it wasn't an issue – I did not look well or healthy. I was so thin and pale and weak, my illness could not be hidden. More recently though, I have tended to look healthier, particularly when I am out and have expended the energy to dress nicely or to put on makeup. So while I may feel horrid, I look okay.

Many serious conditions such as heart disease and cancer are invisible and subject to mis-interpretation, so I wonder why we take offense regarding statements about looking good. When I had a conversation with a healthy friend about this, she also could not understand why a comment about looking good would generate such a strong, negative reaction. I had to think about this and came to the conclusion that it is out of frustration. The lack of knowledge regarding the severity of the disorder, along with the lack of medical care and research, is really what I am frustrated about. For the most part, I assume that those commenting on my looks do not know about ME/CFS. I find it difficult to refrain from educating everyone.

I won't ever forget the time I got yelled at for parking in a handicapped space, even though my disability pass was clearly in view. As I walked to my appointment at a nearby office, the men in the truck beside me yelled out, "You don't look handicapped." I was tempted to use the response I'd seen in a great cartoon from a National CFIDS Foundation newsletter, where one driver says exactly that: "You don't look handicapped," and the lady's response is, "That's funny, because you don't look stupid."

The frustration can happen even when someone is trying to be sensitive. Very recently, a customer of our business visited the house to tend to some things while my husband was out of the country. We remembered each other from more than fifteen years ago, when our children were going to kindergarten. Back then, most of the parents at the school knew I was ill. I told my visitor that I was not with my husband on his trip because I had not recovered from chronic fatigue syndrome and was too ill to travel with him at that time. The man's reply was, "Well, you look good. Maybe you are having a good day." Do I even know what a good day means? It is definitely not the kind of good day I did have when I was well.

There was a disconnect between the emotions I felt when I had to reiterate how ill I was and the one I felt when I heard our customer's response. I know he meant well, but it is characteristic of people who do not comprehend how serious ME/CFS is. There is no doubt I'll need to develop a tougher skin, at least until people have more knowledge.

There are times, I must confess, when I tell people I have MS instead, if I need to tell them anything at all, because they recognize it and understand the possible implications. It just makes life easier, and people respond more sensitively.

An article called "Until We Have a Cure: What CFS Patients Want Well Persons to Know,"[68] based on a 2012 Massachusetts CFIDS/ME & FM Association survey, deals with many of these issues. Included in the article was the following: "Because PWCs (People with CFS) usually look so well, people often comment on that as if to reassure the patient. Patients sometimes take it to mean that you don't believe that they are sick. Better to say something like, 'It must be hard for you to feel so lousy when you look so well.'" I agree this would be a sensitive way around this issue. Personally I am comforted by the compassionate response: "I am sorry you are experiencing this awful illness."

Another reason that the public, and even doctors, may not say the most appropriate things is that most ME/CFS patients I know look young for their age. Many people say time stopped at the start of their illness experience, like a switch was flipped: Maybe aging stopped too. I know that if I were given full health today, I would probably feel thirty years old – not over fifty – as if I became stuck at that age.

---

68   "Until we Have a Cure: What CFS Patients Want Well People to Know – Coping and Hoping," Patricia Larson, article in ProHealth January 4, 2013 based on the Massachusetts CFIDS/ME & FM Association 2012 patient survey. www.prohealth.com/me-cfs/library/showarticle.cfm?libid=17792 (accessed July 29, 2016).

STANZA 24

Dealing with doctors and health care professionals

I deal with doctors who still do not get it,
And if they do, they might rather dismiss it.
Nurses who still think that I am just tired,
"No, I'm not loony or lazy – and you should be fired."

Presenting and sharing the latest in testing,
Hoping the doctors find it worth investing.
The complexity and the difference in views,
Every so often ends up in abuse.

…Educating…
…Can be deflating…
…But how else can they see?…

That's a big burden for someone unwell,
And it can bring me to my knees.

STANZA 24 NOTES

✎ *I deal with doctors who still do not get it* – One of the first things a person with CFS may hear is that he or she should build a team of practitioners for support and care. I've certainly tried to do that over the years.

Unfortunately, many medical and alternative care professionals reject or dismiss ME/CFS patients, because they either don't know the illness or how to manage it, or they misdiagnose it as a psychiatric or other condition. This can lead to "clinically caused traumas" [69] for the person seeking help. Time constraints in the medical system, combined with the lack of medical training to diagnose and treat the illness, leave many ME/CFSers with nowhere to turn for proper care. Patients can become discouraged, and despair can set in, adding insult to injury.

We expect medical establishments to be safe and helpful environments. Unfortunately, this is not always the case. Because my onset was sudden and involved drastic changes over a short period of time, it was obvious that something was physically very wrong. The initial response I had from the medical profession was helpful. However, I haven't always received respectful care. I have had clinically-caused traumas due to responses from many of the healthcare providers I sought out through the years, which added to the injury and suffering of the illness. I recognize that not all of it is specifically related to my illness; some was just bad luck or lack of professionalism, and some of it was due to my own unrealistic expectations, which I learned about much later. Here are a few of my encounters:

(1) A neurologist asked whether I had anorexia because I was weak and thin.[70] I arrived for my appointment in a wheelchair, pushed by my daughter. The neurologist looked at the results of my MRI, which had been done to recheck the areas of my spine that had previously revealed two herniated discs. He pricked my legs with a pin, told me I did not have multiple sclerosis, and said that I did not need to come back – even though I was experiencing numbness, tingling in my body, and extraordinary spinal pain. When I mentioned to him that I had been diagnosed

---

69 Clinically caused traumas – Iatrogenic traumas are hurts that the health-care profession causes you. "When you are disbelieved by a doctor or treated as though a chronic illness is simply a psychological problem, you can suffer a clinically caused trauma." Fennell PA. 2001. The Chronic Illness Workbook. Oakland, CA: New Harbinger Press (Note: A 2012 revised edition is now available). Ms. Fennell notes that other responses can also be impatience or disbelief and that the likelihood of such trauma is increased due to the number of doctors a person with a chronic illness must encounter.

70 I found out much later that I had celiac disease, which probably accounted for some of my very slight appearance. That I was very thin was noticed by the neurologist, but unfortunately he did not know that I did eat a lot, so he had nothing to suggest but anorexia.

with chronic fatigue syndrome, he looked at me like I had two heads. Most neurologists are still not on board with ME or CFS, despite studies revealing abnormalities that are within their areas of specialty.

My daughter was only sixteen or so at the time, but she had the common sense to advise me not to get too upset – to take the good from the meeting and discard the rest. I guess the good was that I was not diagnosed with MS. There certainly wasn't much else. It is so disheartening, when reaching out to find help, only to hear that the people you are supposed to trust have no clue about your illness and even disregard you as a person.

(2)   Another specialist incident was with a gastroenterologist. I had just spent one year with an MD who had a local integrative health clinic. He was offering state-of-the-art testing and treatment for many complex conditions, including CFS. The cost for the year was in the range of $10,000. Many measurable abnormalities showed up in the across-the-border lab work and I was hopeful that this would point the way to treatment.

We employed diet changes, intravenous nutrient therapies, and supplementation. When I didn't show much improvement after ten months, the integrative doctor referred me to a GI specialist on my request, just in case we had missed something. Although I did not have the obvious symptoms for celiac disease such as severe weight loss or diarrhea, I asked the GI specialist if he could test me for it anyway, because I did not know what else to do. During our visit, he was voice recording it and made sure I knew that celiac disease was unlikely because my symptoms did not portray it. I had to request it more strongly because he was hesitant. Eventually he marked the check on the blood work form.

My celiac blood work came back with a strong positive, and because I sat in the office waiting for the next biopsy availability, he did do a biopsy at the hospital that showed severe damage to the lining of my digestive tract from celiac disease. This meant I had not been absorbing nutrients for a long time. Instead of the doctor telling me in an office visit, the diagnosis of celiac disease was delivered to me in a report.

While I asked to be referred to another GI doctor, who ended up being much more helpful and compassionate, my experience with the first one taught me one thing: Never rule out other illnesses that may be traveling together until tested, especially if an easy blood test is available.

(3)   There is a shortage of family doctors in Canada; and over the years, I've had a few difficult family doctor experiences, along with the other major disappointments. When my long-time and very knowledgeable family doctor moved out of the country, I needed to find a new one. I found a young doctor who, after two visits, told me she would rather **not** be my family doctor. She told me she felt ill prepared for a CFS patient and said she did not have time to learn about it despite the resources I brought to our visit (the CCC Overview). She mentioned her busy practice, the fear of a lawsuit, and that my condition was too time-consuming.

She suggested that I go to walk-in clinics or the emergency room for care if I could not find another family doctor. I literally begged to stay in her practice, knowing I would not ever visit a walk-in clinic. We went about regular yearly physicals twice, with an unspoken "Don't Ask – Don't Tell" policy, wherein I did not mention CFS, and she did not ask about it.

Hers was the worst response I've received to date, and it was hard to swallow. In fact, I was shocked that my diagnosis in 1990, by my then family doctor, went smoother than a visit 25 years later with other medical providers. I approached other doctors in her clinic to see if they had an interest in, or familiarity with, other patients with my condition. They all told me they would not receive a patient with ME/CFS either.

It was around that time that my family started to travel to Arizona for parts of the winter. I was so excited because a Mayo Clinic was nearby. I immediately phoned, thinking I had the answer to my doctor search. However, I was told that the clinic had no specialist for ME or CFS, and that I would need to travel to the East Coast to find one. I later learned that the Mayo Clinics have not been helpful to those with this disorder, other than for diagnosing it. Some patients seeking help have told me that the Mayo Clinics in Minnesota and Florida would not see any patients who had been experiencing symptoms for more than six months.

These negative experiences are not exclusive to the Western medical world. They can happen in the alternative, psychological, and spiritual worlds of healing as well.

All of these experiences had deep and profound negative effects on my hope and well-being. Managing my own care, dealing with the medical community's general ignorance and unwillingness to learn about the illness, and at times feeling completely estranged from the medical system, have been discouraging at their best and physically damaging at their worst. Bearing the illness is enough. Having a husband to come home to after each of these debacles, lots of self-knowledge, and a great kid with a good sense of humor have made many of my experiences tolerable, and some of them even funny. But knowing how often this happens to others seeking diagnosis and care for ME/CFS makes it tragic and quickly sours any humor that might be found in some situations.

Clinically caused traumas are not the only traumas chronically ill people face in addition to just being sick:

> There is the trauma produced by a prolonged diagnosis period, as well as the trauma of the actual onset or diagnosis itself. There is the stigmatizing response of family, society, and workmates as they become frustrated by the unpredictability and chronicity of symptoms because the patient never 'gets better' and does not go back to fulfilling former responsibilities. The chronically ill may also suffer from premorbid[71] and comorbid[72] traumas.[73]

Perhaps you are beginning to understand why I end up "back on my knees" throughout this story, both as a figure of speech for surrender and by getting knocked off my feet.

Many years later, I realized that ME/CFS was not recognized in our medical system and definitely was not part of mainstream. I learned that most of the professionals I encountered were not trained in the illness and did not know how to diagnose or treat it. Most did not want to learn about it due to its complexity, and they didn't have a specialist to send me to for treatment. This was the crux of the conflict I was facing, and it amplified my frustration because I thought health care practitioners should know about ME/CFS by this time. Eventually, I came to accept that I was a pioneer in the field, along with many others who are part of the first ME/CFS generation in our country. So I shared information with whoever would receive it and continued to search for the root of why ME/CFS was not part of mainstream yet. This book is one result of that search.

☙ *Nurses who still think that I am just tired* – As recently as 2015, I was getting blood drawn for some special testing at a local laboratory. There were a lot of tubes to fill. The nurse asked, "So do you just feel tired?" Although I used the opportunity to tell her more about my illness, it is exasperating to me that I must continually do so. With rare exceptions, people just do not understand. I am not tired or sleepy in the way she meant it. The fatigue associated with ME/CFS is different for everyone, but what I know is that it is not the same as the fatigue or tiredness I experienced in good health, nor is fatigue the worst symptom for me.

---

71   Premorbid means that it occurs before the development of disease.

72   Comorbid means existing simultaneously with and usually independently of another medical condition.

73   Fennell PA, "Chronic Illness." The Encyclopedia of Social Work, 20th ed. Vol. 1 A-C. Oxford University Press. 2008. 289.

🐛 *Hoping the doctors find it worth investing* – As of 2016, few medical schools in the world have incorporated training on ME, CFS, or ME/CFS into their curricula.[74] There is no specific specialty to which these illnesses belong (e.g., neurology or infectious disease specialties). These conditions require the interest and cooperation of all specialties. This lack of medical education with accurate information means that patients and their families must do their own research and educate their health providers – a significant burden for an already ill and heavily burdened population. Fortunately, some doctors are willing to learn about the illness, and a handful of doctors in each country have taken a special interest in it: They have become the experts within the ME/CFS medical community.

In 2014, Taylor, a Canadian twenty-two-year-old Creative Communications student from Winnipeg, Manitoba, decided to help the ME/CFS community after her mother became ill with the condition. She took the opportunity of a college project and created the video *Mom Needs To Lie Down: The years and lives slept away by ME/CFS*.[75] Taylor's mother's story illustrates how difficult it is to get a diagnosis for the illness among other issues. There are fewer than a handful of ME/CFS-literate doctors in Canada, and none were local to Taylor's mother when she needed them most, nor did she know where to go for proper information. Taylor's mother had an abscessed tooth and was given an unsuccessful root canal which led to the extraction of the tooth. Symptoms appeared and multiplied after this: extreme fatigue, post-exertional malaise, sleep problems, stomach pain, and memory and concentration problems, as well as muscle aches and pains. Without a diagnosis or medical support, she pushed on at her work as an elementary school teacher, and the symptoms became more severe. After taking one semester off, she returned half-time, and then reduced her schedule to three afternoons a week. Eventually she became so ill she had to stop work completely.

Taylor's mom eventually got a diagnosis, but she had to travel many miles to accomplish this.

> I went to Mayo Clinic because I was not getting a diagnosis or medical support in Manitoba, Canada, beyond basic blood work and procedures to rule out discernible physical abnormalities regarding pain, digestive, and weight loss issues.
>
> After ten days of extensive, extremely thorough assessment and testing, I was given a diagnosis of *probable* chronic fatigue syndrome. Sometime

---

74   T. Mark Peterson, DDS, Thomas W. Pertson, DDS., Sarah Emerson, BS, Eric Regalbuto, Meredyth A. Evans, MA, Leonard A. Jason, PhD, "Coverage of CFS in U.S. Medical Schools." Universal Journal of Public Health 1(4): 177-179, 2013. www.hrpub.org/download/20131107/UJPH4-17600991.pdf (accessed July 26, 2016).

75   The premiere screening of Taylor's video was on March 6th, 2014, at the Winnipeg Free Press News Café, and it was a full house.

after returning home from the Mayo Clinic, a woman, who organizes an informal support group for CFS, told me about Dr. E. Stein who practices in Calgary, Alberta, Canada. She offers an E-Team assessment* process for out-of-province patients. It was a 14-hour drive from our home, but after completing the E-Team assessments, Dr. Stein gave me the diagnosis of chronic fatigue syndrome and some treatment recommendations in the spring of 2011. **The diagnosis took four years from the onset of symptoms.** It has been a big learning curve to find strategies to stay within my energy envelope, reduce stress, and cope with all of the losses that a chronic illness such as CFS brings.

*The E-Team assessment is a specialized multidisciplinary assessment for cognitive/ memory symptoms and related problems associated with ME/CFS, fibromyalgia, multiple chemical sensitivity and toxic chemical and mold exposure.

Taylor brings to light many aspects of ME/CFS, including the importance and value of pets to those who are chronically ill. It is true that sometimes a pet is more likely to agree with a CFS lifestyle than another person, and I can testify to this fact: I've had pets throughout my illness – cats and puppies. Every idea is a good idea to my dog, who is now thirteen years old: Let's lie down, let's watch TV, let's go for a scooter ride, let's sit and do nothing. To a loyal pet, there are no bad ideas and no judgments, which is healing on its own.

Taylor gives a perfect example of the kind of initiatives that need to be taken, including ME/CFS education for health care providers. Some other creative ideas to encourage investment by health professionals are from patient organizations and foundations: scholarships to medical students who write the best essays on the subject of ME/CFS; qualified advocates visiting colleges and teaching about the physiology of the condition; or providing an opportunity for them to intern within an ME/CFS expert clinic. These ideas have helped a few soon-to-be doctors, and other professionals, get a chance to review the literature, meet the patients, and get an overview of this growing need in medicine.[76]

In 2016, in my home province of Alberta, progress was made. New Clinical Practice Guidelines for ME/CFS were developed and offered to all family physicians here. These

---

76 See more about these efforts in Part V.

Clinical Practice Guidelines for ME/CFS were developed by an expert committee of Towards Optimal Practice (TOP). TOP is a collaboration of the College of Physicians and Surgeons of Alberta and the Alberta Medical Association. TOP helps Alberta physicians, and the teams with whom they work, implement evidence-based practices to enhance the care of their patients. The committee for the ME/CFS Guidelines was also comprised of one ME/CFS expert, one scientist/researcher, one patient advocate, one psychologist and three family physicians. All had extensive knowledge of, and experience with, individuals with ME/CFS. The site for both the summary and the full guidelines is www.topalbertadoctors.org/cpgs/0242896 (accessed July 26, 2016).

evidence-informed guidelines will help patients and practitioners alike by providing guidelines for diagnosing, as well as offering symptomatic treatment, for people with ME/CFS in Alberta and elsewhere. (See Footnote 76 for more details)

STANZA 25

Treatment trials, cost, and working hard just to exist

IVs and needles and supplements to try,
I do things so that my health doesn't decline.
Bedridden forever, I don't want to be,
I wish there was some form of a guarantee.

Hot moxibustion and T.C.M. 🙠 herbals,
This medicine helpful, getting over hurdles.
Can't try them all at once or *I'll break the bank,* 🙠
Have to try *one by one,* 🙠 see how they rank.

   …This one's helpful…
   …That one's doubtful…
   …This one makes me worse…

I seem to be working hard just to exist, 🙠
How do we remove this CURSE?

STANZA 25 NOTES

❧ *Hot moxibustion and T.C.M.* – Traditional Chinese Medicine (T.C.M.) includes moxibustion, a Chinese medicine therapy that combines moxa, or mugwort herb, with heat. T.C.M. also includes acupuncture and herbal medicines.

I relied on my T.C.M. practitioners for many years, and at times they would come to my home when I was too ill to go out. The treatments always helped me to a degree, but I never improved significantly.

I did occasionally take some of the T.C.M. herbal medicines, but when I later discovered that I had celiac disease, I quit. It was too difficult to discern the source of the starches in them because their labeling was so different from North American labels.

Acupuncture is one modality for which I am eternally grateful because the practitioners I worked with always seemed to understand the seriousness of my health situation and never gave up on me, even after many years.

❧ *I'll break the bank* – Alternative, specialized, or out-of-country care options are very expensive and can become unsustainable over time. I have been fortunate to learn about, and to try, many healing modalities. One part of illness risk management is also financial. There are stages and severities of ME/CFS. Depending on how severely we are affected or which stage of the illness we are in, most of us become desperate at some time or another. I certainly did. Because of the lack of standard effective treatments, I was willing to sacrifice a lot, spend almost anything, and accept some physical risk. "How could it be worse?" I would ask myself. Of course I ended up learning all about that.

❧ *One by one* – Because people with ME/CFS are sensitive to medications, alternative treatments, and even many foods, most health care professionals who work with ME/CFS suggest a "start low – go slow" philosophy for treatments. Starting one new thing at a time or stopping one thing at a time is the only way to test treatments and track the results, positive or negative. Sometimes it is very difficult for a sick person to keep track because he/she is just too ill to do so. I personally have avoided trying certain treatments or medications because I have learned the hard way that when I get too unwell, I am unable to accurately monitor my condition, and things can quickly worsen.

❧ *I seem to be working hard just to exist* – It was a big disappointment for me and my family when we realized that everything I was doing – working so hard at my diet and trying different interventions to manage my symptoms including medications and supplements – was only preventing my condition from worsening and not curing it. It is hard to keep up all the effort for what seems like little to no noticeable reward or relief.

STANZA 26

Treatment disasters, a near-death experience, and the risk-to-benefit ratio

There were some treatments I was really hurt from, ❧
Experimental – they promised me the sun.
Before we understood CFS at all,
I gave them a chance and I took some bad falls.

They didn't care or take responsibility,
A near-death experience ❧ – no accountability.
Others have had the same story as this,
Pushing me deeper into the abyss. ❧

...More months in bed...
...Loss of progress...
...Have I lost my mind?...

If someone else asks me what I have to lose,
The *risk–benefit ratio* ❧ they'll find.

STANZA 26 NOTES

𝕎 *There were some treatments I was really hurt from* – During the many years I have been ill with ME/CFS, I felt I had no choice but to try various treatments in other modalities in an attempt to improve my health. I had four treatment experiences that worsened my condition significantly – and long term. All were alternative or experimental but administered under professional care.

The experimental treatment called Interactive Light Therapy left me badly injured, barely alive, and very disconnected. Some psychologists use this procedure for people who have fibromyalgia and CFS. "What do you have to lose?" the practitioner asked me, while claiming there were no risks or side effects. Little did I know, when it comes to CFS, there is always more to lose. The treatment involved introducing frequencies to influence the brainwave imbalance shown on my qEEG (quantitative electroencephalogram) brain mapping. I knew that CFS was causing alterations and abnormalities in my qEEG because I had explored it with a medical specialist in this field a few years prior. You will hear more about my experiences with the treatment in the next note "A near-death experience."

The other damaging treatments I experienced during my early stages of illness were in the areas of complex homeopathy; a feedback frequency treatment for viruses by a naturopath; and a liver/gallbladder detox involving a lot of lemon juice and olive oil. My family doctor advised me that this detoxification process had left me with temporary liver damage and it also left me with years of excruciating pain in the right ribcage area, for which we never found a reason.

𝕎 *A near-death experience* – Although I did as much research as I could about Interactive Light Therapy, found someone who was doing well from the treatment, and took a slower pace than recommended, my protective measures failed.

After my sixth session, I could barely walk or find my way out of the clinic. I ended up with a very "fried" wiring system, two herniated discs, and was unable to sense normally from the neck down. As a result, I had to stop my yoga practice, and I lost all the progress I had made in the prior five years. "Hell on earth" is how I felt for years after that. I was again bedbound in a darkened room for months. Because of this, I had to hire help to cook and clean for my family, friends coordinated to come to our aid, and my family was further burdened with worry. Years later, I am still experiencing repercussions.

I did not think of asking to sign a consent form because the practitioners had verbally expressed that there were no risks or side effects to worry about. They did give me a form to sign after the damage was done. It was left unsigned but it did explain some possible side effects and risks, and I experienced all of them to the maximum. This led me to call the creators of the Interactive Light Therapy equipment, and after telling them my history and experience, they said I should never have been a candidate for it anyway and that there was no way to reverse what had happened. All too late!

I reported my horrors to the medical authorities and discovered two other people who claimed similar near-death experiences following this treatment. I know of one patient who filed a lawsuit. The clinic is no longer practicing that technique. I learned many hard life-lessons from this, including that not all professionals are trustworthy or knowledgeable about the treatments they offer.

❧ ***Pushing me deeper into the abyss*** – Whether I was very trusting or naive, I am not sure, but it was surprising to me that even the spiritual domain is not exempt from experiences that can be traumatic or damaging to an ill or vulnerable person. Seeking spiritual comfort was something I did to provide support during such a life-altering illness. I experienced many disappointments and abandonments from spiritual seeking, whether they were part of Christian, Buddhism, or other faiths. All of these added to my health crises and created a crisis of faith.

Among these challenging experiences were some wonderful ones with amazing people. I want to acknowledge some of them here: One member of the church congregation, who phoned me periodically over the years, offered his support; my good friend and yoga instructor Elaine, who never let go of our friendship regardless of the state I was in; and my long-time friends and relatives who stayed the course.

❧ ***Risk–Benefit ratio*** – Following these experiences, I learned to calculate the risk–benefit ratio of any treatment or modality: natural, alternative, psychological, or spiritual. Some treatments have the potential for improvement, but I realize that with my fragile system, everything has some risk. As I have learned from the School of Hard Knocks, there is no bottom to the scale of severity for the disease, and getting worse is always possible. I've also learned that I have to consider my family in my decision-making process. If I worsen temporarily or permanently from a treatment, I add further burdens to my loved ones and "carers." So I now know that I have to take into account the potential impact that my health has on everyone.

STANZA 27

Research and confusion about the cause: Lyme disease, viruses, toxins?

From *toxins to mold spores,* harmful heavy metals,
MS to Lyme disease; where trauma settles,
Coxsackie to Epstein, metabolic disease,
In circles we go – *give us one answer, please.*

From body to psyche, from feelings to karma,
Environment, genetics; don't let it alarm ya.
This is the confusion that CFS brings,
No known cause or cure yet, so check out all things.

…Doc, make your mind up…
…What should we treat?…
…Can't it be more clear?…

When dealing with illness with no end in sight,
It's hard not to live with some fear.

STANZA 27 NOTES

✌ *Toxins to mold spores* – Environmental medicine is interested in the role that environment plays on our health. For looking up toxins, mold, and related issues that may affect humans, the National Institutes of Health website lists environmental health topics from A to Z.[77] It includes mold, heavy metals, and many different toxins which can all create health risks. When I was very ill, I became extremely reactive to things like diesel, gasoline, softening sheets for the dryer, perfume, and smoke. I always try to stay in a clean environment due to these triggers that worsen my symptoms. People who have multiple chemical sensitivity (MCS) are very reactive to many chemicals and can become very ill when exposed to them. In Chapter 9, "Trapped: Living with ME/FM/MCS" by J. Samonas, is a detailed example of how challenging it can be to live with MCS.

Mold exposure can be a factor in ME/CFS or can create an illness of its own. The symptoms can be very similar to other diseases.[78] [79] Only certain molds are suspected of creating disease. The most dangerous aspect isn't the mold itself, but the spores, which can end up in the air we breathe or on our clothes and furniture. The spores are invisible. I have personally had two fairly significant exposures to toxic mold in our home due to flooding in the basement. These happened after I was already ill. We had to do mold remediation twice and eventually got everything under control. Without very elaborate testing, I will not know if this has added to the severity or chronicity of my condition.

✌ *MS to Lyme disease* – Both Lyme disease and multiple sclerosis (MS) can appear similar to ME/CFS in signs and symptoms, and all of them can take a long time and be difficult to diagnose. That is why many of us have been sent to specialists to rule out these diseases. Multiple sclerosis, as described on the Mayo Clinic website, "is a disease in which your immune system attacks the protective sheath (myelin) that covers your nerves. Ultimately, the nerves themselves may deteriorate, a process that's currently irreversible. There's no cure for multiple sclerosis. However, treatments can help speed recovery from attacks, modify the course of the disease and manage symptoms." MS is easiest to diagnose once the telltale lesions are visible through testing.

Another illness that has been diagnosed in some of my Canadian and U.S. acquaintances with ME/CFS is chronic Lyme disease (more formally known by the CDC as post-treatment Lyme disease syndrome). Lyme disease can look similar to, and can co-exist with, ME/CFS. Lyme disease was named after the U.S. East Coast town of Lyme, Connecticut, where the disease was first identified in 1975. By 1977, the black-legged tick (also known as the deer tick) was linked to the transmission of the disease. The infection comes from

---

77   www.niehs.nih.gov/health/topics/atoz/index.cfm (accessed July 29, 2016).

78   www.niehs.nih.gov/health/materials/mold_508.pdf (accessed July 29, 2016).

79   www.survivingmold.com (accessed July 29, 2016).

the Borrelia Burgdorferi bacterium, which is carried by a percentage of ticks. The percentage varies by location.[80] The bacteria are released into the blood while the tick is attached to the person or animal. The ticks can be as small as a pencil tip and may go unseen and unnoticed. Not everyone reacts with the characteristic "bulls-eye rash" that is often indicative of an infected tick bite, and a person may not have symptoms until years later. As a result, it may be diagnosed as another illness, for example, rheumatoid arthritis.

There are many co-infections that can also be passed by ticks and other vectors.[81] Some doctors use the term "multiple systemic infectious disease syndrome" (MSIDS) because there is a host of infections, as well as Lyme, in many chronically ill patients.[82]

Each year, thousands go undiagnosed or misdiagnosed, often told their symptoms are all in their heads. Today, Lyme disease is the most common vector-borne disease in the United States – far more common and dangerous to the average American than West Nile virus which is carried by a small percentage of mosquitoes. Ticks are not only carried by deer. Birds and other animals can carry them and drop them off anywhere. For further information on this topic, the International Lyme and Associated Diseases Society (ILADS) is a well-respected organization that deals with tick-borne and related illness.[83]

Canada is not exempt from this problem, and some provinces report more Lyme disease than others. It is not an easy diagnosis to solidify, because once it has moved from the initial acute stages to a chronic stage, Lyme disease is difficult to identify and diagnose. The infection moves quickly out of the blood stream into much deeper tissue, for example the brain and spinal cord. Acute Lyme is easier to diagnose because it is still in the blood stream. However, tests in Canada are often inadequate to achieve accurate results for acute or chronic Lyme and co-infections, so tests are often required from specialty labs in other countries. Unfortunately, even those may give false negative results.

I learned about Lyme disease when I first traveled to an independent treatment center for complex disease in Reno, Nevada, U.S. in the mid 'nineties. It was the first time anyone ever mentioned Lyme disease to me. I had never heard of it before. Although I did not get a concrete diagnosis for Lyme disease from lab work there, the doctor suggested to me that this could be the problem. After I came home, I spent two years trying to prove or

---

80   For example, in British Columbia, Canada, 1% of ticks are reported to carry the bacteria. www.bccdc.ca/health-info/
     diseases-conditions/lyme-disease-borrelia-burgdorferi-infection (accessed July 20, 2016). In certain areas of other
     countries, reports indicate that up to 25% of ticks can carry it.

81   A vector-borne disease is an illness caused by an infectious microbe, which is transmitted to humans by blood-sucking
     insects or spiders.

82   MSIDS is a term used by Richard Horowitz, MD, an expert in diagnosing and treating Lyme disease. Dr. Horowitz's
     website is wwwcangetbetter.com. His book is, "Why Can't I Get Better? Solving the Mystery of Lyme and Chronic
     Disease." St. Martin's Press. 2013. This book represents over 26 years of his work, diagnosing and treating over
     12,000 chronically ill patients with Lyme disease.

83   www.ilads.org (accessed July 29, 2016).

disprove this possibility with different testing. I have never received the additional diagnosis of Lyme disease, but did spend a lot of money and time trying, hoping that I would have more treatment options should I be diagnosed. Since then, I came to understand that even if the diagnosis were made in Canada, finding a doctor to treat it here would be difficult and very expensive.

When it comes to Lyme disease, if one is to have a chance to recover, proper antibiotic treatment should occur within thirty days of infection. The antibiotics can also prevent a fairly benign illness from exploding into a nightmare of an illness that is difficult, if not impossible, to cure. (See Chapter 9, "My Lyme Disease Story" by M. Logan.)

✌ *Coxsackie to Epstein* – Researchers are still trying to figure out why the immune systems of people with ME/CFS do not deal with viruses properly. Many studies have been undertaken to look into the role that viruses play in the illness. Some researchers are focusing on enteroviruses as a cause for the onset of the illness as well as a factor in keeping it active in a subset of patients. After my celiac diagnosis in 2005, I received an additional diagnosis in 2008: enteroviral infection. This diagnosis came by means of a special biopsy, which had been sent to a research lab in California, as well as through blood work at a lab in Utah, which tested antibody levels. These tests were done in the U.S. under the direction of infectious disease specialist Dr. J. Chia, who has a special interest in ME/CFS. This testing and its meaning are still under research.

The enteroviral group includes the polioviruses – some of the ME/CFS epidemics were named "atypical polio" – coxsackieviruses, echoviruses, and a number of others. I was diagnosed with the coxsackie and echovirus variety. Both of these belong to a family of viruses common to the general population and do not normally cause a permanent problem. Non-polio enteroviruses, like the ones I was diagnosed with, are so common that they are second only to "common cold" viruses (rhinoviruses) as the most common viral infectious agents in humans.

I was disappointed to learn that there aren't any antiviral or standard treatments for this type of virus yet; whereas the herpesvirus family does have some antiviral treatment options. Some ME/CFS patients are trying these drugs if they are diagnosed with active herpes viruses.[84]

The most well-known herpes virus is mono, or infectious mononucleosis. Caused by Epstein-Barr virus (EBV), mono is also called human herpesvirus 4 (HHV-4), and in the U.K., it is called glandular fever. It is part of the human herpesvirus (HHV) family, and some ME/CFS patients cite mono as the onset of their chronic illness. That led to CFS

---

84   The Enterovirus Foundation is focused on this specific illness and on finding solutions. It is another great option for channeling your donations or efforts. www.enterovirusfoundation.org (accessed July 9, 2016). Included in Section 3, Ways to Support the Cause of ME/CFS.

being referred to as chronic Epstein-Barr virus in the early 'nineties. This name held until it was proven that Epstein-Barr was not a factor for everyone with ME/CFS, and it was dubbed "chronic fatigue syndrome".

HHV-6 is another virus from the HHV family that is under constant study in ME/CFS. The HHV-6 Foundation supports research and treatment for it.[85]

In its discussion about viruses, the International Association for CFS/ME's *Primer for Clinical Practitioners* (IACFS/ME, 2014) states on page 8:

> A number of other viruses and/or antibodies against them have been found more frequently in patients with ME/CFS than in control populations[86] (e.g. human herpes viruses, enteroviruses). These studies suggest that virus(es) may play a causative role. Alternatively, these viruses may be opportunistic infections.[87] To date, no specific infectious agent has been uniquely linked to ME/CFS.

✒ *Give us one answer, please* – As of 2016, there is no single known cause for ME/CFS. Genetic predisposition and precipitating factors such as infections, environmental influences, trauma, and hormonal shifts are thought to contribute to the development of the illness. Many triggers are known, and lots of puzzle pieces have been discovered and understood, but still no single underlying cause has been identified.

Perhaps there are many causes because every person is a little different. This variability amongst patients, called heterogeneity, is a limiting factor in the research. However, we are starting to understand that there may be sub-populations. We all hope that one day the subsets of patients who have similar illness, but different causes and courses, will be refined. That is the only way to find the best treatment for each individual, much like today's treatments for different types of breast cancer.

Since 1990, I have been trying to understand the cause of my undermined health situation, always believing I would find it. As new options became available, within or outside of Canada, I often participated, whether it was for research or for new diagnostic testing. Many patients participate in treatment trials and studies around the world to help find the answers, even though there is no guarantee that their health will be restored through these methods. One current example is the 2016 NIH clinical study on post-infectious ME/CFS. Professionals, advocates, and researchers involved in this field – as well as patients – are the ones leading us to a better future.

---

85 hhv-6foundation.org (accessed July 17, 2016). Included in Section 3, Ways to Support the Cause of ME/CFS.

86 Bansal AS, et al. "Chronic fatigue syndrome and viral infection." (Rev) Brain, Behavior, & Immunity 2012 J; 26 (1): 24-31.

87 "Opportunistic infections" means that they may be secondary or a consequence of the illness, not the direct or primary cause.

STANZA 28

Scandals and dead-ends

Some say: "What doesn't kill you will just make you STRONGER."
This is one myth that I believe no longer.
For ME/CFS, with this I concur:
"What does not kill you will just make you STRANGER."

Some say: "God doesn't give you more than you can handle."
Not what I see in the case of this *scandal.*
I do think He leaves us with choices to make,
But having CFS is not our mistake.

> ...Just ignore it...
> ...Just work through it...
> ...Change what's in your head...

A lot of advice like this just makes no sense,
When suff'ring at home in your bed.

STANZA 28 NOTES

❧ *Scandal* – The history of ME and CFS is riddled with controversy globally. There has been conflict and scandalous action, and/or no action in politics, the disability insurance business, and medicine.

In the U.S., CFS has had a sordid background. One case of that was in 1999: A report from the U.S. General Accounting Office (GAO) revealed that $12.9 million of funding, which was approved by Congress for CFS research, was reallocated to other illnesses by the Centers for Disease Control and Prevention (CDC).[88] [89] [90] The money was eventually restored to the CDC's CFS research program.[91]

As an example of lack of action, the CDC ignored the initial cluster outbreaks in the mid 'eighties, despite notice from doctors who were inundated with ill patients suffering from a condition they'd never seen before. To add insult to injury, it was the CDC who eventually labeled the illness with the trivial, nonmedical misnomer *chronic fatigue syndrome.*

In the United Kingdom, a group of psychiatrists have claimed a psychogenic model for ME (also called CFS/ME there). "Psychogenic" means originating in mental or emotional, rather than in physiological, processes. In 2011, an influential and highly controversial study called "the PACE trial" was published in the *Lancet.*[92]

One main focus of the PACE trial was on the treatments called Graded Exercise Therapy (GET) and Cognitive Behavior Therapy (CBT). The repeated focus on GET and CBT in research has had an impact on the political, insurance, and medical decisions in most countries. It also influences public opinion, creating a great barrier to forward movement

---

88   General Accounting Office (GAO) report, www.gao.gov/new.items/he00098.pdf (accessed July 1, 2016).

89   To learn more about the political-medical history, "Osler's Web: Inside the Labyrinth of the Chronic Fatigue Syndrome Epidemic." (1996, and updated in 2006) by Hillary Johnson is a must-read that covers the first 10 years of the CFS epidemic in North America. David Tuller's article "Chronic Fatigue Syndrome and the CDC: A Long, Tangled Tale" can be found at www.virology.ws/2011/11/23/chronic-fatigue-syndrome-and-the-cdc-a-long-tangled-tale (accessed July 29, 2016).

90   The GAO investigation was undertaken at the request of Senator Harry Reid and at the urging of The CFIDS Association of America (now Solve ME/CFS Initiative). It followed the release of a report by the Department of Health and Human Services Inspector General. Further information can be seen in the posted article update: "Misuse of CFS funds at the CDC/NIH." www.wicfs-me.org/wi_cfs_-_update_on_misuse_of_cfs_funds_at_nih.htm (accessed July 26, 2016).

91   $12.9 million to Chronic Fatigue Syndrome (CFIDS) Research from CDC, October 25, 1999. www.prohealth.com/me-cfs/library/showArticle.cfm?libid=60 and www.cnn.com/HEALTH/9910/22/sick.tired (accessed July 25, 2016).

92   White PD, Goldsmith KA, Johnson AL, Potts L, Walwyn R, DeCesare JC, Baber HL, Burgess M, Clark LV, Cox DL, Bavinton J, Angus BJ, Murphy G, Murphy M, O'Dowd H, Wilks D, McCrone P, Chalder T, Sharpe M; PACE trial management group. "Comparison of adaptive pacing therapy, cognitive behaviour therapy, graded exercise therapy, and specialist medical care for chronic fatigue syndrome (PACE): a randomized trial." Lancet. 2011 Mar 5; 377(9768):823-36. doi: 10.1016/S0140-6736(11)60096-2. Epub 2011 Feb 18.

for ME and CFS research and treatment. In 2015, David Tuller, a well-respected journalist, wrote "Trial by Error – The Troubling Case of the PACE Chronic Fatigue Syndrome Study." [93]

This led to a letter in 2015 to have the PACE trial reviewed by the HHS in the U.S.[94] In a different development, over 40 clinicians and scientists have requested an independent analysis of the data from the PACE trial.[95]

A good summary of this complex matter was written by Julie Rehmeyer in *Slate* on November 13, 2015, in an article called "Hope for Chronic Fatigue Syndrome: The debate over this mysterious disease is suddenly shifting." [96]

As a result of the influence that CBT and GET-based research has had on the government and health agencies, there have been some frightening consequences: sick children have been taken from their parents' homes and placed in psychiatric hospitals; there has been minimal research into the physical causes of ME; and doctors have been discouraged from treating ME as a physical disorder, with some doctors ending up in legal action because of it.[97] A number of people have worsened in severity due to these inappropriate recommendations for treatment, CBT and GET.[98] The 2012 "Action for ME – Time for Action campaign" in the U.K. states: "We will campaign relentlessly to expose the disgraceful

93   "Trial by Error: The Troubling Case of the PACE Chronic Fatigue Syndrome Study." www.virology.ws/2015/10/21/
       trial-by-error-i/;   www.virology.ws/2015/10/22/trial-by-error-ii/;   www.virology.ws/2015/10/23/trial-by-error-iii/.
       Audio: V. Racaniello speaks with D. Tuller re flaws in PACE trial, July 10, 2016, www.microbe.tv/twiv/twiv-397
       (accessed July 25, 2016).

94   Twelve organizations (including Solve ME/CFS Initiative) sent a letter on November 15, 2015, to the heads of the
       Centers for Disease Control (CDC) and the Agency for Healthcare Research and Quality (AHRQ) asking them
       to examine the issues raised by journalist David Tuller's analysis of the U.K.'s £5 million PACE trial for ME/CFS.
       dl.dropboxusercontent.com/u/89158245/CDC-AHRQ%20Request%20PACE%20Nov%202015.pdf (accessed July
       2016).

95   In view of the PACE trial's many flaws, an open letter dated November 13, 2015, from six top scientists (primarily
       from the U.S.) to the editor of the Lancet, where the trial was published, demanded that there be an independent
       analysis of the data resulting from it. As they note, "the study received international attention and has had widespread
       influence on research, treatment options, and public attitudes." www.virology.ws/2015/11/13/an-open-letter-to-dr-
       richard-horton-and-the-lancet. Update Feb 2016, www.virology.ws/2016/02/open-letter-lancet-again (adding more
       professionals' names to the letter) (accessed July 26, 2016).

96   www.slate.com/articles/health_and_science/medical_examiner/2015/11/chronic_fatigue_pace_trial_is_flawed_
       should_be_reanalyzed.html. (accessed July 25, 2016).

97   Dr. Sarah Myhill before the General Medical Council – from Daily Mail Online. www.meassociation.org.uk/2010/04/
       dr-sarah-myhill-before-the-gmc-latest-from-daily-mail-online (accessed July 20, 2016).

98   "Voices from the Shadows," voicesfromtheshadowsfilm.co.uk (accessed July 29, 2016).

neglect of ME and the institutional discrimination against those who have it, until government commits to putting this right." [99]

The perspectives in the U.K. about ME and its causes can be found in a number of articles by Malcolm Hooper, Emeritus Professor of Medicinal Chemistry, University of Sunderland. [100]

Every country has its own story about how this illness group has been treated and about its label. Canadian authorities have been dismissive and largely unresponsive, despite Health Canada agencies being aware of our large illness population and their unmet needs. For the most part, they have been acting as though ME/CFS and other neuro-immune illnesses do not exist.

99 The book "Lost Voices from a Hidden Illness" (2008) presented by Invest in ME, about severely ill individuals in the U.K.; and the film "Voices from the Shadows" (2011), are part of the advocacy movement for change. As the DVD jacket for "Voices from the Shadows" states, "Hidden away in dark and silent rooms for years on end, men, women and children are suffering. Although severely ill, many are disbelieved and denigrated; their lives shattered by medical neglect and even abuse by the very professionals who should care for them. This desperate situation has been denied for too long."

100 "Magical Medicine: How to Make a Disease Disappear." February 2010. As well, "Professor Simon Wessely's award of the inaugural John Maddox Prize for his courage in the field of ME and Gulf War Syndrome" (with members of the ME community). Nov 12, 2012. More information: "Inquiry into the status of CFS/M.E. and research into causes and treatments – Group on Scientific Research into Myalgic Encephalomyelitis (M.E.)" chaired by Ian Gibson MP. Nov 2006. www.erythos.com/gibsonenquiry/Docs/ME_Inquiry_Report.pdf (accessed Feb 2016). Dr. Ian Gibson is in the process of writing a book in 2016: "Science, Politics and ME" which will explore what the state of ME is since the Inquiry and can be followed at www.investinme.org/IIME-Newslet-1508-01.htm (accessed Feb 2016).

STANZA 29

Enjoying my favorite things, trying alternative treatments

I love nature and music and yoga and psychics,
Humor and beauty and sunshine in the mix,
Angels and family and those who can sing,
These are a few of my favorite things. ❧

Chiropractic treatments and *myofascial release,*
Massage and cranio ❧ and all kinds of therapies,
Acupuncture needles that go up my spine,
These are the things that help keep me aligned.

   …It is costly…
   …Time-consuming…
   …But it's nurturing too…

I know to be grateful to get such a chance
To help myself try to improve.

STANZA 29 NOTES

❧ *These are a few of my favorite things* – I am grateful for many things, despite all the difficulties I share in this story. I love my family and friends, all forms of beauty and nature, sunshine and warmth, music and my spiritual practice. I have an affinity for angels and seeing life's bigger picture, and envisioning change for those with complex illness.

My bedroom closet no longer stores my clothes. It now houses twenty years' worth of file folders and medical records as well as research and history papers, all stored in a somewhat orderly fashion. I stare at the three big storage bins that are under my bed, which are filled with books and other material I have gathered over time. I can't help but see myself as a Sherpa's donkey, with quite a load on her back – a donkey that could not even hold herself up on her legs because of the burden that this illness places on her. For years, my family would say, "Get rid of this junk, this clutter, and you will feel better." For some reason, I just couldn't let go of it and kept gathering material as it presented itself, as if it held the cure for this illness and for my liberation.

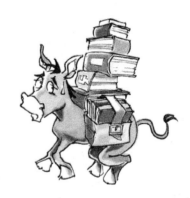

As I began to share my story and all the information I had in hand, the load initially felt heavier, because I still had so much to learn. But eventually, it began to lighten, and I am confident I will completely unpack the twenty-year-plus burden I have been carrying. The time is right to do something useful with these treasures – treasures that looked like junk or clutter to everyone else.

❧ *Myofascial release, massage and cranio therapy* – These are hands-on therapies by professionals that help me manage pain and remain more mobile while living such a sedentary life. Myofascial release and craniosacral therapy are considered by many to be "alternative." While this is anecdotal, I have heard from others that these therapies are also helpful for them. Because there is such variability in individual experiences with these illnesses, it is difficult to gather "gold standard" evidence about treatments such as these. The costs for alternative care are high, and I am very fortunate to have insurance coverage that partially pays for these therapies. Many people with ME/CFS do not have independent insurance coverage, so unfortunately these modalities are out of reach for them.

STANZA 30

Parenting and relationships, disease phases and stages

I think that I've been a *good wife and mother,*
I've completely enjoyed all of our time together.
To let them down is gut-wrenching for me,
Please don't grow impatient – it is a disease.

Phases and stages  of illness keep changing,
Just as in life, constantly rearranging.
It's odd how I'm happy for all the good things,
But *then it comes back, and grief is what it brings.*

   …It's a relapse…
   …No, a bad *crash* …
   …Slow recoveries…

This illness "don't" care if I rest, work, or play,
It still immobilizes me.

STANZA 30 NOTES

❧ ***Good wife and mother*** – I was married for seven years and a mother of one child when I fell ill, so those milestones had been crossed. When I got very ill, parenting became challenging, and my husband and family would help when they could. During the first five years of my illness, I remained relatively functional, though weakened.

The ages of one through five in a child are intense because kids are learning so much and are at home 24/7. I went into a much more severe state of illness when my daughter Jenna started Grade One. I love being a parent, but during my worsening in 2000, parenting at times was impossible. I was grateful Jenna was going to school most of the day when I was resting. I looked forward to her arrival home off the school bus, so we could spend some time together.

As she grew up, I often had to go to bed before her, but my husband was usually close by, working or busy in our yard. When she was about age twelve, I taught Jenna how to get groceries. I would drive her to the store, she would run and get them, and we would unload them together. We all had to work as a team. There is some guilt I carry, even so many years later, for the ongoing help I need from my husband and daughter, although we have done pretty well this way.

I think the hardest phase of parenting for me was when Jenna was very active in school functions, and I often could not attend. She was so young, and I wanted to be there. I shed many, many tears over this. She, however, was fine. Somebody was always around for her, including parents of other children. Other times, I did attend no matter how ill I was, how pale or gaunt I looked, or how close I felt to death, because it was just too important to miss.

Jenna's teenage years were interesting and fun; and then she left home to go to University, followed by entering a career. These years flew by. Jenna has grown into a fine, compassionate young woman who has become an elementary school teacher and health advocate.

Financial stability and good parental care are so important for kids to do well. Being an ill parent just makes it more complicated. On the other hand, this teaches young people to accept others who are sick or different. Raising a child really does take a village, and for ill parents, it is even more important for the village to be there.

I was married at 23 years old, and my relationship with my husband, David, has been such a primary part of my life. We have known each other since we were teenagers. In wellness (until I was 30 years old) it was so easy and fun because we had so much in common and we enjoyed all kinds of things together – in work, in play, and in parenting When ME/CFS arrived on the scene, it became more challenging due to our different energy levels and abilities and because of all the care that I needed. However, even decades later, we enjoy our acreage, our daughter, and the other meaningful people around us. I have tried to stay informed and interested in his life and hobbies since I became ill (although I could not usually participate in much of it), but we have managed to travel a little, enjoying Arizona as a holiday for a few winters.

It can be challenging to maintain close relationships when so disabled with ME/CFS. I appreciate David's ongoing support, which has been life-saving at times; but I do feel sadness when I realize how inequitable the work and financial load has been on him, and that he has had to do so many things on his own. At other times, I feel emotional support is lacking for me and wish that more interest was taken in the illness experience I am having. I know, from my upbringing, the rewards of sustaining a cohesive family unit; but each couple, dealing with serious chronic illness, handles it differently; and it can change over time.

Young people who have ME/CFS are left with big decisions, like whether to marry or have children. I chose not to have more children due to the severity of my illness, but until now, I really never thought about those who have chosen to have children or to add to their family after ME/CFS enters their lives.

A video seminar "Pregnancy and ME/CFS" really opened my eyes to this issue.[101]

Four women with ME/CFS were interviewed about different aspects of parenting. All of them talked about how they felt during pregnancy and how they felt after baby was born. They spoke of how remission is possible for some and relapse occurs for others, and they shared their experiences of raising their children.

They all had to consider things like the weight of the baby equipment purchased, the sleepless nights that come with a breastfed baby, and the onus on partners and parents. These four women expressed their struggles with the lack of ME/CFS knowledge from the medical staff about their special needs before and during the birthing process. See Chapter 1, "Hard Decisions: To Be A Parent With CFS" by J. Turner as an example.

In this video, Dr. R.C. Vermeulen concludes the above-noted seminar: "We still have no definitive idea of the risks involved in pregnancy for women with chronic fatigue syndrome. The suggestion that it's okay to be pregnant is not yet substantiated by science. I will not tell my chronic fatigue syndrome patients to postpone pregnancy. But I must tell them that we don't know enough about the dangers."[102]

---

101 This was presented by Peggy Rosati Allen, CNM, WHNP, MS; Assistant Clinical Professor, University of Utah College of Nursing, BirthCare HealthCare. It was titled: "Chronic Fatigue Syndrome: Experiences of Women During Pregnancy, Childbirth, and the Postpartum Period." www.youtube.com/watch?v=MBk8glip1WU (accessed July 26, 2016).

102 R.C. Vermeulen, M.D., PhD, Chronic Fatigue Syndrome Research Center, Amsterdam.

🐛 *Phases and stages* – I use the word "phases" to describe the changes in my age, roles, and relationships as the illness continues. I use "stages" to describe how living with a chronic illness affects everything; and vice versa. A four-phase model of chronic illness is described in *The Chronic Illness Workbook: Strategies and Solutions for Taking Back Your Life*.[103] The phases are: *(1) Crisis; (2) Stabilization; (3) Resolution; and (4) Integration*. Crisis is the onset and the urgent things that follow such as finding a diagnosis and medical care. Stabilization is when a person with chronic illness begins to understand it is chronic and starts to adapt. Resolution is about coming to terms with the grief and loss, while integration is finding purpose and meaning, weaving the old self and the new together.

Though I do not specifically outline my experience of these phases in this book, my illness process naturally keeps moving through them, and not always in order, nor only one at a time. Sometimes it feels like I go through all four phases in a single day. As you read this section and Section 2, you will see the phases weaving in and out of our many illness experiences.

🐛 *Then it comes back and grief is what it brings* – How can a person have multiple and conflicting feelings at the same time? For me, the most obvious example of this occurred during the earlier years of my illness, when my daughter was young. I would see other mothers doing things with their kids or families, or see someone riding a bike, and immediately I would have the response of being delighted to see this and be happy for them. Within seconds, though, the emotion quickly shifted when I realized that I was no longer able to do or enjoy that experience myself.

Grief then sets in.

These multiple and shifting emotions still happen twenty-two years later, as I write this piece, although I am less exposed to "normal life" now, since my daughter has grown up and moved away from home. Other people with similar illness severities to mine, or worse, ask the same thing: Is it harder to observe life knowing you cannot participate or to avoid it altogether? I try to participate in any way I can and enjoy it when I do, especially when it comes to my family. It does take effort and training to stop this reflection from getting me down: Sometimes I win and sometimes I lose.

There are times when all I can see are healthy people, because those who are ill or injured simply are not visible. Then, I'll see someone in a wheelchair at the mall and immediately feel a bit more at ease. I immediately want to ask, "Hey, how are you? What do you have going on?" I wonder if I am the only one who has this response.

---

103 Fennell PA, "The Chronic Illness Workbook: Strategies and Solutions for Taking Back Your Life." 2nd Edition. Albany Health Management Publishing. 2012.

The other question provoked by this illness at different stages of life is this: Is it harder to long for an experience you have never had (as in the youth who get sick), or to have experienced it and lost it? There are no right answers to these questions, but for me, it is truly difficult to think about all the things I have "loved and lost." A mind trained with wisdom probably would not indulge in these queries, but my thoughts and emotions are not always that disciplined. Ultimately, I just want to join in the world of the healthy, removing the barriers between it and the hidden worlds of CFS and ME.

Crash – As mentioned earlier, PEM or payback refers to a temporary period of immobilizing and worsening physical and/or cognitive fatigue, which seem to be caused by anything – overexertion, allergies, weather changes, or increased stress or emotional states. There are endless aspects to this phenomenon. Many patients have shared with me the irony of wanting to cry due to their suffering or their circumstances, though they do not dare to because of the relapse or crash that it causes. It is hard to appreciate that even emotional highs and lows can cause repercussions for a person with ME/CFS.

Many times, people misunderstand this and will say: "But you are going to a function filled with positive and happy energy, so you shouldn't have a problem after." Many healthy people think that a happy event will not cause the repercussions that a sad or stressful one might for their loved one. But energy is energy, and if it is overdone in a CFSer, the crash looks the same regardless.

At times, we may appear detached or disinterested, but protecting ourselves from these highs and lows can be an important way to conserve any life energy we have. The fact that I have to curb my natural enthusiasm for life and keep such control of emotions is a sad reality for me.

It still immobilizes me – It took me years to understand that the word that best describes this condition is "immobilizing." I may want to do something, but cannot follow through. I may desire to attend an event, but my symptoms may worsen, so I don't go. I may have all the desire and awareness in the world, yet be unable to physically or mentally fulfill the desire. One very immobilizing state I have encountered is what I call the "Sit and Stare" state. This is higher functioning than the "Blink and Breathe" and the "Wishing Death or Wellness" levels of functioning which I have mentioned earlier. In this state, I am just neutral, unable to move or even think, but I am sitting upright. It is strange, and I have heard others describe it similarly. This is just one of many levels of brain and body dysfunction in ME/CFS.

PART IV
ADAPTING TO LIFE WITH CHRONIC ILLNESS
(My Age: 45 to 49)
2005-2009

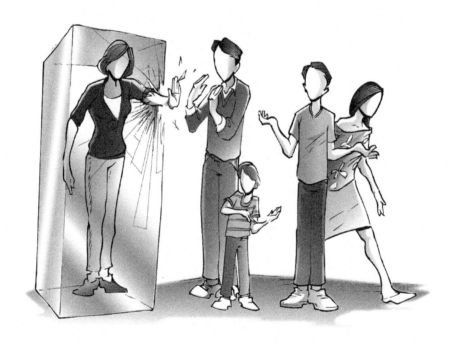

STANZAS 31-37 TOPICS

STANZA 31

Mobility and trying more 'things'

With *scooters and wheelchairs*  for getting around,
Oxygen helps – who knows why – I have found.
Homebound, or bedbound, or carbound I feel.
These are the things I wish were not so real.

Mercury taken out of all my fillings,
Doing it properly, pulling and drilling.
"I'm sure you'll be better – Oh darn, maybe not."
One more thing I learned that does not cure this lot.

   …With the research…
   …With the conflict…
   …With the misinformed…

That's when I give up on healing myself,
But only until the next morn.

STANZA 31 NOTES

❧ *Scooters and wheelchairs* – I've already talked a bit about using a scooter to get around outdoors, but I did not use mobility devices at the beginning of my illness. Even though I was largely homebound, carbound, or bedbound for years after my relapse in 1995, it never occurred to me to use any kind of help to get around more easily, either inside or outside my home. I would make a mad dash into stores or to run errands because the energy clock was ticking, and then pay the price for the exertion.

After reading *Hope and Help for Chronic Fatigue Syndrome and Fibromyalgia,*[104] I became acutely aware that I needed help so I could get out of the house and get around more. When people break bones or have conditions with obvious mobility challenges, their doctors, or others in their lives, usually advise them to seek assistance. ME/CFS limited this aspect of my life severely, so I remained more homebound than I needed to be, but nobody thought about devices such as canes, walkers, wheelchairs, or scooters. Many doctors – and even we as patients – don't realize that we need the help of these things to conserve energy and to help with orthostatic intolerance (the troubles of being upright).

I invested in a lightweight wheelchair for travel and trips to the mall, and a scooter for outdoor activities, and my world opened up a bit. I do not use the wheelchair inside my home, although I did try. My home is small with short flights of stairs, so it did not work out. (As an aside, I thought I might be able to use it while vacuuming my floors, but it turned out to be too cumbersome. Oh well, guess I can't vacuum anymore!) Getting the devices was only the beginning though. I found if I used my arms to move the wheels any distance, I would have a day's-long relapse. Not only did I need a wheelchair, I needed someone to push it! Our loved ones who often wind up being the "pushers" may not always want to accept our need for assistance. Often they have trouble admitting their own feelings about seeing us become so dependent and unable. An electric wheelchair is heavy, and you cannot throw it in the back of a small vehicle like I can my manual, fold-up, titanium wheelchair.

The scooter isn't a simple answer either. If I want to take the one I have off my acreage, it must be disassembled. The pieces are quite heavy to load into the back of the vehicle, and I am often not up to the task. Other options are to get a larger vehicle with a ramp, which is costly both financially and energetically, or to use the scooters available on loan at customer service in large department stores, grocery stores, and malls. If you can stand the snail's pace, the beeping when you back up, and the danger of bumping into a few clothing racks because the aisles are too narrow, loaners are a decent option. The scooter I

---

104 Bested AC, Logan AC, and Howe R, "Hope and Help for Chronic Fatigue Syndrome and Fibromyalgia." Cumberland House. 2008. 2nd ed. Print.

used in Arizona, just like the one I use on my acreage, was much faster and narrower and could scoot around anything, which was fun!

While mobility devices are great, many people with ME/CFS are not well enough to use them often, or at all. Some are expensive, which can be an issue if finances are tight and insurance does not help. Where you live is another factor. On our acreage in Alberta, the scooter is great, but only during the brief summer months. From 2009 until 2014, we have had the luxury of being in Arizona for a couple months during the winters; so with the more agreeable weather, a scooter is useful most of the time.

These devices take some getting used to – not only to maneuver, but in adjusting to the inquisitive glances and questions. I do try and look on the light side when I can; such as when I became the "wheelchair bandit." My daughter and I went to the mall for some Christmas shopping while I was trying out my fancy, new lightweight-wheelchair. I was very self-conscious. I loaded the things we were buying into my lap and we headed to the checkout lane. We paid for our purchases and left the store, my daughter pushing me along. When we were quite a ways down the mall, we noticed a pair of colorful socks, which we hadn't paid for, stuck in the wheel spokes. I still have those socks today, and we laugh about being wheelchair bandits and that stores should be on the lookout.

Using a wheelchair or asking for wheelchair assistance at the airport has been immensely helpful in ensuring that I can manage to travel. Even with the use of a wheelchair, the travel day, for any length of flight, leaves me with at least a four-day relapse. But the wheelchair reduces the stress and strain of it all, and you get a few perks, such as special lines for check-in and security, as well as boarding first.

The scanner at the airport is another place where I've had some "fun". When they see you in a wheelchair, the people who check you through the scanning device often assume that you cannot walk at all, which is true for many different conditions or injuries. But I tell them I can walk a short distance, so they wheel me up to the scanner, I get up and walk through, and they take the chair to be fully inspected (e.g., stripped of cushions). I usually assume they are looking for drugs, but perhaps they have heard about the stocking bandit episode! I walk through the scanner as if it were a high-tech healing vessel from *Star Trek*. On the other side, I joke to myself, *Hallelujah, I have been healed*. If only it were that easy.

❧ *Mercury taken out of all my fillings* – I spent over a year having work done on my teeth in the hopes of improving my health. I had many mercury fillings since I was very young. I worked with a biological dentist who removed and replaced the fillings one section at a time. We also removed two root canals because they were suspected of underlying infection, and did cavitation surgery on the left upper jaw for the same reason. This was a very painful and expensive process, and I was grateful for my health insurance. Unfortunately, it did not improve my overall health.

Heavy metal testing with the use of chelating agents has shown high levels of heavy metals in my body – primarily mercury. I have not had this chelated from my body because it is very costly, as well as time and energy consuming. In addition, there are risks to it and no guarantees.

STANZA 32

An additional diagnosis – celiac disease

A *celiac diagnosis*  so many years later,
Wheat, rye, oats, and barley are grains grown in nature.
An autoimmune disease triggered by these,
Left me with no choice but a gluten-free feast.

Reading the labels and learning the jargon,
Gluten-free food, believe me, is no bargain.
It's just one more thing making my freedoms yield.
It wouldn't be difficult if I had healed.

> …I am still trapped…
> …CFS ruled…
> …No relief was had…

Just more cost and separation to deal with,
How does one not get so mad?

STANZA 32 NOTES

ꙮ *Celiac diagnosis* – As you already know, I received the additional diagnosis of celiac disease in 2005. Other members of my family were also subsequently diagnosed with it. None of us had classical intestinal symptoms, so no one had thought of testing for it. This is sometimes called silent celiac disease.

It is an autoimmune disorder, which is an inherited condition, and it can be triggered any time in life. Celiac disease is described in a brochure by the Canadian Celiac Association (CCA) "Celiac Disease – What is it?" [105] as "a permanent intolerance to gluten, a protein found in various wheats (e.g., durum, kamut, spelt), rye, barley, and triticale. Gluten consumption causes damage to the absorptive surface of the small intestine and can result in malnutrition, anemia, nutritional deficiencies, and an increased risk of other autoimmune disease and some cancers of the gut." Due to cross-contamination of grain fields, oats are also on the list of prohibited foods.

The treatment is a strict gluten-free diet for life. So, unless foods are made with gluten-free ingredients and preferably in a gluten-free manufacturing facility, I can't have my favorites of pasta, bread, pierogi, or muffins, nor some sausages. I am not a beer drinker (more of a red wine buff), but beer is a beverage that contains barley, so it is off the list for those who have celiac.

I need to be on the lookout for gluten in unexpected places, like spices and condiments such as soy sauce because, unfortunately, gluten-based grains are used as stabilizers, anti-caking agents, preservatives, and flavoring. On and on it goes! Aside from food products, I have to refrain from using body and hair products that contain gluten. These include toothpaste, makeup such as lipstick, suntan lotion, or soaps and shampoos, since they may get into my body through my mouth or ears. Unfortunately, the labels for the ingredients on these products are even harder to read than on food because they all look like names of chemicals, but they can be derivatives of grains.

The same CCA brochure clarifies: "Environmental factors such as emotional stress, pregnancy, surgery, or an infection (e.g., travellers' diarrhea, pneumonia) can sometimes trigger the onset of symptoms…The number and severity of symptoms associated with untreated celiac disease can vary greatly from person to person…The similarity of the symptoms of celiac disease to those of other conditions often leads to a misdiagnosis of irritable bowel syndrome, lactose intolerance, chronic fatigue syndrome, or diverticulosis, thus delaying the diagnosis of celiac disease."

---

105 www.celiac.ca (accessed July 29, 2015).

I did not have this knowledge prior to my diagnosis, and I would not have known to ask to be tested until one day I heard someone talking about celiac disease: It just intuitively rang a bell with me, and that is when I requested to be tested.

There are multiple symptoms in celiac disease and many can be very serious, including infertility, anemia, and migraines. There are additional symptoms in children such as irritability and behavioral changes, dental enamel abnormalities, and vomiting.

The day that a nurse advised me about the diet, I learned that even one small bite of bread, or even the host that you receive in church, can trigger an immune reaction for days, which could cause all kinds of symptoms – some that are felt and some that are not! Before I was diagnosed, I don't remember feeling any discomfort that would have indicated my digestive tract was being destroyed. But celiac has more than 300 symptoms, ranging from depression to seizures, to no symptoms at all. It doesn't come as a surprise, then, that some patients don't even feel a thing and remain unaware of the illness.

The skin form of celiac is called dermatitis herpetiformis (DH), also known as Duhring's disease.[106] This form of celiac disease manifests in extremely itchy bumps or blisters. DH symptoms tend to come and go, and the rash is commonly misdiagnosed as eczema. I am glad I do not have this type of the condition, but I have friends and family who do.

As of 2014, one in 133 North Americans has celiac disease, and the rate is much higher within susceptible families. There are many theories on why celiac disease is on the rise. In an interview, expert Dr. Alessio Fasano explained that he believes there are two components of this increase.[107] First, increased awareness; and the second is that there is a true increase in the prevalence over time. He states, "It's not unique to celiac disease or gluten sensitivity; it's what we see in many other autoimmune diseases. We're in the midst of an epidemic."

In this interview, he explains that people have to have the genes and gluten exposure, as well as something else to lead to this problem. "Personally, I believe it is a change in the

---

106 DH affects 15 to 25 percent of people with celiac disease who typically have no digestive symptoms. DH bumps and blisters resemble herpes lesions, hence the name "herpetiformis," but they are not caused by the herpesvirus. It can affect people of all ages, but most often makes its initial appearance between the ages of 30 and 40. People of northern European descent are more likely than those of African or Asian heritage to develop DH. How does a disorder that damages the intestines show up on the skin? "As IgA enters the bloodstream, it can collect in small blood vessels under the skin, triggering further immune reactions that result in the blistering rash of DH." celiac.org/celiac-disease/dermatitis-herpetiformis (accessed July 10 2015).

107 The interview with Dr. Fasano was posted on www.allergicliving.com on April 16, 2014.

composition of the microbiome that can be what tilts you from health to disease," [108] Dr. Fasano proposes.

I took the genetic piece to heart after I learned about it, and I did lab tests to see what my genetics revealed. I have two celiac genes called DQ2; one from my mother and one from my father. Both of my parents have been tested and neither of them have active celiac disease, and they are over eighty years old. This does, however, mean that my daughter has at least one of these genes, unfortunately. She has been tested and will be every few years. She does not have active celiac disease right now, but does have gluten sensitivity. Jenna gets digestive symptoms and fatigue, and feels very poorly when eating gluten, so she refrains from those foods completely. Dr. Fasano explains that gluten sensitivity and celiac disease have many differences but some similarities. "They completely overlap in terms of clinical outcome – you can't distinguish the two just in terms of what kind of symptoms you have."

I grew up in a cattle and grain farming community in Alberta, Canada, where bread and baking were a mainstay of our lifestyle. I don't know if I already had celiac back then, but I suspect it was triggered right after giving birth to my daughter in 1989, as I experienced excessive weight loss, constant hunger, and a new type of fatigue. At the time, I thought it was from hormonal changes and breastfeeding, and we didn't know to test for it then. This was only one year prior to my CFS onset.

Early diagnosis of celiac disease is crucial to prevent complications and certain cancers such as lymphoma, as well as additional immune and autoimmune disease. Associated conditions are Type 1 diabetes, Down syndrome, and unexplained liver enzyme elevations, to name a few. Many of the people I know who are living with ME/CFS have also been diagnosed with celiac disease or gluten allergy/sensitivity. It makes me wonder if there is some sort of link between these as well.

Once I had this very provable autoimmune diagnosis – unlike ME/CFS – I was enthusiastic about learning how to implement the gluten-free (GF) diet because I was sure I would feel better. It didn't happen. Although a biopsy done two years later, in 2007, showed that my digestive tract was healing, I have not noticed any overall health improvements. Over the years, my enthusiasm has waned, and this lifestyle has become more burdensome. Keeping a kitchen safe from gluten cross-contamination requires using separate toasters, not sharing knives in the same margarines or jams, and maintaining vigilance about not

---

108 "The human microbiota consists of the 10-100 trillion symbiotic microbial cells harbored by each person, primarily bacteria in the gut; the human microbiome consists of the genes these cells harbor. Microbiome projects worldwide have been launched with the goal of understanding the roles that these symbionts play and their impacts on human health." Extracted from the paper "Defining the Human Microbiome," by Luke K Ursell et al. www.ncbi.nlm.nih. gov/pmc/articles/PMC3426293 (accessed July 26, 2016).

sharing the same utensil to mix gluten-containing foods for other family members. It has also meant greater expense.

Even though I did not have symptoms of nausea or vomiting while eating gluten before my diagnosis, ten years after it, my celiac reactions are not so silent. For instance, within four hours of mistakenly consuming tiny amounts of gluten, I become dizzy and nauseous, and you'd guess from the projectile vomiting that I'd been poisoned with salmonella.

The supplements and herbals I was using to help with ME/CFS all had to be checked for gluten. I learned that gluten-free products are not always 100 percent gluten free – they can receive such a designation if they are certified to be extremely low in gluten (less than 20 parts per million). This can vary from country to country.

I also learned that regulating laws are different in the food industry than those in the supplement and herb industry. Supplements and herbs are not monitored closely when it comes to gluten labeling. So I bought gluten-testing strips, which I used on my supplements, herbals, and food to check whether they were truly gluten-free. The strips often tested positive for some sign of glutens, despite the way products were labeled. "Free of gluten," "no added gluten," and even "certified gluten free" have different meanings and different thresholds for gluten tolerance in the products. The only way to really know is to talk to the manufacturer about the details, including ingredients and manufacturing practices. When the right questions are asked, the truth comes out and the consumer has a choice to make.

I feel a sense of emotional separation from my friends and family due to food. People have become hesitant to cook for me because they know it is complicated to get it right. And while more restaurants are offering gluten-free fare, I know how difficult it is to keep cross-contamination out of my own kitchen, and restaurants cannot guarantee that it is 100% gluten free. Therefore, we don't go out to eat much anymore, which can be isolating for my whole family.

Celiac disease is a highly studied and researched area. There are exciting findings that are crossing over into many autoimmune diseases, such as the discovery of the human protein, zonulin. It is produced in a certain population with the genetics for it. As I understand it, zonulin can trigger boundaries – also called tight junctions – like those around the gut, blood vessels, and brain, to become more permeable than is healthy. This allows toxins, such as undigested food and viruses, to pass through the boundaries. We need these junctions tight as part of protection and immunity. However, those with one or two zonulin-producing genes do not have the tight junctions required for good gut health, regardless of their diet and efforts to heal.

Zonulin was thought to be related to celiac disease alone, but now Dr. A. Fasano and his team are busy proving that it is a factor in other conditions such as diabetes and Crohn's disease.[109] I believe this will be an extremely valuable piece of information that may tie many of us with serious chronic illness together.

My daughter, Jenna, had a lab test done which detected and measured zonulin levels in order to determine her predisposition to gluten sensitivity or celiac disease and also to learn ways of prevention. She did show a high production of the protein, zonulin. More research will be needed, and the genetic testing will hopefully become available soon, so we can find out who has this vulnerability of zonulin production.

---

109 Fasano A, "Zonulin, regulation of tight junctions, and autoimmune diseases." Ann N.Y. Acad Sci. 2012 1258(1):25-33. www.ncbi.nlm.nih.gov/pmc/articles/PMC3384703 (accessed July 25, 2016).

STANZA 33

Stay independent, prevent isolation, and hypotheses for cause

Try to ... *stay independent; prevent isolation,*
Who wants to think like a CFS patient?
Stay self-sufficient as best as you can,
But 'til there's improvement, you'll need a BIG HAND.

I need help in ways I never expected,
Cannot believe it – I once was perfected.
How could this happen just after a flu,
When 30 and healthy, and shiny and new?

    …Humiliation…
    …And frustration…
    …A pot of emotional stew…

Grief, guilt and fear, anger, jealousy too;
Disappointment, to name a few.

STANZA 33 NOTES

✣ *Stay independent; prevent isolation* – Independence is a wonderful thing and we often take it for granted. ME/CFS etches away at both our independence and participation in society. Isolation can become a reality, adding to the burden.

Social media and the Internet do help; they open up the world for many with chronic illness. We can connect and participate in everyday events, even though we are unable to go out. Everything from banking, to shopping, to building new friendships is possible in this virtual world. However, some are unable to use the computer or technical devices, either because of financial constraints or because the screens can aggravate neurological symptoms and cause migraines or dizziness. So even within this connected world, many remain isolated. Little things make a difference; for instance, newsletter editors from ME/CFS support organizations still mail out paper versions for those who cannot use, or do not have access to, these technological tools.

In the online world, I feel understood, validated, and not alone. In this world, the knowledge and resources related to ME/CFS are vast.[110] However, when I walk out the door and into the physical world – a doctor's office or anywhere else – I am, once again, on my own because no one seems to recognize or acknowledge my condition. These two worlds remain parallel unfortunately, and are not connected – yet.

✣ *How could this happen just after a flu, when 30 and healthy* – It was a shock for me to become so sick so young, especially because of my prior good health. The only health concerns I remember before July of 1990 were a minor car accident where I sustained a mild whiplash, a case of mono at age twenty-two, and occasional anemia. I did not miss more than one day of work for any of these things. But as I came to learn, ME/CFS can affect anyone – all ages, races, and socioeconomic groups – and is widespread throughout at least every developed nation. Though it affects males and females, approximately seventy percent of those afflicted are female. Interestingly, studies reveal that in adolescents, the ratio of males to females is more equal than in adults.

Isolated (known as sporadic) cases of ME/CFS, such as mine, have never been proven contagious. Most patients do not see others around them become ill with it, either immediately or over their lifetime. However, as the International Association for CFS/ME's *Primer for Clinical Practitioners* (IACFS/ME, 2014) notes, there may be a familial connection:

> Predisposing Factors – Female gender is a predisposing factor in adults. In some cases, susceptibility to ME/CFS may be inherited or familial.

---

110 I have included some in the Resource section of this book, Appendix I.

Family studies have shown that 20 percent of patients with sporadic ME/CFS have relatives who also have the illness, and 70 percent of such relatives were not living with the patient.[111] In addition, twin studies have found a CFS-like illness in 55% of monozygotic twins* (identical twins) as compared to 19% dizygotic (non-identical) twins.*[112] A recent report found excess relative risk for developing ME/CFS in first (2.7) second (2.3) and third (1.3)-degree relatives.[113]

* Methods: A classic twin study was conducted using 146 female-female twin pairs, of whom at least one member reported > or =6 months of fatigue.

I wonder which comes first: a virus, other infection, trauma, or environmental factors, and then a dysfunctional immune system, or is it the other way around? Science hypothesizes that the cause is a mix of genetics, environment, and contagion. This combination may explain why only certain people get sick even though others have been exposed. But I also wonder – what was different in the cluster outbreaks of CFS and ME around the world that affected so many over a short period of time? We just don't know.

It is interesting that many women fall ill with autoimmune diseases and ME/CFS close to childbirth. I hope we will, one day, understand the connection between immunity and hormones; perhaps someone already does. I know many CFS patients in their childbearing years who have said, "I got sick after my firstborn," or "after my third," or "after nursing my child." What is the connection?

One thing I have learned about asking questions while writing is that, given enough time, I will receive at least a partial answer.

At a February 2013 patient seminar,[114] Dr. Gordon Broderick, PhD – an engineer by training – demonstrated how they map out immune circuitry differences between men and women by using computational analysis and data gathering technology. The brief layperson version, and the bottom line for me, was that male circuitry took up one square of

111 Underhill R, O'Gorman R, "The prevalence of Chronic Fatigue Syndrome and chronic fatigue among family members of CFS patients." J CFS 2006; 13(1): 3-13.

112 Buchwald, MD et al. "A twin study of chronic fatigue." Psychosomatic Med 2001; 63:936-943.

113 Albright F, et al. Abstract: "Evidence for a heritable predisposition for Chronic Fatigue Syndrome." BMC Neurology 2011 11:62. The numbers in brackets represent relative risk (RR). "Conclusions: These analyses provide strong support for a heritable contribution to predisposition to Chronic Fatigue Syndrome. A population of high-risk CFS pedigrees has been identified, the study of which may provide additional understanding."

114 The seminar was called "A Celebration of Hope and Progress" and was held for the opening of the Institute for Neuro Immune Medicine, which is run by Dr. Nancy Klimas at the Nova Southeastern University in the U.S. Dr. G. Broderick holds a PhD in Chemical Engineering from the University of Montreal, Canada, as well as a master's in chemical engineering and an undergraduate degree in mechanical engineering, both from McGill University. He joined the Institute for Biomolecular Design (University of Alberta) in 2002, where he led a team of computational experts. Dr. G. Broderick is now a Professor/Researcher at Nova Southeastern University in Fort Lauderdale, Florida.

information while female immune circuitry took up four, making it much more complicated. He also said that pregnancy results in an immune and hormonal adaptation (more about G. Broderick in Stanza 44).

In my case, years of unrecognized, long-term stress from an increasingly demanding job, the unfound active celiac disease, the genetic predisposition to ME/CFS (which researchers are in the preliminary stages of understanding), and the timing of childbirth, nursing, and sleepless nights might have all made me vulnerable to the virus from that first flu-like onset. From that point, my body seemed unable to fight it appropriately and things changed. This is a personal hypothesis. I will be very happy to someday understand what happened to my health and, even happier, to regain it.

STANZA 34

What I miss and mourning the loss of my healthy self

I miss ... my power, my confidence, trusting my body,
Learning new things like tai chi and karate,
Planning and knowing that I will be there,
Without all the hassles, without all the care.

I miss ... finances and earning a good solid dollar,
Traveling afar with my husband and daughter.
I miss ... the feelings of fitness, well-being, and strength,
A *predictable day* 'stead of one moment's length.

...To feel solid...
...To feel steady...
...Strong in my own way...

Reliable, skillful, and organized too,
"It" disabled all these in one day.

STANZA 34 NOTES

❧ *I miss* – One day, I asked a friend who is highly functional with ME/CFS, "Despite how it looks, do you ever feel normal?" She said, "No." That really affected me, because I realized that even those functioning at higher levels than myself (i.e. 70 or 80 percent) may not feel the normalcy of good health and that it may never return. Why did I not know to appreciate the normalcy of good health?

At the time of writing this note, I am fifty-four years old, and after reflecting on this book for five years, I am actively and deeply mourning the loss of my past healthy self. Although I have been in and out of this phase for years, it now feels like the death of a very close friend. It is horribly painful and sad at times. I miss and long for my old self and have trouble seeing a future with my new self who I don't even like very much. She is needy, vulnerable, and fragile. I realize that my loved ones also lost the prior version of me and they are left to cope with, and adjust to, a changed person in their lives.

I have quoted and referred to the work of Patricia Fennell MSW, LCSW-R, author of *The Chronic Illness Workbook: Strategies and Solutions for Taking Back Your Life* (2nd edition). The way she explains one of the phases of her four-phase model of chronic illness describes some of what I feel in 2014. (p.136).

> **Deep mourning for your lost self.** When you finally recognize that you've got a chronic – a permanent – illness, it throws into stark relief everything that you've lost. You now must consciously acknowledge that your old life is never coming back. You can't perform your old roles in the way you used to. Your partner may have left you because she or he can't adjust to your changed life. If you've got children, they may be confused, perhaps even scared of the person you seem to have become. You've doubtless lost some old friends who used to mean the world to you. You've assuredly lost many of your old activities, to say nothing of your sense of vibrancy and vitality. You've often lost your old personality. These are huge losses, and it's urgent in phase three that you grieve for them. You can't move forward if you don't express the intense feelings that so much loss occasions…

She then advises us to ask the hard questions pertaining to when our old self dies and our old life ends, which creates great dread and confusion and which she refers to as the "dark night of the soul": Who am I now? Why should I live? Why me? She recommends immediate medical help and support if someone is desperate or suicidal, and lets us know we will eventually come out the other side. "You're going to emerge from the dark night, the tunnel…as a new self, as a person who combines qualities from both your past self and your present explorations."

I sure hope she is correct, and that I'm going to emerge from this stage, because I am not feeling it right now. I do believe that acceptance is an ongoing process, but accepting an illness that affects all of me, all of the time, doesn't seem like something I will ever be good at. I realize that Patricia Fennell is not encouraging us to give up, but rather to surrender and accept the experience as it is now, while working toward improvement and regaining some happiness and quality of life within the boundaries that exist.

It is not always possible or a priority to do the emotional work to get through the tunnel that Ms. Fennell speaks of. By that, I mean that there have been times when I have been so ill that I can't do the grieving and emotional work required. Survival and/or basic activities for family care are all I can manage due to the severity of my symptoms, lack of stamina, as well as cognitive and emotional dysfunction.

Aging is also a factor that I sometimes forget. It is natural for my perspective and experience to change with my age and stages of life. It is one of the reasons I have incorporated my ages in the five parts of "The Chronic-Call." Being over fifty years of age feels very different than thirty.

While cycling through the phases of chronic illness and moving toward a meaningful life, despite debility, I am also working toward effective treatment and hope for the future through advocacy, writing, and educating. That is where my heart is – progress and improvement. I do not believe the grieving will ever stop completely unless there is a vast improvement in my health, but maybe it will lessen one day.

❧ *Predictable day* – ME/CFS renders many things unpredictable, even our own bodies and minds. For the most part, I cannot know what a day will be like until it is over. Without knowing my level of health and well-being, I cannot make plans: If I do, I am often unable to follow through with them. This leads to many disappointments for me, my loved ones, and friends. It also leads to isolation and loneliness. A level of health is imperative to plan life, for successful relationships, and to be part of society.

The illustration on the front of this part, "The Glass Box," depicts the invisible boundaries we face. Everybody's glass perimeter is different. Some are more confining than others, but they will always be there. In this illustration, the other people around the CFSer cannot see this boundary and encourage her to come with them and do things. Some of those people get frustrated with her, as you can see, and walk away; others do not understand and shrug their shoulders. Living in a glass box is not easy, and breaking through it only creates physical and psychological damage to those who live within it. It is hard for people to spend time in the glass box with an ME/CFS patient, but it can be done. Just being part of our world is so helpful.

Over many years, the relapses and increased suffering from exceeding my energy envelope, while trying to stay within safe boundaries, have diminished my desire to do things and to make plans. I asked my ME/CFS doctor whether this was a sign of depression or a sign of intelligence. She said, "It is a fine line, and perhaps a bit of both."

I sometimes think about my past healthy life. Predictability was pretty much a given in all areas: family life, work, counting on my body and mind every day for walking, thinking, socializing. It seems like the only predictable thing for me now is that I will be predictably unpredictable.

STANZA 35

How I live, affecting my loved ones, and what I fear

Acceptance, I try to, but how can I do that?
Affecting my loved ones, ✻ I hate what that feels like.
Fear of leaving all I care for behind,
Makes it so hard to let go with my mind ...

Kindness and caring are soul food for me;
Compassion and healing with simplicity.
Slowly and gently I pace out my life, ✻
Keep a loving perspective amidst all the strife.

...Where it's honest...
...Where it's joyful...
...Where it's peaceful too...

That's where I do well to survive my mess,
And where you might do well too.

STANZA 35 NOTES

❧ *Affecting my loved ones* – The guilt that results from being ill and disappointing loved ones and friends is challenging. In the early years, there was often a blame-the-victim mentality for illnesses that were not mainstream. I know it is not anyone's fault I have ME/CFS, but I still find it hard not to feel blame or shame for becoming ill, mostly because it is such a misunderstood disease. When the illness is so long-standing, it is also difficult for loved ones not to feel all kinds of uncomfortable emotions for having to deal with it. Accurate information and communication helps.

This chronic illness has made it difficult for me to be the equal and independent partner I would like to be. My husband has had to do a lot on his own: Thankfully, he is a very focused person with creative ideas, hobbies, and ongoing projects. No one expects or plans to have a spouse who needs such unique and ongoing care and who is unable to participate in life in the most normal ways, especially during their young adult years. Financial responsibilities as well as physical help, in the home and yard, end up one-sided for long periods of time, which can create resentment and strain on any relationship.

We need to acknowledge the difficulties faced by people who love and care for us. Caregivers or carers also need emotional and physical support at times. These are not only spouses, but can also be children or parents of the person with ME/CFS. Keeping families together and supported is a beautiful goal. This can be done by educating families about the illness and also educating the patient on how to live within a family while suffering with the illness.

From the opposite point of view, one of the things I do worry about is that I will be unable to respond to the needs of those I love in the case of an emergency or if they were to fall ill. It is one of the most fearful aspects of disability for me. My parents are aging gracefully and healthily, but I feel concerned that I may not be there as they need me or when things become more difficult. I watch both of my sisters act as able, stable grandparents, and I have concerns about how I will get through the same role, should my daughter have children one day. I need so much quiet and alone time to care for the little health I have. What will happen if my husband should fall ill or need care and I cannot provide it? These thoughts have become more front and center in my life because I am getting older, as are the people around me. I can see now that the safety net I have relied on is getting thin.

❧ *Slowly and gently I pace out my life* – I have learned I need to pace, rest, conserve energy, do things differently and try different techniques and treatments for relief of symptoms. I rely on compassion, gentleness, and love – for others and for myself – and trust that all will work out somehow. On the days I feel most fragile or afraid, I vow to treat myself like a lamb. This changes my attitude toward my condition and my situation, as well as how I relate to others. These are keys to survival and peace despite external circumstances. However, they do not replace the longing for a healthy body and mind.

STANZA 36

What I need, give, and share

I need ... patience, and courage, more stamina for bearing,
More faith in my spirit, to keep up the caring;
More perseverance to press for a cure, ❧
More insight to heal; love to keep my heart pure.

I give friendship and nurturing, I help where I can,
I'm happy, when able, to massage feet or hands.
I share info and prayers and a meal now and then,
Encouraging words to my family and friends.

  …Set just small goals…
  …Value each step…
  …Do simple things to please…

This is not what I expected at all,
But this illness brings humility.

STANZA 36 NOTES

❧ *More perseverance to press for a cure* – Until I started working on this book, I was unaware that activists for many other illnesses, like autism and HIV/AIDS, had to advocate and engage the public and government health agencies for years in order to advance the political and medical changes they required. I have learned that medicine is highly intertwined with politics, as well as with pharmaceutical and insurance companies.

Despite the heroic efforts of some, ME/CFS advocacy is still lacking in power, money, and energy. Advocates of other illnesses like cystic fibrosis and Duchenne's muscular dystrophy, which are considered rare, have integrated the political, medical, pharmaceutical, and public pieces to benefit their causes. Over the years, advocacy groups have made a real difference in the quality of lives for their young people with these conditions. ME/CFS is not a rare condition, so I hope that it is also possible to attract more interest and action from the pharmaceutical industry for us.

However, inadequate resources make it difficult for the leaders of support organizations in any country to press for the necessary changes. Some advocacy strategies include: forming patient registries; encouraging researchers at universities and within industry, including pharmaceutical companies, to take an interest in ME/CFS; and better informing the public for added strength and power. Advocacy organizations need help so they can take these steps.

My hope is that we will start to find solutions for this illness. With sustained effort and focus, we will have Centers of Excellence for complex neuro-immune disease in all countries.[115] The stigma, neglect, and ill regard will be things of the past. This won't happen on its own but will take the awareness and hard work of many. Meanwhile, the lives of people with ME/CFS are affected every day to different degrees, and they are waiting for signs of real hope and action. This issue deserves priority and urgency.

---

115 Centers of Excellence are medical facilities which combine research and treatment to care for ME/CFS patients. For more on Centers of Excellence, refer to Dr. D. Peterson's presentation in Sweden at Section 2: Chapter 12 – Science, Research and Progress.

STANZA 37

What I can do, what does the future hold?

I can do…light household tasks and errands that are drive-thru,
Arrange things for others; make lists for them to do,
Work on the computer for short spurts of time,
Take care of "my healthcare" and make these words rhyme.

Pay bills, chat on Facebook, do the research needed,
Write articles 'bout things I think should be heeded,
Shop in the mall; travel once in a while,
That wheelchair and scooter let me go in style.

> …To worsen, easy…
> …To improve, hard…
> …Which way will it go?…

Take nothing for granted with CFS,
'Cause the future we do not know. ✎

STANZA 37 NOTES

☙ *'Cause the future we do not know* – We know a lot about ME/CFS as of 2016 compared to ten years ago. In the Foreword of the International Association for CFS/ME's *Primer for Clinical Practitioners* (IACFS/ME, 2014),[116] Anthony L. Komaroff MD, professor at Harvard Medical School and senior physician at Brigham & Women's Hospital, states:

> In my view, research of the past 25 years has identified many underlying biological abnormalities that are present more often in patients with ME/CFS than in healthy control subjects or in subjects with other fatiguing illnesses, including depression, multiple sclerosis, and Lyme disease.

He then outlines the areas where science has revealed abnormalities found in ME/CFS, including: neurological, energy metabolism, infectious triggers, immune activation, and the genetic component.

Although it is true that we do not know what the future holds for ME/CFS, we are learning more every day. There is every reason for hope.

---

116 iacfsme.org/portals/0/pdf/Primer_Post_2014_conference.pdf p.3 (accessed July 26, 2016).

PART V
HIDDEN NO MORE
(My Age 50+)
2010 to the Future

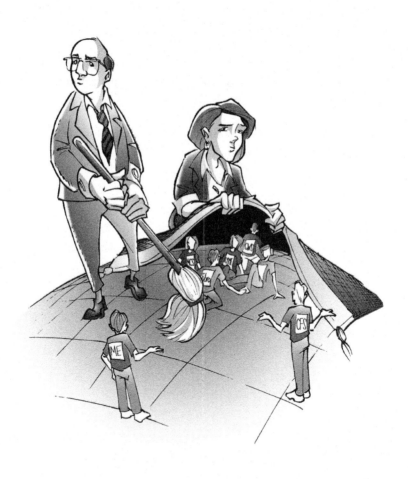

STANZAS 38-44 TOPICS

STANZA 38

Concerns, frustration, and the need for a place

Who will clean the house and make enough income?
Who will pay the bills and raise all the children?
Who will take care of our everyday lives,
While we're out of commission; trying to survive?

It's easy to say: "Only do what you can,"
But who does the rest until we take a stand?
People don't need any more on their plates,
Who is to take care of us all with this fate?

    ...No place for it ...
    ...Need to get well...
    ...What's the other choice?...

Most do not think 'bout how this life would be,
Until we all give it a voice.

STANZA 38 NOTES

❦ *But who does the rest until we take a stand?* – Most ME/CFSers need support from well people to complete the tasks that they cannot. Meanwhile, in the larger picture, the advocacy community is working to change the political, medical, and societal landscapes. This community is comprised of individuals, some organizations, a few dedicated researchers and scientists, and a small number of steadfast health care providers. I was surprised to learn that some have been fighting for decades to better the quality of life for those with ME/CFS in many countries. The way that I am practicing advocacy and activism is by writing this book.

❦ *No place for it* – One day after I became ill, I was on a drive with my family, and I noticed a homeless man on the street. All of a sudden, I had a scary thought: *I am not well enough to be homeless. What would I do if my family was not here to help?* I was not mobile enough to get from point A to B, I didn't have enough energy and, along with other limitations, I was not able to sustain enough mental power to get help. I have heard of people who have ended up living in their cars for financial reasons or because they didn't know what else to do.

Among other concerns, many with ME/CFS have a real fear of going to a hospital for any type of surgery or procedure, and they are also reluctant to go for emergency care. Often, the medical staff doesn't know much about our illness. Some people have been sent to psychiatric wards because doctors didn't recognize or understand the presentation of the illness and its similarities to, and differences from, mental illness. Appendix F is a chart which demonstrates the similarities and differences.

The International Association for CFS/ME's *Primer for Clinical Practitioners* (IACFS/ME, 2014) recommends that patients contemplating surgery talk to the surgeon and anesthesiologist beforehand to make sure they understand the special considerations such as depleted blood volume, orthostatic intolerance, pain control, and sensitivity to medications. However, many report that surgeons and medical staff disregard their diagnoses or special concerns, and some have worsened in hospitals or long-term care facilities as a result. (See Chapter 4, "From Six to Thirty: A Life with ME" by E. Collingridge as someone who did experience this).

In Canada, in 2012, a petition was started by Liisa Lugas and sent to the Ministers of Health, both nationally and provincially, to create dedicated care units in hospitals with appropriate services for patients with ME/CFS. To my knowledge, no action has been taken to deal with this request.

There are patients like my friend Patricia who, despite their young age, have to go to senior facilities or nursing homes. Senior facilities and nursing homes can be difficult environments for ME/CFS patients because not only do they have to deal with nurses and staff who lack knowledge on the condition, but the environment may not be optimal for sensitivities to light, sound, and smells like cleaning agents. People with severe ME/CFS may have added medical needs for IV fluids and major pain medications or require care for their seizures or paralysis. Patricia told me in a recent phone call:

> I am very sick now, living in a Seniors Lodge where I know no one after six months. These people are all in their nineties. I am so very alone and miserable. My health is very bad, and I have dropped down to bedridden. But there is no nursing care that can help me, so I have only my doctor. I have so few visitors. So many of my friends have moved away, died, or become ill themselves.

STANZA 39

Hidden illness, those who have died, media, and numbers impacted

This *hidden illness,* its enculturation
Is taking too long and is hurting the patients.
The functional, bedbound, and a restored few,
Each has a story worth listening to.

Teens who cannot school and *adults who can't work;*
Mothers who can't lift the children they have birthed.
People from complications who have died;
And *some who took their lives* from suffering denied.

…*Where's the media?* …
…*Affecting millions* …
…Needing social change…

No proper care, and few doctors who know,
There is so much to rearrange.

STANZA 39 NOTES

❧ *Hidden illness* – ME/CFS is a hidden illness as well as an invisible condition.[117] Conditions such as diabetes and cancer can't be seen from the outside either, but they have been accepted for quite some time in mainstream medicine, have more developed research and treatment, and are largely recognized by society. However, as the illustration for Part V shows, ME/CFS and associated illnesses have been swept under the rug for decades by politics and medicine.

In a clever blog at Free Ideas!!! the blogger writes: "Here are some aspects of privilege associated with having a recognized illness as opposed to a non-recognized, maligned, stigmatized, or doubted illness. Many autoimmune diseases fall in the latter category, as well as chronic Lyme disease, MCS, ME, fibromyalgia, and a variety of other conditions."[118]

The list of aspects of privilege associated with having a respected, official, non-stigmatized illness includes:

> 1. You can expect to have a straightforward process of diagnosis with clear diagnostic criteria or accurate tests…8. You can expect to receive treatment for the diagnosis if you happen to be hospitalized. 9. You can typically expect not to be mistakenly interpreted as being a drug addict or having a mental illness if you seek care for an aspect of your illness…15. You can share about your diagnosis with friends and acquaintances and expect to receive sympathy rather than arguments about whether you actually have the disease.

❧ *Teens who cannot school* – Too many children with the illness lack proper diagnosis and treatment, which ends up barring them from getting an education. Children and teens with ME/CFS often cannot handle regular, full-time schooling. I have spoken to several mothers of children or adolescents with ME/CFS who have opened my eyes to the difficulties. It seems the problems – getting an accurate diagnosis and then getting special needs met for education – are the same irrespective of country. Accommodations for home instruction or part-time schooling are difficult to obtain. Training needs to be given to medical providers, parents, teachers, school nurses, and the patients/students

---

117 Dorothy Wall wrote a wonderful book about this entitled, "Encounters with the Invisible: Unseen Illness, Controversy and Chronic Fatigue Syndrome." Southern Methodist University Press. 2005. Llewellyn King, the creator, executive producer and host of the White House Chronicle, takes this further. He often refers to the ME/CFS situation as being "hidden in plain sight." Also a 2010 film, "Invisible," deals with these issues. The film is by Michael Thurston, a filmmaker, and Rik Carlson, the founder of the Vermont CFIDS Association. www.prohealth.com/shop/product.cfm/product__code/N0524 (accessed July 25, 2016).

118 You can find the blog post at freeideasblog.blogspot.ca/2014/06/list-of-recognized-illness-privileges.html. It was published on June 18, 2014 (accessed March 30, 2016).

themselves. Pediatricians trained in ME/CFS are needed. They can diagnose and recommend appropriate management, and with that, provide protection in all areas of their young patients' lives, including the education and social systems.

To learn more about how ME/CFS can affect children and their families, refer to Chapter 2. Documents are available from support associations[119] to help educators and social services learn more about the illness and how to accommodate young people.

☙ *Adults who can't work* – Although ME/CFS affects people of all ages, the majority are those in the middle of their working lives. Just as I did, many adults lose their ability to work at regular employment after their ME/CFS onset. Some are able to work off-and-on, and some can work if they are able to change their jobs to low-stress or part-time positions. Those who return to work are sometimes described as "the working ill." That is because, although they can go to work, most are unable to continue other aspects of life such as parenting, socializing, or even helping around the house. Everyone is different, and one's ability to work can change over time.

Flexible hours, part-time schedules, and working from home are examples of accommodations employers might make for those individuals who are able to consider working.

☙ *People from complications who have died* – Dr. Leonard Jason[120] and others at DePaul University in Chicago examined the causes of death of people with ME/CFS in a 2006 study.[121] They found CFS patients are more likely than healthy people to die prematurely due to heart failure, suicide, or cancer. This is an area where further research is needed and Jason's team has another study underway.[122]

---

119 Including Massachusetts CFIDS/ME & FM Association – The children and youth section is available at www.mass-cfids.org/pediatric (accessed April 2016) and National ME/FM Action Network – Teach-ME sourcebook is available at www.mefmaction.com/index.php?option=com_content&view=article&id=288&Itemid=356 (accessed July 26, 2016).

120 Leonard A. Jason, PhD is a professor of clinical and community psychology at DePaul University and a well-respected member of the ME/CFS community.

121 "Causes of Death Among Patients with Chronic Fatigue Syndrome" Health Care for Women International, Volume 27, Number 7, August 2006, 615-626 (12). The abstract reads in part: "…there are few studies that have investigated causes of death for those with this syndrome. The authors analyzed a memorial list tabulated by the National CFIDS Foundation of 166 deceased individuals who had had CFS. There were approximately three times more women than men on the list. The three most prevalent causes of death were heart failure, suicide, and cancer which accounted for 59.6% of all deaths."

   More recently a 2016 study released in the Lancet: Roberts E, Wessely S, Chalder T, Chang C, and Hotopf M. 2016. "Mortality of people with chronic fatigue syndrome: A retrospective cohort study in England and Wales from the South London and Maudsley NHS Foundation Trust Biomedical Research Centre (SLaM BRC) Clinical Record Interactive Search (CRIS) Register." The Lancet. Summary Feb. 16 at https://batemanhornecenter.org/increased-suicide-risk (accessed July 25, 2016).

122 Abigail Brown is the principal investigator. https://redcap.is.depaul.edu/surveys/?s=DHxuYxScEn (accessed July 28, 2016).

🌿 *Some who took their lives* – The factors that increase the risk of suicide among patients of chronic illness like ME/CFS are high levels of unmanageable pain and suffering, lack of family and financial support, depression, social alienation, and medical estrangement.[123]

Certain medications and combinations of medications can be a factor. Some people experience worsening of their physical and mental states while on antidepressants. In fact, studies show that antidepressants have not been reliably effective in ME/CFS, and most doctors advise a lower dose and working up for effect.[124]

Tom Hennessy,[125] founder of May 12 Awareness Day, took his own life in 2013, after many years of what some of his friends say was unmanageable pain and suffering. And I was saddened to learn of the February 2015 death of Vanessa Li, the originator of the crowd-funding appeal for Dr. Ian Lipkin's ME/CFS microbiome project at Columbia University. She was thirty-four and had been living with ME/CFS since she was fifteen.

I personally lost one of my best friends, Lisa, to suicide in 2015. She had been ill with ME/CFS for seventeen years. You can read more about Lisa and others in Chapter 4: Those Who Have Died.

Other sources for learning more about ME/CFS and suicide are: Lisa Lorden Myers' 2007 article, "*Killing Me Softly: FM/CFS & Suicide*"[126] and Action for ME in the U.K., a special report devoted to the subject in their InterAction publication Winter 2009.[127]

Although most ME/CFS organizations I am familiar with are not staffed around the clock, some have information lines. One example is the PANDORA Org website,[128] which has phone numbers and information about outreach and crisis calls.

🌿 *Where's the media?* – As with any controversial, conflicting, and ever-changing subject, the information relayed to the public by the media regarding ME and CFS has sometimes been good, sometimes bad, and at times, downright ugly. Many aspects have

---

123 In a 2012 Blog Talk Radio show, "In Short Order," host Sue Vogan led a discussion about CFS, Lyme disease and other neuro-immune conditions entitled "Let's Talk about CFS and More." One of the subjects was suicide. www.blogtalkradio.com/in-short-order/2012/08/05/in-short-order--pandora (accessed July 25, 2016).

124 Bliss Sandra; "Antidepressant Therapy of No Benefit For Chronic Fatigue Syndrome." University of Michigan Department of Pediatrics. You can find the summary at www.med.umich.edu/pediatrics/ebm/cats/cfs.htm (accessed July 28, 2015). Vercoulen JH et al; "Randomised, double-blind, placebo-controlled study of fluoxetine in chronic fatigue syndrome." Lancet. 1996 March 30;347(9005):858-61. www.ncbi.nlm.nih.gov/pubmed/?term=Randomised%2C+double-blind%2C+placebo-controlled+study+of+fluoxetine+in+chronic+fatigue+syndrome (accessed July 28, 2015).

125 Refer to Chapter 4: "My Brother by Choice – a Goodbye to Tom Hennessy" by Cort Johnson.

126 www.cfidsselfhelp.org/library/killing-me-softly-fmcfs-suicide (accessed July 25, 2016).

127 www.actionforme.org.uk/get-informed/publications/interaction-magazine/read-selected-ia-articles/living-with-me/special-report-on-suicide (accessed July 28, 2015).

128 pandoraorg.net/Support_Chapters.html (accessed July 25, 2016).

been minimized, or the reporting has relied on partial or outdated information.[129] There hasn't been much reporting on the significant underfunding of research by government agencies. There have been some exceptions thanks to journalists like Miriam Tucker, David Tuller, and Llewellyn King. Some 2015 articles in *The Washington Post*[130] and *The Atlantic*[131] are encouraging to read.

Often in media, the illness is referred to as **chronic fatigue**, instead of **chronic fatigue syndrome**. Chronic fatigue refers to long-term fatigue that can be caused by many things. Examples might include a new mother's sleepless nights or the exhaustion of a cancer patient. However, this fatigue is a *symptom*, completely different from "chronic fatigue syndrome," which refers to a distinct, biological, clinical disorder. **General fatigue** is the term most healthy people refer to in everyday life as normal tiredness.

Another misrepresentation regularly seen in the media is a visual one – perhaps the fault of stock images[132] or poorly chosen representations for television news. I have never seen media coverage of an ME/CFS patient with a walker, cane, or wheelchair, nor one with IV tubes in their arms, an oxygen tank by their side, or with dark sunglasses and earplugs, lying in a dimly lit or dark room to avoid the pain of overstimulation. A photo of a very tired person does not set the illness apart from the healthy.

The only television media I know that dealt with CFS in a realistic way was the hit sitcom *The Golden Girls,*[133] and this was due to writer/producer Susan Harris who has CFS. She is also known for her work on *All in the Family, Benson,* and *Soap.* In the two episodes called "Sick and Tired," actor Bea Arthur portrayed the character Dorothy as a person struggling with CFS. I think these episodes are brilliant: They managed to take this serious subject, maintain its importance, and yet lighten it up with funny, everyday events. More importantly, the struggles that Dorothy faced back in 1989 on TV are still familiar to us now

---

129 In 2011, advocates posted a petition on change.org addressed to members of the media. It set out ways in which the media could get up to speed about ME/CFS efficiently and encouraged them to use current studies and statistics to cover the illness accurately.

130 The Washington Post, Miriam E. Tucker October 5: "With His Son Terribly Ill, A Top Scientist Takes On Chronic Fatigue Syndrome." www.washingtonpost.com/national/health-science/with-his-son-terribly-ill-a-top-scientist-takes-on-chronic-fatigue-syndrome/2015/10/05/c5d6189c-4041-11e5-8d45-d815146f81fa_story.html (accessed August 6, 2016).

131 The Atlantic, Olga Khazan, October 8, 2015. "The Tragic Neglect of Chronic Fatigue Syndrome." www.theatlantic.com/health/archive/2015/10/chronic-fatigue-patients-push-for-an-elusive-cure/409534 (accessed August 6, 2016).

132 If community members including Jennifer Brea (director of the documentary Canary in a Coal Mine) have their way, this will change. In March 2015, Jen floated the idea of producing stock photos that "authentically portray the experience of living with ME" and putting them on a popular stock photography site for newspapers and magazines. The call for volunteers has gone out. It would be wonderful if this meant the real impact of the disease could be accurately visualized.

133 Golden Girls: "Golden Moment". www.youtube.com/watch?v=Zovd9eKvy8s (accessed July 25, 2016).

– difficulty getting a diagnosis, medical dismissals, referrals to psychiatrists and specialists that didn't go so well, gender issues and the lack of treatment or cure.

✨ *Affecting millions* – In the United States, higher and lower estimates have been published with prevalence numbers as high as four percent of the population. This range occurs, in part, because of the different diagnostic criteria used in medicine and in research studies. The most commonly accepted estimate is 0.42 percent of the adult population[134] – that comes to 1,314,666 people (using 2012 U.S. population numbers of 313 million) or one person in every 240.

In Canada, the 2014 statistics from the Canadian Community Health Survey (CCHS)[135] show prevalence numbers for CFS as 1.4%. Canadian health agencies are aware of these numbers but have done very little to further investigate their accuracy or to deal with this population's unmet medical, social, and financial needs.

I have always found the results of the Dubbo study to be interesting. The Dubbo Study,[136] published in 2006, revealed that, ***"Eleven percent of those presenting with different acute infections met the diagnostic criteria for chronic fatigue syndrome at six months."*** This study took place in the township of Dubbo in rural Australia. It concluded that CFS occurred in similar numbers whether it followed acute infection with Epstein-Barr virus (aka mononucleosis or glandular fever), Coxiella burnetii (Q fever), or Ross River virus. The severity of the infection onset was a large factor in determining who developed CFS over time. Where people lived in the township, their state of mind, or the type of infection they started with were not determining factors.

---

134 Jason LA, et al. "A community-based study of chronic fatigue syndrome." Arch Intern Med. 1999. Oct 11; 159(18):2129-37.

135 "Canadians reporting a diagnosis of fibromalgia, chronic fatigue syndrome or multiple chemical sensitivities; by sex, household population aged 12 and older." www.statcan.gc.ca/daily-quotidien/150617/t002b-eng.htm (accessed July 20, 2016).

136 Hickie I, Davenport T, Wakefield D, et al. "Post-infective and chronic fatigue syndromes precipitated by viral and non-viral pathogens: Prospective cohort study." doi:10.1136/bmj.38933.585764.AE. The criteria used to diagnose CFS in this study was the 2004 CDC criteria commonly referred to as the Fukuda definition.

STANZA 40

Suffering as fuel, Awareness Day, and advocacy

To each person I've met, I have asked the same question:
"What do I do with this *suffering* 🕊 damnation?"
I'd get "the look" and not much would be said.
I thought, "Someone must know this." No comfort was led.

Years later, I heard the answer to my query.
It came from inside me, not from Madame Curie;
"To change things for you and for the others too, 🕊
You use the *suffering as a source of fuel,* 🕊

　　…For *speaking out* 🕊 …
　　…*Awareness Day* 🕊 …
　　…*Advocacy* 🕊 times"…

The next generation 🕊 depends on us now,
Not to fight for them would be a crime.

STANZA 40 NOTES

❧ *Suffering* – Human suffering is a universal experience. Almost anyone can relate to suffering stemming from physical, mental, emotional, and/or spiritual pain. For those of us with unrecognized complex illness, the illness brings pain and losses in all these areas. Besides the obvious, an aspect of suffering rarely acknowledged is knowing that those close to us have to be exposed to our ongoing struggle.

I have some control over the physical pain and the inner suffering, especially when I am well enough: I adapt my lifestyle by energy conservation, pacing, and doing things differently; I adjust my attitudes and beliefs about myself and about being chronically ill; and I try to manage my symptoms through medication or alternative care.

But there is another type of suffering – one that stems from the actions and reactions of those outside of us, like the doctor who does not know the illness is real, or the general feedback from society as I am out in the world. This *outside-in suffering* is out of our control and has many sources, including the inaction of government health and funding agencies, as well as inadequate access to medical care, effective treatment, or a cure.

❧ *To change things for you and for the others too* – As I fought for care and for treatment, I sensed that something was missing. I didn't know what it was, but I certainly felt relieved when I was introduced to Ken Wilber's Integral Theory work.[137] In his paper "Introduction to Integral Theory and Practice: IOA Basic and the AQAL Map," [138] Wilber describes what I instinctively knew was needed: the whole picture. His theory provides a way of recognizing and then dealing with suffering that arises from the outside as well as from the inside. It provides some insight into how and why we have had our hands tied behind our backs for so long with ME/CFS. Society has a role to play, and his theory provides us with ideas as to where we can focus for solutions.

In Integral Theory, everything is connected. Wilber posits that there are four quadrants or perspectives that create a whole:

I – the inside of the individual (personal subjective experiences), like our thoughts;

It – the outside of the individual (objectively viewed), like our genetics;

---

137 Ken Wilber is an American author who has written extensively about philosophy, ecology, developmental psychology, and mysticism. In 1998, he founded the Integral Institute for the purpose of teaching and applying his Integral Theory. As synchronicity would have it, Ken Wilber was one of the people who became ill at the first cluster outbreak of CFS at Incline Village, U.S. in 1985 with what he labels CFIDS/REDD*/ME (*REDD – RNase-L Enzyme Dysfunction Disorder).

138 AQAL stands for All Quadrants, All Levels. www.terrypatten.com/sites/default/files/files/other_files/AQAL_intro.pdf (accessed July 25, 2016).

We – the inside of the collective (cultural – collective subjective shared experiences), like attitudes of friends and family; and

Its – the outside of the collective (objectively viewed), like government funding.

INTEGRAL THEORY (Simplified diagram, as applied to medicine)[139]

	INTERIOR/Subjective	EXTERIOR/Objective
INDIVIDUAL	• Meaning • Thoughts, beliefs, attitudes • Emotions and feelings • Exteroception (i.e., the five senses) • Personality style I	• Genetics • Biochemistry • Structural issues • Atoms, molecules, organs & systems • Physics of the energy body IT
COLLECTIVE	WE • Doctor/patient communication and relationship • Attitudes of friends and family (e.g., supportive and understanding or skeptical and dismissive) • Cultural understanding and beliefs/prejudices around the illness • Cultural beliefs around treatment modalities	ITS • Government funding for research • Government funding for treatment • Support from insurance companies • Proven etiology of ME/CFS • Environmental toxins • Access to information (e.g., the Internet)

Integral Theory has been likened to a camera lens zooming in and out on its subject to see each of the perspectives more clearly. Since they interact, none of these quadrants exist on their own. It is easy to see why ME/CFS remains largely in Square 1.

🌿 *Suffering as a source of fuel* – Because I am curious and compassionate, the inequities I've seen and experienced motivate me – provide the fuel – to write, advocate, and try to help make positive changes for me and for others. These inequities also spur on the actions of advocates everywhere: Carol Head, President of the Solve ME/CFS Initiative, had these powerful words to say, "This is a moral issue. The fire in my belly leads to passionate, respectful words. But that fire is burning." (Spring 2016 Chronicle).

---

139 This is my adaptation of information from two sources: K. Wilber's paper already mentioned and a chart from "The Application of Integral Medicine in the Treatment of Myalgic Encephalomyelitis/Chronic Fatigue Syndrome." Howard A, and Arroll M. www.theoptimumhealthclinic.com/wp-content/uploads/2012/01/OHC-Research-Paper-December-2011.pdf (accessed April 2016).

Although it felt like I might be engaging in the ultimate David-and-Goliath battle in even thinking that I could influence the outside environment, including the general population, political, and medical systems, I soon realized I wasn't alone – that there are many others already working hard to improve the situation.

First and foremost, there is an urgent need for more objective research and replication of study findings in the field of ME and CFS. We need millions, if not billions, of dollars, and governments need to offer more than just verbal reassurance. After all, addressing societal health concerns is part of their purpose and a promised use of taxpayer dollars.

A paradigm shift is needed in the medical field itself. The mistake of medicine holding fast to one way of thinking has been seen in the case of stomach (gastric) ulcers. These ulcers were thought to be the result of stress until 1984, when a physician and pathologist discovered their association to the bacteria *Helicobacter pylori,* and as a result, its relationship to certain cancers. This discovery had important consequences for the way ulcers are diagnosed and treated.

As an example of the need for a paradigm shift in the case of ME/CFS, patients plead for policymakers to stop recommending cognitive behavioral therapy (CBT) and graded exercise therapy (GET) to doctors as primary treatment options and request policymakers to put a black box with an X on these treatments just as they do for dangerous or toxic drugs.[140] This issue is often included in presentations to the Chronic Fatigue Syndrome Advisory Committee (CFSAC) in the United States.

Fortunately, not all protocols labeled CBT or GET are the same. Some practitioners are able to properly protect and monitor their patients and use CBT and modified exercise in beneficial ways – as coping tools and management strategies – with the patient guiding the pace. This is how these treatments are used for other serious illnesses.[141] However, it is difficult to find the practitioners who know how to administer these treatments without causing more harm than good.

✎ *Speaking out* – Some of the ways to be proactive all year include letter writing, blogs, rallies, demonstrations, and speaking at meetings. Social media and the Internet are speeding up advocacy efforts by making it easier for people to connect.

In common with other social movements, sometimes we see isolated flares of activity, but we are also seeing some longer-term steps and actions such as those taken by ME/

---

140   Tom Kindlon, "Reporting of Harms Associated with Graded Exercise Therapy and Cognitive Behavioural Therapy in Myalgic Encephalomyelitis/Chronic Fatigue Syndrome," Irish ME/CFS Association. iacfsme.org/PDFS/Reporting-of-Harms-Associated-with-GET-and-CBT-in.aspx (accessed July 26, 2016).

141   An additional concern is that CBT is shown on some government websites as a primary treatment, unlike other serious illnesses where it is shown as an adjunct.

CFS activist Rivka Solomon.[142] Rivka has accomplished amazing things while bedbound, inspiring women across the world as well as members of the ME/CFS community.

❧ *Awareness Day* – One way to speak out is with an awareness day/week/or month. May 12th has been ME/CFS and FM Awareness Day for almost twenty-five years. The idea originated in 1993 with the late Tom Hennessy,[143] an American patient-activist. May 12th was chosen because it is the birth date of Florence Nightingale (also known as the Lady with the Lamp). She was the famous English army nurse, from the mid-1800s, most of us learned about as schoolchildren. She became chronically ill in her thirties with an illness resembling ME/CFS. Her poor health did not prevent her from being a tireless crusader for improving sanitary medical conditions and advancing the profession of nursing.

Ms. Nightingale was one inspiration for my book cover – the candle. She carried her lamp from soldier to soldier so that she could care for them. The other influence for the cover is the indigo blue color which represents the ME/CFS awareness ribbon. Most people are not even aware there is a representing color for the illness. (See Chapter 9, "From a Blue Ribbon to a Pink One" by D. Fleck.)

To this day, May 12th remains "the Awareness Day few are aware of." Fortunately, there are some signs this is slowly changing: Activities are growing in number and variety and are more consistently done year after year. People have gone on a hunger strike, had one-person marathons, walks, bike racing events, held vigils, have parachuted out of a plane, and have even produced an opera to further the cause of ME/CFS research, awareness, and cure.

Two of my favorite recent May 12th events were "Light Up the Night" and "The Big Sleep for ME."

"Light up the Night" is when public buildings, landmarks and homes are lit up – from Australia, Canada, Germany, Japan, Northern Ireland, Puerto Rico, U.S.A. to the U.K.

---

142 Rivka Solomon has had ME/CFS since 1990 and is known for her one-woman protest in front of the Department of Health and Human Services and Red Cross headquarters in Washington, D.C. and for a comedic protest video demanding – via song – ME/CFS clinical trials. She also has created a how-to guide for ME/CFS demonstrations that has inspired others to action. phoenixrising.me/resources/taking-a-stand-a-how-to-guide-for-mecfs-demonstrations. April 12, 2012 (accessed July 26, 2016). Rivka is the author of That Takes Ovaries! now in its sixth printing, and it still inspires action with its essays by women telling their true stories of "being bold and brazen, outrageous or courageous." "Rivka Solomon Acts Up, Chronic Fatigue Be Damned," Ms. Magazine blog. msmagazine.com/blog/2011/06/02/rivka-solomon-acts-up-chronic-fatigue-be-damned (accessed on June 20, 2016).

143 You can see Tom Hennessy in the news piece "Too Tired" by correspondent Fred de Sam Lazaro, which appeared on The MacNeil/Lehrer NewsHour in late 1992 or early 1993. It was uploaded by May12.org and is followed by the 1993 documentary "Living Hell: the Real World of Chronic Fatigue Syndrome" by Lennie Copeland and also by footage from a Larry King show from 1992 on CFS. The program is available at www.youtube.com/watch?v=SyB49g_l9Sg (accessed on July 9, 2016).

The photos of this event are breathtaking and inspiring.[144] I'm particularly fond of the one showing the colored lighting of Niagara Falls for our cause.

"The Big Sleep" involved wearing pajamas so that even bedbound patients could participate, and it was part of Invest in ME's "Let's Do it for ME" fundraising campaign for a Centre of Excellence.[145]

Since 2012, I've marked Awareness Day in my home province of Alberta, Canada, by doing something other than putting on an awareness ribbon and resting at home. I, along with my daughter Jenna and a good friend, have organized a small event at a local health food store to raise awareness with the help of promotional items including T-shirts, ribbons, and candles. Each year I've predictably relapsed after the event, but I am so glad we can help to break ground in our city.

Severe ME has a different day for awareness – the 8th of August, recognized for the first time in 2013. Severe ME day in 2013 focused on those who had "lost their battle to this dreadful disease," with the theme "Understanding and Remembrance." In 2014, the theme was the "ME Cover Up." This was a clever idea, using photos of people with ME covered by a sheet and holding up an awareness slogan to depict four things: the invisibility of the most severe patients to the outside world; that ME is not taken seriously; that sufferers want and need to be seen, heard and recognized; and lastly, that they refuse to be ignored or invisible. As they state: "We want the medical profession and general public to understand the seriousness of the illness and recognize that beneath the sheet there is still a human being." [146] The theme of Severe ME day in 2015 was to raise awareness for the significant home care needs of this group.

Advocacy – Chuck Smit, President of the ME Society of Edmonton, Alberta, Canada, once wrote an article regarding advocacy: "What's the point? We as a community must stay on top of current ME news from around the world. We as a community must advocate for change however we can – whether it's here in our backyard or another country. We will determine our success or failure in bringing ME to the forefront and thus finding a cure." [147]

I have become an advocate almost by accident. In order for me to be able to answer my own questions about the history, current state of affairs, and what was missing, I had to dip my toe into the shallow end of the political/medical pool. Before I knew it, I was knee

---

144 The photos are posted on May 12th – International ME/CFS and FM Awareness Day's Facebook page www.facebook. com/media/set/?set=a.10152010333857161.1073741830.220534562160&type=3 (accessed July 2016).

145 Invest in ME announced on February 21, 2015 that their biomedical research campaign had surpassed £½ million (U.K.) www.investinme.org/IIME-Newslet-1502-01.htm (accessed March 4, 2016). Updates available at Idifme.org.

146 www.25megroup.org/campaigning_Severe_ME_Day.html (accessed March 4, 2016).

147 Newsletter of the ME Society of Edmonton, Volume 6, Issue 1, February 2013. www.mesocietyedmonton.org/ uploads/9/5/8/2/9582199/volume_6_issue_1.pdf on June 23, 2014 (accessed July 28, 2015).

deep. It would have been easy for me to get in over my head, gasping for air, because there is a lot to learn and do and so little time and energy for it.

Erica Verrillo is the editor for ProHealth ME/CFS Health Watch and Natural Wellness Newsletters. She is an active advocate and writer in the field of ME/CFS.[148] Erica became ill during her travels to Guatemala in 1992 and has battled ME/CFS since then. E. Verrillo's 2014 outlook for ME/CFS was that it would be the "Year of the Advocate."[149] As she noted, people who have been sick for thirty years are growing impatient.

Although 2014 has come and gone, advocacy action has been continuously growing: The May 25, 2016 "#MillionsMissing" action was an encouraging united event –

> ...dedicated to the millions of Myalgic Encephalomyelitis (ME) and Chronic Fatigue Syndrome (CFS) patients missing from their careers, schools, social lives and family due to the debilitating symptoms of the disease. At the same time, millions of dollars are missing from research and clinical education funding that ME should be receiving. And millions of doctors are missing out on proper training to diagnose and help patients manage this illness.

> ... #ME Action is sponsoring a community organized protest at the Department of Health and Human Services (HHS) in Washington D.C. ME patients, advocates, caregivers, and allies will join together to protest the lack of government funding for research, clinical trials, and medical/public education, leaving ME patients without relief.

> The protest has now gone global, with participation in the United Kingdom, Australia, and Canada." Millionsmissing.action.net.

❧ *The next generation* – As has been introduced, there can be many complications when children with ME/CFS are involved. For example, they can be removed from their homes and allowed limited parental visitation due to misdiagnoses and/or a lack of understanding about ME/CFS. Experts and advocates try to help in these cases.[150] (See Chapter 2, "A Child's CFS, Misdiagnosed as Munchausen's by Proxy" by Dr. D Bell.)

---

148 In 2012, Verrillo published an updated second edition of her book "Chronic Fatigue Syndrome: A Treatment Guide" which has been endorsed by many prominent ME/CFS experts and researchers.

149 "A Year We Will Never Forget," Erica Verrillo. December 30, 2013. www.prohealth.com/me-cfs/library/showarticle. cfm?libid=18567 (accessed July 26, 2016).

150 The Young ME Sufferers Trust in the U.K., is promoting a recent publication called "False Allegations of Child Abuse in Cases of Childhood ME." www.tymestrust.org/pdfs/falseallegations.pdf (accessed July 12, 2016).

Dr. Nigel Speight,[151] a pediatrician for over thirty years in England, and a medical advisor to the U.K.-based ME Association, has dealt with hundreds of cases of pediatric ME, and has been involved in over thirty child protection cases. He feels the situation is not improving in the U.K. and might be getting worse. He notes that once child protection proceedings begin, they are very difficult to reverse. His interventions have mostly been successful, but the process can take immense financial resources, lawyers, and a great deal of time.

One of the ongoing cases in 2016 is that of Karina Hansen (Denmark), who became ill in 2009 at age sixteen. At age twenty-four, on February 12, 2013, she was forcibly removed from her home and placed in a psychiatric facility. It has been very difficult for her as well as for her family. People from around the world have been trying to help in any way they can, for example by petition and the updated book by Greg Crowhurst[152] titled *Severe ME featuring Justice for Karina Hansen.*[153]

Sadly, on April 20, 2016, the General Medical Council, which is the U.K. body that sets standards for doctors, imposed conditions on Dr. Speight's ability to practice medicine, including refraining from any work – paid or unpaid – in relation to Myalgic Encephalopathy/Chronic Fatigue Syndrome.

For the sake of our children and of our children's children, we need more people to take initiatives like Dr. Speight did, to ensure quicker and better outcomes.

---

151 Dr. Speight is one of the experts interviewed in the Science to Patients video series I mention in Appendix I.

152 Crowhurst, Greg, "Severe ME featuring Justice for Karina Hansen." Stonebird. Jan. 1, 2014.

153 Book website: www.stonebird.co.uk/severemebook/severeme.html (accessed July 28, 2016).

STANZA 41

Writing my story and choosing action

So, I'm telling my story at twenty years ill.
Child grown, husband travels, gives me time to kill;
Writing and research when *"on"* and awake,
Gives purpose for me when my health is at stake.

This illness community, global and strong,
It needs so much help but I'm glad to belong.
Thank you to everyone working so hard;
Many are ill, but they still hold these cards;

    ...*Choosing action* ...
    ...And compassion...
    ...Connecting ME to you...

I believe there is a voice that you can hear now;
The outcome will be what we do.

STANZA 41 NOTES

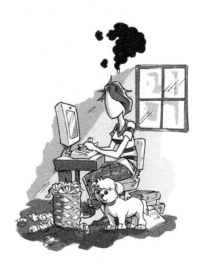

❧ *"On"* – Since I became ill, I have only rarely felt "on". I try to write while sitting when I can, but I also write lying down, in a resting position, or in my sauna where I am warm and feel better. Any sort of mental work is difficult, and I have trouble concentrating on more than one thing at a time. If I do mental work for any length of time, my brain hurts, and I know if I keep at it, I will "crash" or have more symptoms later.

A brain that hurts when it's thinking, as depicted in this illustration, was a very new phenomenon for me. In spite of this, when I'm in a creative space or have an idea that's taking off, I don't like to stop – although I know a payback will almost inevitably occur.

❧ *Choosing action* – I used to take social change for granted. I never really considered how it came about, who was involved in making it happen, or that years of effort were required to bring these changes to fruition. Now I appreciate that these improvements for society don't happen on their own – or overnight.

Dr. Leonard Jason's book, *Principles of Social Change, 2013*, reflects on five basic principles that are necessary for policy change to occur in society: [154]

1. Determine the nature of the change desired. Is it a cosmetic, short-term fix or does it address the root of the problem?

2. Identify power holders – know who your influential friends are, who your foes are.

3. Create coalitions. Identify and work with others who share your goal.

4. Learn patience and persistence. Small wins are crucial to attaining long-term goals.

5. Measure your success. Know what you have accomplished and what is left to achieve.

---

154 His presentation at the 2013 conference of the Society for Community Research and Social Action "Principles of Social Change: Community Partnerships Promote Social Justice" gives a clear explanation of the five points. www.youtube.com/watch?v=Gy1BsgBYb5Q on June 19, 2014 (accessed July 12, 2016).

Dr. Jason[155] points out that because those who take on these jobs to create change often endure many assaults, they must have ***dogged optimism, community support, and spiritual beliefs*** as their shields. In a Webinar[156] interview in the "Science to Patients" series, Dr. Jason had more specific things to say to the ME community:

> … Ultimately it's endurance, it's staying committed to something over long periods of time, it's basically having community coalitions that work and try to really deal with the power abuses that occurred. And it's really looking at some other structural issues that need to be faced. We need to organize. We need to be more effective. We need to basically be able to change the status quo, because the status quo is not working for patients with ME. It's only by us collectively being involved in action that the situation is really going to change.

Many doctors who have shown interest in ME and/or CFS – and who have been helpful to the community – have the condition themselves or have experienced someone close to them who is afflicted. Ultimately, we hope more doctors will choose to take part in diagnosing, treating, and researching ME/CFS as well as related complex diseases.

155 Dr. Leonard Jason is one of the preeminent figures in the ME/CFS world and has taken action to influence positive change for us. Over the years he has discovered some of the answers, and these answers are applicable for many areas, not only ME/CFS. Dr. Jason had ME/CFS as a young man, but with forced rest, care, and accommodations as a university professor, he became very functional and hasn't stopped his valuable work since. An extensive list of Dr. Jason's ongoing research and group publications spanning more than two decades are found at http://csh.depaul.edu/about/centers-and-institutes/ccr/myalgic-encephalomyelitis-cfs/Pages/publications.aspx (accessed July 19, 2016).

156 www.me-cvsvereniging.nl/english-page. Webinar 56, "Population and Social Impact" (accessed July 12, 2016). Video at www.youtube.com/watch?v=lsXze-Qw6Q8&index=7&list=PLsQ0FZQ_5JXQSlHbE68aISSbyGtwCmlB. The complete transcript can be read at www.meresearch.org.uk/wp-content/uploads/2014/10/Prof.-Jason.-Population-and-social-impact.pdf (accessed July 12, 2016).

STANZA 42

Cost to society, getting to know the ME/CFS community, and underdog no longer

The public, the systems, the funding too slow;
Cost to society? Billions, you know. 🌱
You're meeting patients from all walks of life
At different stages and phases of strife.

So now that you know the "new" illness on the block,
And know some people who have to "walk the talk," 🌱
If everyone can move toward the same goal,
Better outcomes, a cure, and some rest for our souls.

    …A worthy cause…
    … Justifiable…
    … Money, time, energy…

Underdog no longer 🌱 with you by our sides,
We will have a winning team.

STANZA 42 NOTES

ᔧᔭ *Cost to society? Billions you know* – The economic burden to all countries for the consequences of ME/CFS is exorbitant. Lost productivity and income – which includes being unable to help in the home – along with increased health and other costs, add up to billions of dollars per year. The dollar range from the 2008 study (L. Jason et al.) "The Economic Impact of ME/CFS: Individual and Societal Costs" is $18 billion to $23 billion (U.S.).[157] So a $6 million/year investment by the U.S. NIH, and less in other countries, does not seem to make any sense.

ᔧᔭ *And know some people who have to "walk the talk"* – Aside from all the stories that you will get to read in Section 2 of this book, we put together a list of some books, documentaries, and videos in Appendix I which span time and distance.

ᔧᔭ *Underdog no longer* – My dad often cheers for the underdog in any sports event, and one day I asked him why. He said, "Somebody has to." He has a big heart and is a wise man. I think he wants people who are in a less powerful position to do well. ME/CFS and related illnesses have been the underdogs in care and research for decades now. To my mind, it feels we have been oppressed and marginalized[158] by our political, medical, and social systems.

Most research done so far for ME/CFS is the result of independent private or corporate funding. Without widespread public support, the sums have been too small to move science quickly.

Donations, small or large, add up quickly when numbers of people participate. This was demonstrated by the "March of Dimes," established back in 1938 by President Franklin Roosevelt (who had polio). The March of Dimes was a grassroots campaign, run primarily by volunteers. Over the years, millions of people gave small amounts of money to support care for people with polio as well as research into prevention and treatment. Those contributions financed Jonas Salk, Albert Sabin, and the other researchers who developed the polio vaccines that children around the world receive today." [159]

Roosevelt's initiative is a great example of motivated leadership, the coordinated efforts of agencies, and full participation of the public. Imagine the years and lives lost if, instead of being treated as an urgent health concern, polio had been treated with rehabilitation alone.

---

157 The research can be found at www.ncbi.nlm.nih.gov/pmc/articles/PMC2324078 (accessed July 28, 2016).

158 Oppression means to "dominate harshly" or "inflict stress on." To marginalize means "to prevent from having attention or power."

159 amhistory.si.edu/polio/howpolio/march.htm (accessed June 17, 2016).

STANZA 43

Official apologies, the bottom line, needing to increase funding, righting the past wrongs, and creating a new future

With science and politics working together,
An official apology  to help remember,
That *research, education, and good patient care,*
Can follow our efforts: Speak up if we dare.

There's *so much more now that is understood,*
About why we're ill and what's under our hoods.
With your help and ours, in cooperation,
The future is hopeful for all of the nations.

    …*Fund the research* …
    …Talk to government…
    …Help to move us along…

We can do more now than ever before,
To right the many past wrongs.

STANZA 43 NOTES

🐛 *An official apology* – I continue to struggle with my health, so as I learn and write, I sometimes imagine someone of influence in the political and medical arenas telling me and others: "We are sorry for our mistakes and dismissals. Things are going to change. This is the plan." Clearing the past makes room for the new. In part, I have gone into our illness stories to address this past and focus on what is to come. An apology does not change the past, but it may, to quote from a paper on the power of apologies, "restore dignity, trust and a sense of justice." [160] I am not alone in believing that apologies are important. Both the Norwegian government and Dr. Jose Montoya from Stanford University have made statements to the patient community. In addition, respected scientist, Ron Davis, PhD, has expressed a similar sentiment.

The apology from Norway came after research findings – involving the administration of the cancer drug Rituximab in ME/CFS patients – revealed some benefit.[161] Cort Johnson discussed the apology by the Norwegian government in the October 2011 issue of *Phoenix Rising* as follows:

> The Norwegian Directorate of Health ... apologize[d] for the poor treatment that ME patients have received at their hands. ...we have not cared for people with ME to a great enough extent...it is correct to say that we have not established proper health care services for these people...[162] [163]

The numbers of medical providers who believe their ME/CFS patients and who recognize that they are facing a real biomedical illness are slowly increasing. But not everyone does. We can take solace from the words of Dr. Jose Montoya from a lecture on chronic fatigue syndrome at Stanford University: "...my dream is that our medical community

---

160 www.ombuds.unc.edu/downloads/The%20Power%20of%20Apologies.pdf (accessed June 17, 2016).

161 "A Drug for Chronic Fatigue Syndrome (ME/CFS)? The Rituximab Story." Phoenix Rising. Cort Johnson, December 15, 2010. phoenixrising.me/archives/1977 (accessed on June 17, 2016).

162 "Treatment Breakthrough (and Paradigm Shift) For CFS? Rituximab Trial Promises Hope." Phoenix Rising. Cort Johnson. October 28, 2011. phoenixrising.me/archives/6157 (accessed on June 17, 2016).

163 In 2011, after Norway's admission of inadequate care, a petition was created on change.org aimed at the Assistant U.S. Secretary of Health and Human Services and other HHS officials. The petition contained suggestions for change, such as increasing NIH research funding and removing outdated and harmful information from the CDC's CFS website, including CBT and GET recommendations. Its message "Apologize for not responding appropriately to the ME/CFS epidemic" resonated with many in the ME/CFS community – although it hasn't produced any apology, as yet. www.change.org/petitions/apologize-for-not-responding-appropriately-to-the-me-cfs-epidemic (accessed June 17, 2016).

will produce a formal apology to the patients for not having believed them all these years – that they were facing a real illness." [164]

Dr. Ron Davis ended his discussion with C. Johnson with this strong statement: "The millions of suffering ME/CFS patients are owed an apology and a concerted urgent effort to find effective treatment." (Chapter 12, " 'End ME/CFS' Mega Chronic Fatigue Syndrome Project Begins".)

✍ ***Research, education, and good patient care*** – Apologies are a great start, but action speaks louder than words. The mantra ***"research, education, and good patient care"*** is the focus for integration of ME/CFS into all parts of society.

As previously mentioned, education on these illnesses does not occur in most medical schools. A study [165] looked at a sample of U.S. medical schools and showed that in 2013, little was being taught about CFS in three areas: in the classroom, in the hospital, and in the lab (Peterson M, et al.) If what Peterson found in his research still holds true today, it is no wonder that doctors do not know about the condition: They are simply not being taught.

Lori Chapo-Kroger was an intensive care charge nurse before she fell ill from *clostridium difficile toxin B*, a bacterial infection. It was a nosocomial infection, meaning it was acquired in a hospital. This infection triggered her severe case of ME/CFS, leaving her bedbound for four years. Despite the fact that she was part of the medical community, Lori was first misdiagnosed, prescribed harmful treatments, or dismissed entirely. She says she felt betrayed and abandoned by her own profession. She eventually found a doctor who was knowledgeable in ME/CFS and experienced some improvement. Lori was then determined to help other patients and became an advocate for them.

PANDORA Org, which is under the direction of L. Chapo-Kroger, knows it helps when advocacy is directed at a particular aspect of the illness. For instance, focusing on education and training for health care professionals about neuro-immune illnesses will make a big difference to patients.

---

164 Address on CFS by Dr. Jose G. Montoya (then Associate Professor of Medicine, Division of Infectious Diseases at Stanford University School of Medicine). March 11, 2011. www.youtube.com/watch?v=Riybtt6SChU (accessed on June 17, 2016).

165 "Coverage of CFS in U.S. Medical Schools," T. Mark Peterson, DDS, Thomas W. Peterson, DDS., Sarah Emerson, BS, Eric Regalbuto, Meredyth A. Evans, MA, Leonard A. Jason, PhD. Universal Journal of Public Health 1(4): 177-179, 2013. www.hrpub.org/download/20131107/UJPH4-17600991.pdf (accessed July 28, 2016).

Some initial efforts have been made in this area by organizations across the globe. PANDORA has made such advocacy a priority.[166] The work to educate professionals is being done at hospitals, health fairs, career fairs for medical students, and in biology classes. It includes education about ME/CFS, as well as other diseases such as fibromyalgia, chronic Lyme disease, Gulf War illnesses, and environmental illnesses.

The following are examples of other organizations that encourage medical students to learn about these conditions:

- Immune Dysfunction.org, Vermont, provides a scholarship for a winning essay by a medical student at the University of Vermont when funds permit, as does FM-CFS Canada.[167]

- The Blue Ribbon Foundation, associated with the Forgotten Plague documentary, is raising money to offer internships to first and second-year medical students to work with some experts in the ME/CFS field.

There have also been some positive steps in putting research, education, and good patient care together:

- The Open Medicine Institute. (California, U.S.)

- The Institute for Neuro-Immune Medicine at Nova Southeastern University. (Florida, U.S.)

- Simmaron Research. (Nevada, U.S.)

- The National Centre for Neuroimmunology and Emerging Diseases is a research team at Griffith University (Australia). They opened an ME/CFS clinic in summer 2014.[168]

- The European ME Research Group (EMERG) – Invest in ME – Inaugural meeting, October 2015. (London, England)

Across the world, others are working to develop research and care facilities, including the ME/CFS Centre in Norway at Oslo University hospital[169] and a Complex Chronic Diseases Program which opened in British Columbia, Canada, for research and treatment into ME/CFS and other complex diseases.

---

166 PANDORA stands for Patient Alliance for NeuroEndocrineImmune Disorders Organization for Research and Advocacy Inc. PANDORA also takes the lead in creating collaborations in U.S. advocacy efforts and in providing some helpful practical and emotional assistance for patients in need.

167 Funds dispensed in 2009, 2012 and 2013. FM-CFS Canada has offered a monetary award for many years since 2011 to medical students who write the best essays on preselected titles.

168 www.griffith.edu.au/health/national-centre-neuroimmunology-emerging-diseases (accessed July 12, 2016).

169 ous-research.no/home/dgm/ME%20CFS%20Centre/12921?submenu=1 (accessed July 12, 2016).

⚘ ***So much more now that is understood*** – Thanks to conferences, anyone with an interest – including patients – can understand more and more about these conditions. Well-informed patients are known as E-patients. E-patients and E-caregivers are "individuals who are **e**quipped, **e**nabled, **e**mpowered, and **e**ngaged in their health care decisions." [170] This describes many ME/CFS patients and their caregivers.

Although I am not well enough to attend the following events to stay updated, there are summaries and videos available to everyone after their conclusion. Following is a partial list from a growing and ever-changing array of important gatherings.

- The biennial IACFS/ME conferences, with their professional and patient seminars, attract attendees from around the globe. The eleventh conference[171] was held in March 2014 in San Francisco, CA, U.S. It was called "Transforming Science into Clinical Care." The next conference will be held October 2016 in Fort Lauderdale, FL, U.S.

- Stanford University hosted a one-day symposium on ME/CFS in conjunction with the 2014 IACFS/ME Conference.

- Invest in ME Conference[172] London, U.K., May 2015. It was preceded by a bio-medical colloquium. The 2016 conference and colloquium was held June 2016.[173]

- UK CFS/M.E. Research Collaborative – The 3rd annual conference will be held Sept 28 - 29, 2016, in Newcastle, England.[174]

- Gold Coast Conference (Australia) – 2nd International Symposium for CFS/ME,[175] December 2013.

- European ME Alliance (Sweden) – "The invisible ones: A conference on Severe ME/CFS and the Way Forward," [176] October 2015.

---

170 "e-patients: how they can help us heal health care," Tom Ferguson, MD and the e-Patient Scholars Working Group 2007. www.e-patients.net/e-Patient_White_Paper_with_Afterword.pdf (accessed June 19, 2016). The term includes friends and family members of the patients too, sometimes known as e-caregivers.

171 Summary of the conference by Dr. Anthony Komaroff (slides and audio). www.youtube.com/watch?v=nyyjRdbvPj0 (accessed June 17, 2016). OR audio only – www.dropbox.com/s/vame7msb9h6nnfs/DrKomaroff.MP3 (accessed April 17, 2014).

172 Dr. Rosamund Valling's report on Conference 10 – www.investinme.eu/IIMEC10.shtml#report.html (accessed March 12, 2016).

173 www.investinme.eu/IIMEC11.shtml (accessed June 2016).

174 www.actionforme.org.uk/research/uk-cfsme-collaborative (accessed March 12, 2016).

175 Dr. Rosamund Valling's report – sacfs.asn.au/news/2014/02/02_08_the_2nd_international_symposium_for_cfs_me.htm. (accessed May 20, 2016).

176 www.euro-me.org/news-Q32015-002.htm (accessed March 12, 2016).

℘ *Fund the research* – When you take the number of people who have an illness in any country and divide that by the government health agency funding allotted to it for research, the result is the amount spent per person with the illness. The following table outlines the funding in dollars per patient, as well as the number of research studies per illness. It is an excerpt from the "CIHR Funding for Research Into Chronic Conditions." [177] (CIHR stands for Canadian Institutes of Health Research.)

1 ILLNESS	2 ANNUAL AVG. PER-PATIENT FUNDING 2012-2015	3 CANADIANS AFFECTED (CCHS 2010)	4 CIHR FUNDING 3 YRS. 2012-2015	5 NUMBER OF STUDIES FUNDED 2012-2015
PARKINSON'S DISEASE	$428.16	39,000	$50,094,279	234
ALZHEIMER'S DISEASE	$287.05	111,500	$96,016,737	433
MULTIPLE SCLEROSIS	$66.46	108,500	$21,631,220	106
DIABETES	$37.11	1,841,500	$205,010,686	1024
HEART DISEASE	$24.21	1,431,500	$103,971,956	475
ASTHMA	$6.59	2,246,500	$44,425,625	212
ARTHRITIS	$4.63	4,454,000	$61,807,451	352
FIBROMYALGIA	$0.89	439,000	$1,166,409	11
CHRONIC FATIGUE SYNDROME	$0.52	411,500	$645,925	2
MULTIPLE CHEMICAL SENSITIVITIES	$0.00	800,500	$0	0

In the United States, funding spent per patient is also very low and inequitable. During a U.S. CFSAC meeting May 10, 2011, Robert Miller, who is a long-time patient and advocate, really drove this point home by slamming $3.64 on the table in front of him,

---

177 Excerpted from the CIHR (Canadian Institutes of Health Research) funding decisions database using keyword searches by M. Parlor, statistical analyst and president of the National ME/FM Action Network. Funding provided by CIHR April 2012 - March 2015. Source: Quest 101, Winter 2014 page 3 at www.mefmaction.com/images/stories/quest_newsletters/Quest101.pdf (accessed March 2016). (Column 4 divided by 3 years = Annual $; divided by Column 3 = Column 2, Annual $/patient).

which is the amount spent on U.S. National Institutes of Health (NIH) funding per patient per year. He stated that he was worth more than that! His dramatic demonstration was powerful to watch. At that same meeting, Robert recommended that they increase their funding to $100 million annually for CFS research, beginning in 2014, versus the current $6 million.

A similar situation exists in Australia. In a February 26, 2016 posting on "Junkee" (an Australian pop culture title which covers film, TV, politics, comment, tech, online and everything in between), author Naomi Chainey made the situation for Australians with ME/CFS very clear. The post was titled *Getting by with "Bugger All": The Invisible Suffering of Australians with Chronic Fatigue Syndrome*. The title references comments made by Senator Scott Ludlum to an Australian parliamentary committee on February 10, 2016. During committee hearings, Senator Ludlum explored the amount of funding provided by the Australian government for ME/CFS research and found (quoting from the post) that the "initial figure of $2.4 million over 14 years was revised down to $1.6 million when challenged."

In addition to research, Senator Ludlum also highlighted the need for increased governmental support for improved medical care and patient advocacy. The Junkee post notes, "Estimates of how many of us there are range from 92,000 to 242,000." [178]

➤ *To right the many past wrongs* – Unfortunately, misinformation and stigma persist. This has been an intense six years (2010-2016) for advocates – including organizations, professionals, patients and their carers. Contributing to a better future for people with ME/CFS can seem complicated at first. It requires foundational knowledge about political and medical issues, but luckily, people naturally develop this as they become more interested. Sometimes, advocates have to try to right past wrongs to get things on track, and sometimes they are able to participate in creating something new.

Following are examples where the ME/CFS community tried to influence decisions but were unsuccessful. They did raise the concerning issues, and hopefully these will end up as building blocks for the future:

1. Somatic Symptom Disorder (SSD) was a category created and included in the DSM-5, (*Diagnostic and Statistical Manual of Mental Disorders*) which became effective in May 2013. This manual is used by clinicians and researchers to diagnose and classify mental

---

178 junkee.com/the-invisible-suffering-of-australians-living-with-chronic-fatigue-syndrome/73998 (accessed July 25, 2016). Another source reporting on the work of Senator Ludlum is Russell Logan's website Shoutoutaboutme.com, which contains the "latest news, opinions and extensive resources about myalgic encephalomyelitis."

disorders. Concerns were raised that the overly broad category of SSD could be interpreted to include many with ME/CFS.[179]

2. The American Academy of Family Physicians (AAFP) provided information in 2012 on the diagnosis and treatment of chronic fatigue syndrome[180] [181] to physicians.

   The information within it, and the absence of other information, upset some ME-literate professionals.[182] Since then, the AAFP website contains information about the more current IOM report including its recommendation to rename and redefine chronic fatigue syndrome as "systemic exertion intolerance disease." However, the AAFP website continues to suggest that further information can be obtained from the 2012 AAFP article.[183] [184]

3. The Food and Drug Administration (FDA) made the decision to decline the approval of Ampligen.[185] [186] [187] [188] Rintatolimod (trade name, Ampligen) is manufactured by Hemispherx BioPharma. It is a drug administered by some experts in the field for certain subsets of ME/

---

179 www.psychiatry.org/psychiatrists/practice/dsm/dsm-5 (accessed August 6, 2016).

    Allen Frances, MD has a blog "DSM5 in Distress" on Psychology Today. Two of his blogs related specifically to the harm he saw would come with the SSD category. They were his December 8, 2012 blog "Mislabeling Medical Illness as Mental Disorder," www.psychologytoday.com/blog/dsm5-in-distress/201212/mislabelingmedical-illness-mental-disorder (accessed August 6, 2016) and his January 16, 2013 "Bad news: DSM 5 refuses to correct Somatic Symptom Disorder," www.psychologytoday.com/blog/dsm5-in-distress/201301/bad-news-dsm-5-refuses-correct-somatic-symptom-disorder (accessed August 6, 2016).

180 It refers only to chronic fatigue syndrome – not to ME/CFS – and references the Fukuda and Oxford definitions.

181 "Chronic Fatigue Syndrome: Diagnosis and Treatment," American Academy of Family Physicians. October 15, 2012. www.aafp.org/afp/2012/1015/p741.html (accessed August 6, 2016).

182 "Article on CFS Does Not Reflect Current Best Treatment Practices," letter to the editor of the Journal, American Family Physician. April 1, 2013. www.aafp.org/afp/2013/0401/ol1.html (accessed August 6, 2016).

183 "Chronic Fatigue Syndrome Renamed and Redefined" – article on the IOM report, which starts with the lack of information in medical schools. For further information, this sends you to the 2012 article. www.aafp.org/news/health-of-the-public/20150302newchronicfatigue.html (accessed August 6, 2016).

184 Update on the background and findings of the IOM report, www.aafp.org/afp/2015/0401/p425.pdf (accessed August 6, 2016).

185 Article on the history of Ampligen and the clinical trials done by Hemispherx "Rintatolimod, aka Ampligen on Trial," Suzanne Vernon, Scientific Director (Solve ME/CFS Initiative). March 21, 2012. solvecfs.org/rintatolimod-aka-ampligen-on-trial (accessed July 25, 2016).

186 "Rintatolimod for Chronic Fatigue Syndrome gets FDA panel's 'No' vote." Miriam Tucker, December 21, 2012. www.medscape.com/viewarticle/776562.

187 "Chronic fatigue syndrome patients need an effective therapeutic, leading expert argues," January 24, 2013. Source: Nova Southeastern University. www.sciencedaily.com/releases/2013/01/130124183448.htm (accessed August 6, 2016).

188 Llewellyn King, White House Chronicle, "A Drug Goes Down in a Perfect Storm," February 7, 2013. whchronicle.com/?p=1316 (accessed July 1, 2016).

CFS patients, and over many years, they have had some good results. The story continues to evolve.[189][190][191] More recent developments are that the price is set to rise and that it will be available in Europe under an early access program.[192]

And following are important U.S. Health and Human Services initiatives which have forged a new path for progress. The ME/CFS community has been giving their input and feedback to influence the outcomes from these valuable documents:

1. The "Patient-Focused Drug Development Initiative - CFS and ME," yielded a well-regarded "Voice of the Patient[193] Report" dated September 2013, as well as the "Draft Guidance for Industry – CFS/ME: Developing Drug Products for Treatment," dated March 2014.

2. The Institute of Medicine (IOM) was contracted to create a diagnostic criteria for myalgic encephalomyelitis/chronic fatigue syndrome, and a report was delivered on February 10, 2015. The report was entitled "Beyond Myalgic Encephalomyelitis/Chronic Fatigue Syndrome: Redefining an Illness." It proposed new diagnostic criteria and a new name, "systemic exertion intolerance disease," or

---

189 Hemispherx Biopharma Press Release, Feb. 4, 2013. "Hemispherx Biopharma receives complete response letter from FDA on Ampligen New Drug Application for Chronic Fatigue Syndrome." "…Hemispherx will seek an end-of-Review-Conference with the FDA." www.hemispherx.net/content/investor/default.asp?goto=746 (accessed August 6, 2016).

190 The FDA response letter regarding the approval of Ampligen for ME/CFS and related information which can be linked to from this page regarding drug development for Myalgic Encephalomyelitis/Chronic Fatigue Syndrome (ME and CFS), www.fda.gov/Drugs/NewsEvents/ucm337750.htm (accessed August 6, 2016).

191 The Ampligen story is not over yet. C. Johnson has created a resource on Health Rising that contains the most recent updates on Ampligen and ME/CFS. Updates can be followed on www.healthrising.org/forums/resources/chronic-fatigue-syndrome-me-cfs-ampligen-resource-center.334. A recent post was "New president of Hemispherx says Ampligen approval is top priority" (accessed May 20, 2016).

192 Hemispherx enters into an agreement with myTomorrows for an Early Access Program for Rintatolimod in Europe August 10, 2015. http://forums.phoenixrising.me/index.php?threads/hemispherx-enters-into-agreement-for-early-access-program-for-ampligen-in-europe.39204 (accessed May 20, 2016).

193 The Voice of the Patient report on ME and CFS, www.fda.gov/downloads/ForIndustry/UserFees/PrescriptionDrugUserFee/UCM368806.pdf (accessed May 20, 2016). For responses to the report see "FDA's Voice of the Patient report on Chronic Fatigue Syndrome reveals disease impact and areas for progress." October 3, 2013, press release from PANDORA, www.prohealth.com/library/showarticle.cfm?libid=18390. Draft Guidance document, www.fda.gov/downloads/Drugs/GuidanceComplianceRegulatoryInformation/Guidances/UCM388568.pdf (accessed May 20, 2016).

SEID.[194][195] IOM has disseminated this report through medical journals and other means, although it has not been formally approved by the U.S. Health Agencies who charged the IOM with this task.

3. 2015 published reports: The report from the Pathways to Prevention ME/CFS Workshop held December 9 and 10, 2014; the background systematic evidence review reports from the Agency for Healthcare Research and Quality (AHRQ); along with a review article by Anthony Komaroff, were published in the *Annals of Internal Medicine* in June 2015.[196][197][198]

Although I live in Canada and these events are occurring in the United States, I realize that powerful health agency decisions influence all countries. The processes, and the results, have been of great interest to patients worldwide. Some patients watch and participate as much as possible, either in person or via webinar. Regardless, it always seems to be two steps forward and one step back in advocacy.

A lot of the research and decisions that I am writing about are ongoing.[199] By the time this book is published, we should have a better understanding whether these initiatives have had a positive or negative effect. Will they move our cause and cure backward twenty years, or will they move the system and patient care forward?

---

194 The report "Beyond Myalgic Encephalomyelitis/Chronic Fatigue Syndrome: Redefining an Illness" from the Institute of Medicine and supporting documents, including an ME/CFS Clinicians' Guide, Key Facts, and the Diagnostic Algorithm, can be found at iom.nationalacademies.org/Reports/2015/ME-CFS.aspx (accessed July 25, 2016).

195 An article authored by Ellen Clayton JD, MD, "Beyond Myalgic Encephalomyelitis/ Chronic Fatigue Syndrome: An IOM report on Redefining an Illness," appeared in the Journal of the American Medical Association on March 17, 2015. AMA. 2015;313(11):1101-1102. jama.jamanetwork.com/article.aspx?articleid=2118591 (accessed July 20, 2016).

196 The final report, and other material from the P2P workshops, are available at prevention.nih.gov/programs-events/ pathways-to-prevention/past-workshops/me-cfs/workshop-resources#finalreport (accessed July 25, 2016).

197 Information about the Pathways to Prevention program can be found at prevention.nih.gov/programs-events/pathways-to-prevention. The AHRQ report is at https://effectivehealthcare.ahrq.gov/ehc/products/586/2004/chronic-fatigue-report-150505.pdf (accessed July 15, 2016).

198 An article by Miriam E. Tucker was published in Medscape following the publication in the Annals of Internal Medicine "Chronic Fatigue Syndrome Report: More Research Needed," June 16, 2015. www.medscape.com/ viewarticle/846597.

199 Recommendations from the HHS Chronic Fatigue Syndrome Advisory Committee, following publication of the IOM report and the NIH P2P report, August 2015, are at www.hhs.gov/advcomcfs/recommendations/2015-08-18-19-recommendations.pdf (accessed July 15, 2016). There were fifteen recommendations made covering a wide range of issues, although no consensus was made on a recommendation for the name of the illness. They did note that: "A meaningful and sustained commitment by the Department of Health and Human Services is needed at this time to identify biomarkers, reproduce important research, address identified gaps, overcome institutional barriers, promote accurate medical education, and offer hope to patients and their loved ones through better diagnosis, treatments, and access to care from knowledgeable providers."

STANZA 44

Devoted scientists and researchers, looking forward to the pieces coming together

Some family and good friends and doctors keep sharing,
Scientists who research  and really are caring.
They keep the hope up for us to hang on,
Without them, it would be hard to belong.

So I say thank you to all those beside me,
Can't always tell you the good that I do see.
I'm still sure you know how much that I care,
But for the illness, I'd always be there.

   …ME/CFS…
   …Neuro-immune disease…
   …These are hidden no more…

Some day they'll put all the pieces in one,
And then all of us… WILL SOAR.

STANZA 44 NOTES

᷈ *Scientists who research* – Some past scientific ventures into the cause of ME/CFS have failed but have brought attention and worldwide interest. A notable example is xenotropic murine leukemia-like retrovirus (XMRV). It was discovered in late 2009 and was reported to have a link to CFS and certain cancers. In 2012, after many studies and millions of dollars spent, XMRV proved to be caused by cross-contamination in the research process – completely unrelated to the illnesses. Science works by proving or disproving hypotheses and moves forward from there. Even though the initial hypothesis regarding XMRV proved false, the attention it garnered resulted in a huge leap forward for the ME/CFS community. That was the silver lining.

One of the scientists at the center of the XMRV research was Judy Mikovits, PhD. She has written a book co-authored with Kent Heckenlively. It is called *Plague: One Scientist's Intrepid Search for the Truth about Human Retroviruses and Chronic Fatigue Syndrome (ME/CFS), Autism, and Other Diseases.*[200]

One of my favorite more-recent stories of commitment and hope by a researcher and his team is that of Gordon Broderick, PhD. This story comes from journalist Ryan Prior, my friend, who is a fellow patient. Ryan experienced this while interviewing and filming for the documentary *Forgotten Plague: M.E. and the Future of Medicine* (more about Ryan and the documentary in Chapter 7: The Good Fight).

> You know it's a really special day when you hear a scientist, Gordon Broderick, PhD, who can't stop talking about the passions that animate his soul: 40 teraflops (or 11,000 personal computers), sorting out the mysteries of ME/CFS and its infinitely complex interactions of the nervous, endocrine, and immune systems. The one thousand high-powered supercomputer fans in this room leave everyone's hair blowing with the air current, and the drone of the machines at work made it almost impossible to hold a conversation.

> This scientist and other brilliant researchers will deliver truths far faster than one might think about the underpinnings of the disease. These are the wild dreamers undertaking the noble pursuit of bringing solace to those who've suffered so deeply...

---

200   Mikovits, Judy. "Plague: One Scientist's Intrepid Search for the Truth about Human Retroviruses and Chronic Fatigue Syndrome (ME/CFS), Autism, and Other Diseases." Skyhorse Publishing. 2014.

PERSONAL UPDATE

(Summer 2016)

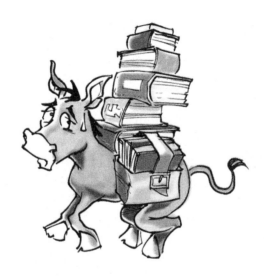

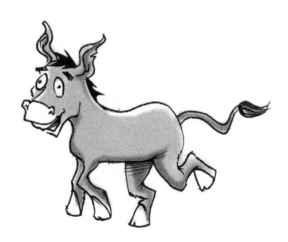

Back to the Heart

Valerie Free

You are probably glad to know I will not do this update in song/poem. I was beginning to feel like the Dr. Seuss of ME/CFS and related illnesses. I call this update "Back to the Heart" because it comes back to my personal story and my vision and aspirations – this, after spending so much time in Part V with a broader focus. As you see from the illustration on the title page of this update, I believe at this point I have unpacked both my personal experiences of living with, and learning about, ME/CFS...and more. That load is feeling a bit lighter, and if you look at the second little donkey, she is no longer weighed down and has a grin. She is even giving a little ME/CFS kick of relief.

From what you've read so far, you are probably aware of the ever-changing landscape surrounding ME/CFS and that most patients cannot participate in advocacy for very long – if at all. The progress and pitfalls in this field are apparent, although I do feel there is a pull forward since 2015. Unfortunately, this does not mean that we are receiving better care or that there is treatment that is effective for everyone.

Now at age fifty-five, I am entering a new stage of life. My health is stable between 30 and 50 percent, and that is because I lead a very quiet, adapted, and sedentary lifestyle. I have been filling my days with meditation, finishing this project, and basic daily tasks. Even now, it is not easy to accept the constraints when I see the healthy hustle and bustle of people around me. The phases and stages of life keep changing, as do my relationships. I have not traveled to Arizona for two winters but hope to go back again to enjoy the beauty and the warmth.

Knowing that things have advanced a lot in ten years, I did invest $12,000 in more testing from a local Integrative Clinic. We did all the tests to get a basic view of how my body is working and came up with three pages of abnormal results. These tests are done largely through specialty labs in the States. They include genetics, biochemistry, nutritional tests, celiac and digestive function tests, and all the blood work available, including toxic elements.

We pursued the basic treatment for the things that we could, but to look deeper into the cause would have required more testing for mold toxicity, detailed heavy metal testing, multiple panels for Lyme disease, viral panels, sleep assessments, and immune testing. These tests would add significantly to the amount I have already spent. Between original testing sent to the U.S. and then re-testing as needed, the physician fees, along with treatment trials, supplements and IVs, the cost would easily reach between $70,000 to $100,000 in the first year; and who knows how much it would take to sustain. This frustrates me because I think that the testing and treatment could help (even if just in understanding the illness better), and I wish everyone had access to them. The stress of the cost and increased effort after all these years is beyond what I am capable of handling – always keeping in mind that none of this comes with a guarantee.

I look forward to the future when this book is complete and when you are reading this material and hopefully finding it beneficial in some way. Then I will return my focus to other things and pursue the options that make the most sense within my energy – and our financial – abilities. I can see, through my own writing, that I may benefit from some support to deal with the losses due to this hidden chronic illness. I look forward to exploring that. Neuroplasticity is something that I am looking into because the science in that area is advancing quickly: People are getting some benefits with different brain plasticity programs for pain, multiple chemical sensitivity, and other conditions.

In the future, it is my true hope to tell the stories of how people with neuro-immune illness – myself included – find effective treatment and the support needed to restore our health and our lives. It is a vision I hold daily.

Please take the time to read Section 2: The Global ME/CFS Community – Voices of Struggle and Strength. It contains poignant portrayals of many aspects of health and illness including compassion, commitment, courage, patience and faith. Every story is important and gives perspective to the overall picture.

Best,
Valerie

SECTION 2
The Global ME/CFS Community

Voices of Struggle and Strength

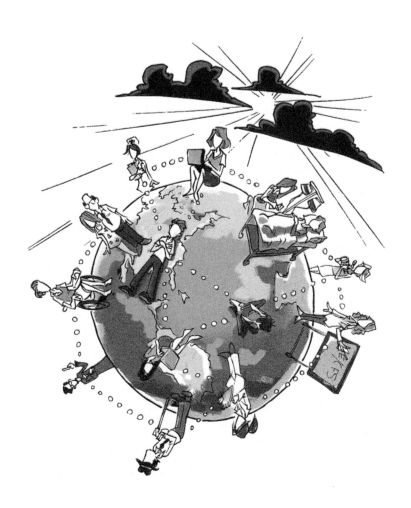

Some names have been changed to protect privacy

INTRODUCTION

Hannah and The Gift of Connection

Valerie Free | June 2011 | Alberta, Canada

One rainy afternoon, the pain levels in my body were just too high to tolerate, so I made an appointment at my local chiropractor to see if a treatment would help. As I sat in the waiting room, two young children were playing quietly.

The older of the two began to visit with me. Her English accent made her curly-haired perfection even more endearing. We chatted about all kinds of things, including her name, Hannah. Her little sister remained close by and semi-interested. Hannah told me how they had both been happy in the morning, but had had a little accident at the pool earlier that day, leaving the little one with a minor bump. This had made them sad, but they had both returned to being happy by that afternoon. How smart and observant I thought she had been to sort all that out and remember it.

The shy, smaller girl would pop over to say one or two words and then disappear around a corner with her dolly under one arm.

It was soon time for me to move on into the treatment room, but my new acquaintance decided she should come along – and she did. Her mom poked her nose into the room once in a while, since I was still waiting for the doc. I told her we were fine, just visiting. No problem.

Hannah and I sat sideways on the chiropractic adjustment table, her legs swinging back and forth as she spoke of everything she could think of.

All of a sudden, she became still, and her demeanor changed as if she had just had a brilliant idea. Her eyes looked up directly into mine, her voice got quiet, and she said, "Do you want to be friends?"

At that moment, I imagined a halo over her head and wings on her back. The pain in my body dissipated for a second, and pure joy filled my heart as I said, "Of course."

"Okay then. What is your house number?" she questioned me.

I thought she meant an actual neighborhood house number, but because I live on an acreage in the country, I said, "I live in the country. I don't have a house number. Sorry, honey."

Her common-sense reply was, "What country do you live in, then?"

I chuckled. "I mean in the countryside, where the horses live."

She thought for a moment, trying to figure this out, and then insisted, "But what is your house number?"

At that point, her mom was ready to go, and the doctor was coming in. Hannah hung on the doorframe in my appointment room, pleading again, "Your house number."

I finally realized she was probably asking for a house phone number, which, of course, I wouldn't have shared without first talking to her mom; and secondly, how would she remember it anyway? So that is how we left things.

But something very special happened that day.

Children are probably the closest thing to angels we have on this earth, and for days I felt very bad for not finding a way to stay connected with Hannah, since she had asked for the commitment of friendship so seriously.

Who was this little girl? I realized two weeks later, as I was working on this book, that her angelic presence reminded me of a photograph that I had taken in my dear neighbor's yard in Arizona. It was of a beautiful angel statue holding a dove and she was settled into a background of bougainvillea smothered in rich pink flowers. I have reminded myself of this statue's effect on me while writing. I even had it illustrated as a representation of divine presence who had a message to be sent and carried, with the hope it will be heard. I'd never thought of naming the angel statue that had become so inspirational to me, but now it became clear – her name would be Hannah.

How pure, innocent, open, and honest this little girl was. She did not see the pain in my body, the wince on my face, or the broken-hearted sadness I carry from dealing with a debilitating chronic illness – or maybe she did. But I am so thankful that she reminded me of who I am and how important connecting with one another can be.

Thanks, Hannah.

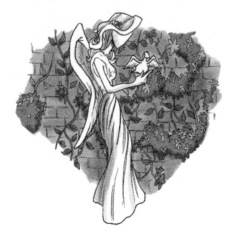

The Early Days: A Mystery Illness
Arrives in Lyndonville, New York

David S. Bell, MD, FAAP | July 2012 | New York, U.S.
Introduction by Valerie Free

Dr. Bell practiced both in his specialty of pediatrics and in general family medicine. He has published research papers and books on ME/CFS, and he has lectured widely. His book "Faces of CFS: Case Histories of Chronic Fatigue Syndrome" published in August 2000,[201] remains a classic. In each of the ten case histories of the book, he illustrates a different aspect of the illness. One of the cases, "A Child's CFS, Misdiagnosed as Munchausen's by Proxy," is shared in the CFS Kids chapter of this book.

In April 2011, Dr. Bell gave a lecture to the Massachusetts CFIDS/ME & FM Association where he spoke about both his thirteen-year follow-up study[202] and his twenty-five-year follow-up research. A report on his lecture can be found on the CFIDS/ME & FM website.[203]

Dr. Bell served on the Board of the American Association for Chronic Fatigue Syndrome/ ME (now the IACFS/ME) and chaired the Chronic Fatigue Syndrome Advisory Committee (CFSAC) in the early 2000s. Although he is now retired, he has maintained his interest and his intellectual curiosity regarding ME/CFS.

I am grateful for the request by Ms. Free to describe the early days of my experience as a doctor treating and studying chronic fatigue syndrome (CFS). It is a topic I have not thought about much since I retired.

People have assumed that what happened in Lyndonville, New York was an epidemic like the plague. Because of this misperception, people, particularly those who have the illness, are bewildered when they hear that the majority of medical providers still do not recognize CFS. It was not like a ravaging bubonic plague; instead it was subtler – subtle, but very real.

While I did not see my first case of what would later be called chronic fatigue syndrome until 1983, I opened my solo, rural general practice in 1977. Life could not have been

---

201 "Faces of CFS" can be viewed at web.archive.org/web/20140213014605/www.mecfs-vic.org.au/sites/www.mecfs-vic.org.au/files/Resource-BellFacesOfCFS.pdf (accessed July 15, 2016).

202 Bell DS, Jordan K and Robinson M, "Thirteen-year follow-up of children and adolescents with Chronic Fatigue Syndrome." Pediatrics Vol 197 No. 5, May 1, 2001. 994-998 (doi: 10.1542/peds.107.5.994). www.ncbi.nlm.nih.gov/pubmed/11331676 (accessed July 15, 2016).

203 "25-Year Follow-up in Chronic Fatigue Syndrome: Rising Incapacity." www.masscfids.org/resource-library/3/311 (accessed May 20, 2016).

better. I had quickly come to terms with leaving the sterile, academic world of Boston and had relaxed into the completely unfamiliar role as a rural family doctor in Lyndonville, New York.

⟡

Academic medicine teaches you that, in order to be a worthwhile person and physician, it is necessary to specialize and sub-specialize. So that is what I did: Harvard University, then medical school, then straight into pediatric training. Five years of pediatric residency, and I never saw or treated an adult except for the occasional neurotic neighbor in Boston.

I sub-specialized in pediatric behavior disorders and developmental disabilities and found that in order to be really specialized I needed to have family therapy training. This meant another year or two. It was then (when I was finished with all the exams, applications, and degrees) that I realized I had no idea what I wanted to do with my life.

And that wasn't the only problem. With all the training, the only role open to me was to go on and become a professor of behavioral pediatrics. There were openings in the inner cities of Boston, New York, Philadelphia, Chicago, and several other places. I hated the inner city, and it had never occurred to me that I would have to spend my life in one. My wife, Karen, was in the same position; she being in internal medicine sub-specialized in infectious diseases. So we took a year off to think things over.

One day, we drove by a huge, rundown farmhouse in the middle of upstate New York and bought it. The first year there, we did not tell anyone we were physicians, and I picked apples for a living. Our neighbors brought over fresh pies and raspberries. It was the best year of my life. After a while, the mailman noticed that the mail was addressed to two MDs, and he told the local Lions club, who told the local hospitals. The quiet days were over: It was time to get to work.

⟡

I decided to open a pediatric practice. There was one little shop in Lyndonville that was vacant, and the town offered to pay the rent. I started to fix up the office, as it was pretty run down.

It was a lovely, cool summer evening in July, and I was painting the walls. Although I didn't know it at the time, I was about to have my first patient (one who had nothing to do with CFS). I heard a strange sound and looked down from the stepladder and there, crawling into the building on hands and knees was a middle-aged lady, covered in bruises of a type never caused by physical injury. I knew she had a bleeding disorder – a disease called idiopathic thrombocytopenic purpura, or ITP. As I watched from the third step of the ladder, she slumped down to the floor.

My academic training immediately came into gear: "Call someone else." This is the first rule of academic medicine. I was a pediatrician, and this lady was probably in her late thirties – well out of my range. But there was no phone to call an ambulance, and there were no other physicians in town. I knew what she had – kids get the same thing – and the treatment was probably the same. So I drove her to the hospital.

My idea of a pediatric practice hadn't lasted long. I became the town General Practitioner (GP) and saw whoever walked into the office. At first, most of my adult patients were people with very advanced cancer who wished only for palliative treatment and to stop the chemotherapies. I realized I could help them in their final days, for I had been a resident on the children's cancer ward.

In a nearby town, there was an internal medicine specialist who helped me with the adult patients who had standard internal medicine illnesses, such as heart attacks, gout, and the like.

☙

My first contact with what would later be called chronic fatigue syndrome was in 1983. I had been following a neighbor named Mrs. Tomlinson, who had a large number of problems. She was housebound, and the first thing that struck me was that none of her previous medical providers knew why she was disabled.

I had collected all her old records and read through them; they sat in a pile that weighed more than fifty pounds. Later, this became the first diagnostic criteria I was to devise for this mysterious illness: *"When the patient's medical records weigh more than fifty pounds and you have no idea of the diagnosis, consider chronic fatigue syndrome."*

She had been diagnosed with anxiety, depression, bipolar disorder, chronic pain, migraine, arthritis, and numerous other ailments, but none of these explained why she was unable to leave her house. She was a shut-in, spending most of her day in bed, and the remainder of the day on the couch or doing light activity.

On one early visit, I asked her why she could not get out of the house. She said it was because she felt so sick; sick and exhausted. I already had lists of specific symptoms she would have at different times, but in all the records, no one had ever written down that the disability she suffered from was "feeling sick." This would turn out to be quite important.

So I went back to my training and did the academic thing: I sent her to specialists. The first specialist was a neurologist in Buffalo who said she had Huntington's disease, and she would die soon. He did not make a return appointment for her.

Neither Mrs. Tomlinson nor I liked this diagnosis much, so I sent her to another neurologist who said she had multiple sclerosis. But he made no return appointment either. He had no suggestions as to tests or treatments, although Buffalo was the center for MS treatment with the interferon trials going on at that time. That told me that he was not sure about the diagnosis.

The third neurologist made the diagnosis of anxiety and somatization.[204] In short, he felt that Mrs. Tomlinson was a fruitcake. But I had come to know the Tomlinson family, and I had years of training in behavior disorders. Whatever was causing her to feel sick was not something she was making up. She would try different tasks, and if she exerted too much, she would become worse. I did not think she was a fruitcake. Yes, she was depressed, but that was not causing her difficulties; it was the result of them.

Her worst symptom was "feeling sick," and after that came exhaustion, headache, joint pain, muscle pain, lymph node pain, and sleep problems. After these, there were about twenty more symptoms, and these symptoms would vary in severity and prominence. But while the intensity of the symptoms varied, the pattern did not. That meant that she could not have somatization disorder.

One of my biggest regrets is that while I tried to help Mrs. Tomlinson, her visits to me and to the specialists did not help. They merely added to her burdens.

∽

At this time, I began to see other patients who had the same thing that Mrs. Tomlinson had. They usually had no diagnosis for their ailments either. The severity of individual symptoms varied, but the pattern was the same. All had impaired ability to function in everyday life. Those with milder illness were limited by "fatigue," and those more disabled felt "very sick along with the fatigue." In my reading, I came across nothing like it.

In 1984 and 1985, there seemed to be a huge increase in the number of people with this illness. I began to see the early stages of it in healthy persons I had come to know. Initially, it looked like mononucleosis, and in a few, it was true mono, but they just didn't get better. The illness evolved from an acute infectious-appearing illness to a chronic smoldering of fatigue and pain and other complicated symptoms.

Around October of 1985, I referred one of the teens who developed the illness to a pediatric specialist who said, "This kid is just trying to get attention."

I was stunned.

I knew this teen well and had seen her over several years for minor ailments and school physicals. She was a good soccer player, was on the girls' varsity team, and never complained about her soccer injuries. Now the specialist who saw her for forty minutes diagnosed her with somatization disorder. As a specialist in behavior disorders myself, I knew this to be an absurd diagnosis.

This young lady was deeply injured by the specialist's treatment and diagnosis, and I do not think she has ever gotten over it. The doctor is supposed to be one who is trusted

---

204 "Somatization is a tendency to experience and communicate psychological distress in the form of somatic symptoms and to seek medical help for them. More commonly expressed, it is the generation of physical symptoms of a psychiatric condition such as anxiety." – Wikipedia.

to give help and use his or her knowledge to remove or reduce suffering. In CFS, to this day, the medical profession is the second leading cause of suffering, after the illness itself.

❧

And this is how our search for answers for this mysterious illness began.

Around this time we contacted the Centers for Disease Control (CDC), and talked with a Dr. Gary Holmes there. Although we did not know it at the time, he was advising Drs. Cheney and Peterson from Incline Village, Nevada, on a similar situation with their own cluster of the same illness. I regret that Dr. Holmes did not tell us this because I would have called the Incline Village physicians for their views. As it turned out, I did not get to talk with them about our shared experience until three or four years later.

The CDC eventually said they would send the New York State Health Department to investigate the cases. I was thrilled. By then, it was clear to me that this was an unknown illness to us, although cases had been described in Iceland and England as early as 1950.

On the day of the New York State Health Department investigation, I closed the office and laid out about fifty charts of those persons – adults and children – who had the illness. The officer came, and I left him in the room for about ten minutes while I prepared coffee and made myself available for questions. He left the office, and I thought that he was going to get something from his car or get a sandwich for lunch. He never came back.

About two months later, I received a letter saying that the cases were due to "mass hysteria." Among the really dumb things I have heard physicians say, this one takes the cake.

After talking with the CDC a few more times, they offered a suggestion. One of the very prominent symptoms of this illness in children was tenderness in the lymph nodes. The CDC suggested that if we did lymph node biopsies on the children and did not find the answer, they would come and investigate.

So we lined up eight young patients with CFS and tender lymph nodes and took out an axillary (armpit) lymph node. We sent pieces of these lymph nodes for every test imaginable, and all the samples came back with the diagnosis "reactive hyperplasia." One node was positive for a spirochete suggestive of Lyme disease, but only one. Reactive hyperplasia is the term used when a lymph node is swollen from a viral infection, but in my patients, no virus was found.

When the CDC heard these results, they concluded that no illness was present.

They never did return to investigate. I relate this with some bitterness because now, twenty-five years later, the CDC still does not know what is going on, and my patients have felt betrayed by the years of apparent inaction and dismissal.

❧

I learned several important things from these early days and from my patient Mrs. Tomlinson. The first was that the specialists knew absolutely nothing about what was causing her illness, yet none of them would admit that. They invented diagnoses that were so obviously false they were ludicrous.

Secondly, I learned that whatever disease she had, it was not diagnosable yet – return appointments were never made. Physicians did not want to be confronted with their own ignorance.

I may have had an advantage here. I was completely ignorant of internal medicine. Six years in pediatric training, and not one day with adults. So I had no problem admitting that I had no idea of what her diagnosis was.

A third thing I learned is that patients with this illness suffer tremendously. There is a difference between suffering and pain. Many people have pain from cancer and other illnesses, but because of the compassion of family and medical providers, treatment is offered, and the suffering is reduced.

With CFS, there is no compassion from the medical industry; even family and friends sometimes come to doubt the reality of the illness. I have been told that doctors will tell family members to treat the patient with CFS as if there were nothing wrong because it helps recovery. For Mrs. Tomlinson, the suffering was done alone and in silence.

A fourth thing I came to learn was that CFS was a really interesting disease. I had to read books about arthritis, headache, and fatigue. It became a real challenge, and I took it on. Much of primary care is pretty boring stuff, and while I enjoyed seeing my patients with sore throats, they were not that difficult to treat.

∾

By 1987, 214 people, adults and children, were ill with the "Lyndonville mono" – as we were calling it then – all within a fifty-mile radius of my clinic.

After that, patients showed up from all over the country seeking diagnosis and care. There were very few places for patients to go in the country that would acknowledge CFS and attempt to treat them.

In 1988, we published the criteria we were using for diagnosing these cases.[205] These criteria were similar to what was published as the first CDC criteria.[206]

The illness was given the name "chronic fatigue syndrome" by the CDC. This was unfortunate because it implied that patients with this illness were just tired. People who are tired can still do stuff. Mrs. Tomlinson was not tired. Her malaise and exhaustion were in an altogether different category.

We did not know the cause. We did not know if it was contagious (and if it was, how it spread), so I began to take more interest in research and education for CFS. For one

---

205 Bell D, Bell K. "Chronic fatigue syndrome: diagnostic criteria," (Letter). Ann Intern Med. 1988; 109: 167.

206 Holmes G, Kaplan J, Gantz N, et al. "Chronic fatigue syndrome: a working case definition." Ann Intern Med. 1988; 108: 387-9.

thing, I began exploring post-infectious arthropathies,[207] such as the one caused by the bacteria *campylobacter*, as the possible mechanism of the illness.[208]

This "mysterious illness" turned out to be the start of something big in the medical world and has led me to a very interesting life indeed.

---

207 Diseases of the joints.

208 Dr. Bell said, "Drs. Cheney and Peterson (the Incline Village physicians) were pursuing other routes including persistent infection with Epstein-Barr virus in their own patients with the illness. This is the virus that causes the majority of cases of mononucleosis. I knew that EBV was not the cause because in kids, only half of them have antibodies to EBV, and with the kids who had CFS in my practice, half had no antibodies to EBV. The symptoms were identical in those with and those without these antibodies."

CHAPTER 1

Experiences of Adults with ME/CFS

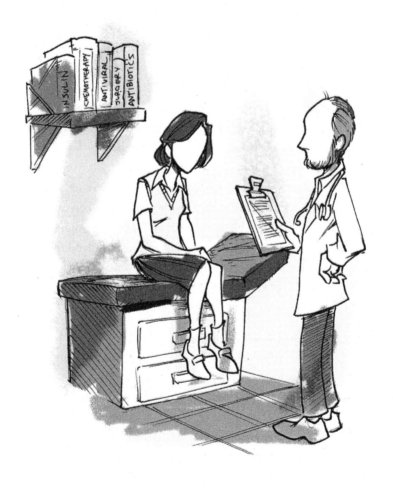

Corinne: A Fortunate ME/CFS Patient?

Corinne[209] | July 18, 2013 | Arizona, U.S.

The window to my left frames a spectacular view typical of the American Southwest. The scenery begs to be explored, but instead, due to chronic illness, I'm relegated to my usual spot: my overstuffed recliner, with my feet elevated to combat persistent light-headedness.

For six months, I have been experiencing new symptoms: electric shock sensations down my legs, numbness, and hypersensitivity in my extremities, jabbing pain and pressure in my mid and lower back, and worsening of dizziness. A recent abnormal MRI of my neck area highlighted a spinal cord lesion, and so new investigations are under way.

Though I have been ill with ME/CFS for almost twenty-three years, this recent battle inspires me to look through one of my many photo albums that record my very active, pre-chronic illness life. I grab the one dated 1986-87. I haven't opened it for a long time but, like all the others, it chronicles the many memorable travels with my husband in our RV, as we hiked, biked, and explored. I tentatively turn the pages, expecting to feel a hint of sadness. Instead I'm smiling, in awe of the incredible beauty I was so blessed to have been able to visit and capture on film.

I feel extremely fortunate – that is, until I find myself looking at the photos of my husband. Happiness radiates from his image. In the snapshot where we appear together, I am reflected in his proud and admiring eyes – a fit and tanned woman and the epitome of health at age thirty-three. I sigh. His radiance and inspiring reflection of me are things I have not witnessed in years. It isn't long before my smile transforms to tears.

As a fitness professional and personal trainer, my days were filled with plenty of activity. However, at age 37, in 1990, just over three years after these photos were taken, I came down with a "flu" that has yet to depart. Though they called it "sudden onset" – one day well, the next extremely ill – I often wonder, was it really? I remember having some minor health issues when I was younger, including Bell's Palsy in 1979, which exhibits as facial nerve paralysis. It was unusual because the paralysis occurred on both sides of my face, but I did not feel ill with it, and it healed within one month. In the late fall of 1982, I got a flu; tender lymph nodes in my neck, non-restorative sleep, muscle weakness, worsening after exercise, low-grade fevers, and brain fog. Though I recovered within six weeks, I continued to experience unexplained low-grade fevers that came and went.

---

209 For more on Corinne's journey and treatment, go to Health Rising. www.healthrising.org/blog/author/corinne (accessed July 25, 2016).

The flu I got during the fall of 1990 followed a recovery from an intestinal infection called giardia. It was similar in symptoms to the one in 1982, only much more disabling; I struggled just to complete the simplest of tasks. I relapsed back to bed with each attempt. There were days when I felt so weak that I had to talk myself into mustering up the energy to crawl to the bathroom to empty a bladder that had reached its limit over an hour ago. It was a chronic and unrelenting version of the illness I experienced eight years earlier.

In the ME/CFS world, suffering for years before being diagnosed is quite common. Because my doctor happened to be a member of my fitness class, witnessing first-hand my decline – and she also happened to have a colleague with the illness – I got diagnosed within one month. Subsequent searches for second opinions denied there was anything physically wrong with me, including one from a well-respected, world-renowned clinic.

Diagnosis or not, validation or not, fortunate or not, according to the medical community, there was no treatment and nothing anyone could do to help. So I stayed home to deal with the consequential suffering without medical support.

୬୨

My husband was not unlike many partners in this situation. We'd been married seven years, and he was ill equipped to handle the loss of a young, vibrant, and independent wife to such sudden disabling circumstances. Grieving his loss, and overwhelmed by the weight of additional responsibilities and my growing dependence on him, he became increasingly distant emotionally.

We also had moved from California to Arizona in 1989, so my family was not close by. Both of my parents passed away within two years of my illness onset. So I managed the forced reinvention of my life virtually alone. In doing so, I undoubtedly made mistakes. I did not have a clue how to cope with so many unfamiliar symptoms as well as confusing emotions such as anger, fear and grief.

Fast-forward sixteen years to 2006: At fifty-three years of age, I was a far cry from the physical specimen captured in the photos I mentioned earlier. My health had slowly declined, and I had become officially homebound, with many days spent bedbound. The reflection I saw in the mirror was one I myself no longer recognized – pale and frail, with the appearance of "wasting away." What I saw in my husband's eyes was no longer pride and admiration but, painfully for me, the worn-out, detached look of someone who has had to deal with chronic illness in a spouse for far too long.

Most activities had become mentally and physically overwhelming with a worsening of symptoms with each attempt. My headaches worsened and were, at times, unbearable; so much so that my brain felt too tender for me to move – afraid that even gently doing so might result in the sensation that it was slamming against the inside of my skull. It literally hurt to think.

Personal hygiene was an effort – showers were few and far between. Social interaction was very limited. Even using the computer or speaking too long on the phone triggered dizziness and a relapse of symptoms. As a result, being this ill was very lonely. Because of the chronic nature of this illness, most people around me had given up on asking me how I felt, but if they did, I would answer, "poisoned."

There was no other way to put it – I felt sick and poisoned. There were nights I was so weak, I wondered where the energy for my next heartbeat was going to come from. I began to think that this illness, without a doubt, was killing me.

❧

Thankfully, hope entered in the form of a physician, an ME/CFS expert who practiced a state away – 800 miles to be exact. His name was well known to me because he had dedicated his life to treating patients like me for twenty-two years. I had never considered traveling so far. How would I manage with the traveling? How expensive would it be? Being this ill, how difficult would it be to perform the required diagnostic tests? But I had become too desperate to lie here and do nothing. So I went on his waiting list and three years later, in June of 2009, I had my first appointment with Dr. D. Peterson in Incline Village, Nevada.

I have visited this dedicated doctor ten separate times since 2009. Each visit involves a one-week stay, during which I see him three days of the week and perform multiple tests, which keep me busy from 8:00 a.m. until the staff clocks out at five. Testing examples include, but are not limited to, exercise stress tests, extensive blood work, MRIs, as well as scans and spinal taps. Each time I return home, having pushed beyond my limits, I need anywhere from two to four weeks to recuperate. I am always left wondering if the difficult effort to complete this medical obstacle course will sabotage any positive results.

❧

It took the first two years of traveling and testing to fully develop my treatment protocol. This was partly due to the complication of finding a physician in my community who was willing and able to implement the treatment locally. Despite how difficult it was, the resulting payoff was a gradual thirty percent improvement in functioning, which commenced in mid-2010. I was able to do things that I wasn't able to do in years: going out to a restaurant for lunch one week; shopping for a pair of jeans the next; and walking daily to the end of a short driveway to get the mail. Though I still had to remain seated to shower, it became more regular. Sure, my activity continued to be severely limited. I still could not do much without triggering flu-like symptoms. I still had to take daily naps in addition to getting twelve hours of sleep each night. But at least I could sit and watch a movie without feeling so sick and so poisoned. What a healthy person might consider a measly thirty percent improvement was, to me, a jump-for-joy accomplishment.

One of the highlights was the ability to travel to visit family in California. Because it was the first time in seven years that I had been able to reunite with them, it was quite a joyous occasion. My improvement was especially timely because my husband was no longer able to stomach the rollercoaster ride of the illness. He finally expressed his disconnection from me with heartbreaking and gut-wrenching words. Though he remained at home (and traveled with me to California), his need for "more space" made it critical for me to be able to function better and do more for myself.

My treatment protocol was extremely expensive financially, physically, and time-wise, but I felt it was worth the gains I had made. I felt very fortunate! It soon became clear that to describe myself as a fortunate ME/CFS patient would prove to be an oxymoron. I'd forgotten that ME/CFS is highly unpredictable.

Just two weeks after my short trip to California, the new level of well-being that I had for a year and a half came to an abrupt halt. In February 2012, I awoke one morning, surprised to see my extremely pale reflection in the bathroom mirror. The next day, I was in a full-blown relapse from which I have not yet fully recovered: bedbound, aching, weak, and once again too sick and poisoned to function. I was devastated.

It is 2013, and I am now fifty-nine years old. I was hoping to spend the last year of my fifties having a little fun, perhaps celebrating my sixtieth birthday by going out for an evening meal, since I have had a bedtime of 5:00 p.m. for so many years.

But instead, the next months are booked with appointments, which include CT scans, PET scans, neurology exams, another spinal tap, and another MRI, in an attempt to determine a cause for the cervical spinal cord lesion I have developed. Now, as these new and additional serious symptoms have emerged, I will, yet again, be spending my days ruling out malignancy, multiple sclerosis, and other autoimmune diseases. As I write, I am awaiting the results of tests which will confirm whether or not I have neuromyelitis optica, a disease that often results in blindness and paraplegia.

I am forced to dip into my retirement funds. My medical bills far exceed my monthly Social Security Disability check, even with the health insurance I have had in place.

My husband and I have been married for thirty years and still live under the same roof. Though I am grateful for his assistance with some of the more physical demands of everyday life, as well as for driving me to some local medical appointments, he remains separated from my illness experience. He justified this by referring to the story of the boy who cried "wolf" one too many times when he stated, "After a while, you just don't pay attention anymore." This leaves me feeling vulnerable and afraid, making continuous difficult medical decisions on my own.

This wolf that is ME/CFS, is real, alive, and well – and it preys on my health daily. My husband's rationalization makes it evident that it is not only the patients who are affected. Their loved ones, family, and friends are neither well supported nor educated enough to deal with the consequences of this illness. This increases the suffering for everyone.

❦

So am I a fortunate ME/CFS patient?

It is a difficult question to answer. I don't believe anyone is fortunate to get ME/CFS. I am, however, one of the privileged few who has been validated and treated by a physician/expert in the field. My illness road has been a difficult one with suffering mixed with hope and blessings.

I often question whether there is purpose to such suffering. When patients with ME/CFS approach treatments of any kind, it is experimental and not without risk, even with the experts to guide us. I opted for the protocol I now follow because there was a chance for improvement in my health, as well as an opportunity to help with data collecting and research. My expert, and the neurologist that he has referred me to, are very competent in their respective fields. They are desperately hoping these tests will reveal something that they understand and can treat more specifically.

As my improvement has faltered and complications have occurred, I now feel more like a sacrificial lamb for ME/CFS research on the one hand and a guinea pig for the general medical community on the other. All of this because not enough is known about ME or CFS, even after all these years. As a person of faith, I know that if my journey contributes to increased understanding and resolution of ME/CFS, in that respect, I will indeed be fortunate.

❦

One day, in frustration, feeling overwhelmed by my latest health crisis, I sat down and wrote a letter. I will share it here because it best sums up the way I feel about my ME/CFS journey of over two decades:

To Whom It May Concern (Whom might that be?)

I consider myself a grateful person, but I am also angry and understandably so. It should never have come this far. More tests, more stress, more money, more consultations, more second-guessing – years of the same old thing as my illness progresses and manifests itself with a new set of attention-getting symptoms demanding a different diagnosis. If this follows the same path as the episodes of the past twenty-two years, there will be no official explanation, no effective treatment, no relief, and no acknowledgement of the severity of this illness as it continues, over the years, to progress.

None of this would have happened if the Centers for Disease Control and Prevention (CDC) had recognized this disease as serious and life-altering (often times life threatening) thirty years ago, when they issued me, and so many others, the "kiss of death" by naming it (my illness) chronic fatigue syndrome. With that title came disrespect and abandonment, not only from the medical community, which includes researchers and drug companies, but from many friends, family and the rest of society in general – all who pre-judge or misunderstand me because of a name that suggests merely a frivolous sort of tiredness.

I have a neuro-immune illness – what the rest of the world might call Myalgic Encephalomyelitis. I sincerely wish everyone would recognize its severity and treat me accordingly. I send out a heartfelt "thank you" to the too few doctors, nurses, family, and friends who have done just that. For this I remain so grateful. I also pray that each of you may be blessed with the gifts of incred-ible wisdom, knowledge, insight, and compassion when dealing with those of us suffering from this devastating disease so that we, who struggle day-to-day to survive, may one day actually thrive again.

ೲ

Update | March 2015 | Corinne

After continued testing and visits to numerous doctors who were all searching for a rec-ognized illness to attribute the lesion to, we still do not have a diagnosis that explains it – other than ME/CFS. Without a definitive diagnosis, I do not have a treatment option for the post-exertional flares that worsen my neurological symptoms and pain. Dr. Peterson did put me on a six-month protocol involving a potent antiviral drug, hoping it would help. It has improved my overall functioning, but the lesion remains unchanged. We are currently working on managing pain, because it increases with the flares.

Mark's Invisible Prison: From Military Service to ME/CFS

Mark | August 1, 2013 | Illinois, U.S.

My ME/CFS journey began in 1991, when I was nineteen years old. It was the summer before sophomore year of college. Before that, I was a healthy young man who could do whatever he wanted. I was hard working and was involved in extracurricular activities and sports. I was the valedictorian of my high school and worked manual labor jobs during the summers.

My dream since I was in the eighth grade was to become a naval aviator. And when I saw the Blue Angels at an air show, I was hooked. So I joined the Naval Reserve Officers Training Corps (NROTC) at my university at the beginning of my freshman year, and I did well in the program.

We spent parts of our summers at sea training with the navy. I received my dream assignment – an aircraft carrier that was deployed overseas. Then, while I was there, I talked them into letting me work on the flight deck. I worked with the "Crash and Salvage" crew. We stood just feet away from where aircrafts were launching and landing at over 150 miles per hour. It was our job to put out fires and to save the aircrew in the event of an accident. The noise levels and heat were incredible, and it is considered to be one of the most dangerous jobs in the world. I was in heaven.

At some point during my time aboard ship, I got a bad case of diarrhea. I may never know how it all started. I figured it was traveler's sickness that I picked up from food on one of our port visits. It was strange that none of the guys I went ashore with got it, but they all drank more alcohol than I did – maybe that killed it for them. I did have a cut on my foot at the time as well, and we did have to wade through some pretty nasty water at one point to get to the boats that took us to the ship – so maybe it was that. I just took some over-the-counter medicine that one of my buddies had and kept working.

Eventually, it came time for me to head home, and I had three weeks with my family before I had to head back to school. The diarrhea kept getting worse, and my mom insisted that I go see a doctor. They immediately hospitalized me, put me on IVs, and took away all oral food and liquid intake. It continued to get worse. At one point, I had thirty bowel movements in a day that were filled with blood and some sort of discharge. Without the IVs, I certainly would have died. I wish I had been sent to a research hospital at the onset, but I was probably so sick that they did not want to move me.

It is so long ago now that I cannot remember all of the infections they looked for, but none of the test results showed anything. The doctor finally prescribed a drug called

Flagyl, which seemed to help. Even though there were no test results for him to go on, he told my mother, "We have to try something."

⚬

With my health situation more under control, I insisted that I be allowed to go back to school. Classes were starting soon, and I was in a very rigorous degree program at the time. I didn't want to get behind. With some reluctance, the doctor discharged me the day before classes started, and I traveled back to school.

Other than the fact that I met my future wife on the first day back, returning to class was a bad idea. Although the diarrhea had slowed, I still had bouts of intestinal troubles and serious problems with fatigue. I was barely hanging on in school and was failing some of my classes. A doctor at the hospital near the university continued to run numerous tests with no luck.

One morning, a month and a half into the term, I woke up and my skin was jaundiced. I called the nurse at my new doctor's office, and she said I should get in there right away. I said I had a class I needed to attend first – she told me, "If you don't get in here, you may never go to class again." That finally got my attention. They ran more tests, and the doctor said I needed to drop out of school for the semester and focus on recovering. The next day, my parents picked me up and took me home.

I woke up at about 2:00 that morning, shaking so badly, my whole bed was vibrating in sync. I was running a high fever, and the doctors told my parents to take me back to the hospital. I was admitted, put on IVs, and tested extensively – again.

I started vomiting frequently, including blood, even though I was not eating. The nausea was so severe despite receiving medications for it that I wanted to be knocked unconscious. My throat was so sore it literally felt like it was on fire. My glands became so swollen that I almost couldn't speak – I could only make guttural sounds at times. The nurses were telling my family not to leave the area – they didn't know what was wrong with me and didn't know how much time I had left.

⚬

Eventually, the tests showed that I had a severe case of Epstein-Barr virus, which causes mono and hepatitis. They never did find the original organism that started it all. I was eventually discharged from the hospital and spent the rest of that semester at home recovering. My parents and my brother helped me with daily activities as I slowly regained some strength.

The fatigue stayed. The doctor said that after an illness like this, it was normal to get more easily exhausted; but I should be able to live a normal life.

I changed to a less demanding program of study and managed to finish my degree. I was also able to earn my commission as an officer in the navy and was selected to be a student naval aviator – one of its most elite positions. Other than my wedding day, this was probably the proudest day of my life.

But my health problems were far from over. In addition to the lack of energy, I gained weight more easily and was having a much more difficult time staying fit. I would occasionally get flu-like spells with sore throats, nausea, headache, and difficulty concentrating. They were infrequent enough that I thought I was just getting touches of the flu. A doctor told me that I should be okay, so I just kept pushing and trying to work harder. My emotional and physical drive, as well as energy, were never what they were before I first became ill.

Eventually, the demands of active service and training were just too much. I ended up receiving a medical discharge from the navy in 1996, after over one year of active duty. Although it was an honorable discharge and not my fault, the amount of shame and self-blame I experienced was devastating. I felt like I had failed my shipmates, the navy, my country, my family, my fiancée, and myself.

⁓

I managed to get civilian jobs in the Information Technology (IT) field in the years that followed. I switched back and forth from full to part-time work as my health allowed. Luckily, I was able to find some understanding and kind supervisors who were willing to work with me. It was a struggle. The flu-like spells became more and more frequent. I would see various doctors, hoping to get help. One of them diagnosed hypothyroidism, and the medication seemed to help a bit. But then I got worse. Another one mentioned a "chronic fatigue-like syndrome" at one point, but he was a gastroenterologist, and it wasn't his area of specialty. I took some vitamins and supplements that seemed to help for a little while. But then, I got worse. Again. This extreme illness caused me to become anxious and depressed, so I received medication for that as well.

In 2002, at age thirty, my health was undermined so much that I couldn't work at all. In the months and years since, I've essentially been housebound. We finally found a doctor who was a recognized expert in CFS, and he officially diagnosed it.

This was eleven years after the first bout of illness on the ship. Years later, I ended up receiving full disability benefits from the Veterans Administration and Social Security.

⁓

We started to get some abnormal test results that explained some of my symptoms and allowed some level of treatment. We have found that I have low or non-existent levels of LH and FSH, the pituitary hormones that tell your body to make testosterone and sperm. This meant that I had to be on testosterone replacement shots. This also meant I was essentially sterile.

My second CFS specialist had the idea of testing me for IGF-1, which came back very low. This is a test that helps measure, indirectly, the level of growth hormone in your body. I then failed growth hormone stimulation testing by the endocrinologist, which indicated that my pituitary gland didn't make growth hormone. I was diagnosed with Adult onset Growth Hormone Deficiency (AGHD).

The endocrinologist I still see is from a leading university hospital. He thinks I've been dealing with this problem since I first became sick, and the most likely explanation is that the severe infections damaged my pituitary gland. The growth hormone I have been taking has helped me improve in several areas: cholesterol levels, thyroid levels, liver function levels, and body fat around the waist.

I was given a tilt-table test, which checks for abnormalities of blood pressure regulation based on posture and other factors. Medical research has linked CFS to abnormal results on this test. When I was administered the test and given the drug, my blood pressure dropped so low that they couldn't even measure it. They said I should have become unconscious, but the doctor performing the test said I must have just adjusted to the problem enough to prevent passing out.

My CFS specialist also noticed orthostatic intolerance symptoms when my blood pressure would drop when standing. I've used atenolol (a type of blood pressure drug called a "beta blocker") to help with this, as well as with tachycardia. Unfortunately, beta-blockers also have fatigue as a side effect, so I've had to deal with increased fatigue from that.

Strangely, I also have high blood pressure, so it seems that my body just can't regulate that.

I've had abnormal ANA and C-reactive protein tests – these are tests for autoimmune activity and general inflammation in the body. The drug Plaquenil (given for lupus and other autoimmune diseases) seems to help and keep those test results more in line. I don't get the "feverish" symptom quite as often. A bunch of abnormalities did show up on an extensive neurological exam. I've also had several chronic reoccurring viral and bacterial infections, including reactivated Epstein-Barr virus and chlamydia pneumonia.

Despite receiving the hormone injections and other helpful medications, I really struggle with what is called "post-exertional malaise." Unfortunately, anything more than a minimal amount of exertion makes things much worse. That is why I am still considered to have CFS by my doctor, despite all the abnormalities and helpful treatments.

On average, I am at about ten percent of the activity level I was at pre-illness.

Any kinds of activities with real exertion are out. I used to love to play basketball, but I haven't done that in fifteen years. I can do some things that a normal person can do, just at a greatly reduced level. For example, I can sometimes visit friends for quite a while, but I can also quickly develop what we've come to call "sensory overload," which is when the interaction with people brings on one of my flu-like spells. In recent years, I have driven for an hour or two a day (on a good day) without bringing on symptoms. In my worst years, the most I could drive without losing focus was about fifteen minutes.

I help out with the laundry, but I break it up in very small chunks over the course of a week or more. I can only prepare meals that require short preparation because I find it very difficult to stand for lengthy periods most days. On bad days, I'm essentially housebound, and sometimes bedridden. On those days, if I try to do much of anything for more than five minutes, everything starts getting worse. Sometimes, I can't even take the sensory input or muster up the concentration required to watch simple TV programs – I just have to lie in a quiet, darkened room. If there is any kind of big event planned, I often have to rest for several days to make sure I can be there and several days to recover from it.

❧

Throughout this whole process, I've had to come up with a new definition for what "being a man" is. I am incapable of doing the traditional things by which society defines manhood. I'm incapable of working and supporting a family. I'm incapable of having a family without help due to the sterility caused by the hormone issues. I'm even too physically weak to take care of a child for any length of time. I've tried watching the kids of our friends, and even if I'm having a good day, the exertion causes the flu-like symptoms to kick in after a short time. There's no way I could do it day after day. My wife works, so this has prevented us from even thinking about adopting children.

Over time, I've learned that what makes a real man is treating others with kindness and compassion. I've also learned that a real man doesn't judge or quantify someone else's pain and suffering, because despite how the person looks externally, you have no idea what it is like to be in their shoes – the terror of not knowing what is going on in your body that makes you feel so horrible; the terror of others not understanding, and how you are going to deal with that in all its forms.

Anyone who has experienced this illness, either in person or as a caregiver, knows how serious this is. Sadly, research for it is woefully underfunded.

❧

What has carried me through these years is the love and support of family and close friends, especially my wife. As I mentioned, we met early on in my illness, and her love and support has never wavered. I wouldn't be alive today without her. She has always been the one bright spot that I could look to no matter how dark the days got. Our lifestyle is so limited because of my health, and yet she never complains or bats an eye. She just accepts it as something we have to work with.

I am one of the lucky ones in that regard – I've heard of, and talked to, many people with this illness who don't have a supportive partner. I can't imagine the despair and sometimes outright terror they must go through living with this.

Even with the fulfilling relationship I have with my wife, my life is a shadow of what it should be. It often feels like living in an invisible prison: It's like I have a temperamental and unstable prison guard watching over me all the time, allowing different levels and types of activity based on his mood that day. If I try to get away with too much, he beats me down so severely that I can't get out of my "cell" for days.

I'm in my early forties, and there is so much I want to do. I want to go back to school and have another career of some kind. I want to play basketball again. I don't want to constantly plan how to expend what little energy I have. My dreams used to be so big.

Now I just dream of being able to work a regular workday, play a little basketball in the evening, and be able to get up the next day without it affecting me.

Hard Decisions: To Be A Parent With CFS

Jessica Turner | August 2014 | Utah, U.S.

Two p.m., I'm in bed – I'm there most days. My baby girl, Gracie, is standing on the other side of my bedroom door, and she's calling for me, lovingly at first. "Mommy. Mommy! MOMMY!"

The nanny eventually comes and picks her up. I hear the desperation in Gracie's voice. "No! NO! MOMMY, MOMMY, MOMMY!" As the shouts diminish, so does my sense of self-worth. I take a look at my life.

I'm thirty years old, my husband and I have two kids, and we're living in my parents' basement. We don't have enough money for a place of our own, and I'm in bed. We pay for a nanny to watch our kids all day every day, and I'm in bed. My baby girl wants her mommy to hold her and love her, AND I'M IN BED!

How did I get here? Why do I stay here? Why can't I move?

I remember being sixteen years old in high school. I was part of the track team, and I laughed, ran, and traveled all over the state. And then I got a headache.

It wasn't a normal headache: It never fully went away and ultimately spread through the rest of my body like sap oozing from a damaged tree. Then it affected my ability to think, focus, and act. I was referred to a specialist who then referred me to a neuro-surgeon. Test after test, the conclusions were the same: I was a healthy young lady, and everything was fine and dandy.

So why did I feel so wrong?

It took four years, a handful of doctors, and a jaw specialist to finally figure it out. My jaw was fine, the ENT (eye, nose and throat) doctor said. "But what you're saying sounds a lot like chronic fatigue syndrome," he added.

Fatigue? I didn't feel tired. I felt in pain. Still, my mom and I had exhausted all other explanations, so we followed the CFS path and did all sorts of tests. As it turned out, there was something in CFS that resonated with my symptoms. I started to drag, and the pain started to hinder my ability to function. I started to sleep longer each day. Every time I exercised, my body would shut down for a day or two before I felt well enough to exercise again. I started to understand the real meaning of "chronic fatigue."

The fatigue affected my physical and mental well-being. I cut down on work. And then, I met a boy.

I waited until our fourth date to tell him about my CFS diagnosis. As we spent more time together, he understood the extent of my inabilities. But he proposed, and we married in the spring of 2006.

With little money in our pockets, my in-laws let us live in their basement during our newlywed phase. My husband worked full-time in a neighboring city, and I found a part-time job delivering Meals on Wheels to the elderly folks in our little town. I did not keep that job for long – a mental, physical, and spiritual pain was eating away at me.

∞

The days wore on. Each day, the pain grew and it became a twenty-four-hour experience. "Why can't I break free of this? What am I supposed to do with my life? How am I supposed to have a life under these conditions?"

My husband and I both wanted a family. But I wondered, "How am I going to function if I'm carrying a baby inside me for nine months? How about giving birth? Will I recover from that exertion? And how will we manage after the baby is born?" We were scared and worried, but our wonderful CFS doctor comforted and prepared us to take this giant leap of faith. She said, "You cannot put your life on hold for this illness. You might get better, but you might not. The key to finding happiness despite this illness is to choose the one thing you want most in this life and find a way to make it happen – even if it means making major accommodations."

I became pregnant shortly thereafter, and during my pregnancy, we consulted with various therapists, including doctors, homeopaths, and gluten-free advocates. We didn't know which remedies would help the most, so we tried the ones that we could afford and that seemed sensible.

To help offset these medical costs, my husband applied for a new job in Salt Lake City, and we moved to my parents' three-bedroom home. My days were very lonely. My parents didn't come home from work until after 8:00 p.m. The effects of the pregnancy made me feel like my soul was breaking. By the time my due date arrived, I was spent. My body was crumbling, and my mind was a blur. I didn't know if I would have the energy to deliver a baby. I thought a C-section would make the process easier. But my doctor told me the recovery process would take much longer. She advised against it.

Eight days later, I was admitted to the hospital. My baby boy took twenty-seven hours to come out into the world. I expected him to scream and be frantic. But he was quiet, calm, and patient. I thought, *This precious child has a golden heart. And with all the trials we'll have to endure as a family, he's going to need it.* We named him Benjamin Golden.

The first few hours after the birth were a whirlwind. We told the medical staff I wanted to breastfeed our baby, so we had lactation specialists hounding us at all hours of the night. They constantly talked about the health benefits of breastfeeding and how breast milk enhances brain development in infants. They told us it was a bad idea to let an infant drink from a bottle because then the baby wouldn't want to put forth the effort to nurse.

We got home two days later, and I tried to breastfeed Benjamin during the night. I was too exhausted to teach him how to latch on properly. We broke down and purchased a breast pump, and in spite of what the lactation specialists had advised, my husband volunteered to feed our son with a bottle when I was asleep.

All the pain and desperation I felt leading up to the delivery was nothing compared to the week following the delivery. On the fourth day, my husband came into our bedroom and collapsed on the bed. Neither one of us had the power to move as we listened to Ben screaming in his crib.

As we cried together and held each other, my husband and I hit the lowest point possible. We were shattered. Our lives had spiraled out of control, and we admitted defeat. "We can't do this," we sobbed.

∽

Enter my sister-in-law, a nurse in the making, who was working the night shift at the university hospital four times each week as part of her program. She asked if she could take care of Ben when she wasn't working at the hospital. This simple question – this simple act of love – was the turning point. It gave us time to recoup and to rest. It gave us time to heal and to mend. We had friends, family, and neighbors who cared about us and helped us as much as they could. But we didn't have an organized support system until four years later when my husband and I decided to have a second child.

My husband saved up time off work, and when our little girl Gracie was born in 2012, he was able to spend the first month at home taking care of her. While my husband cared for the baby, family members cared for Ben and for me. We had a schedule set up, and we all knew the schedule was flexible. It wasn't set in stone, and we were all okay with that.

The second pregnancy wasn't a walk in the park either. It was a tremendous undertaking, and we were confronted by new challenges that we didn't anticipate. It was a huge lifestyle change. But we had a support system, which made it manageable. Having our children was, and is, wonderful.

∽

But right now, it's 2:00 p.m., and I'm still in bed. I can't move. My body hurts when I move, and my body hurts when I don't move. My baby girl is standing on the other side of my bedroom door. She's knocking softly, and she's calling for me. The nanny picks her up, and Gracie's voice grows softer. My doubts and worries slowly vanish. I have parents and a husband and children who love and think the world of me; I have neighbors who are watching out for us.

We're going to make it. I'm going to make it. Everything is going to be okay – some day, somehow.

Tina's Perspective: Acceptance, Purpose, and Joy

Tina Tidmore | November 2013 | Alabama, U.S.
Introduction by Valerie Free

Tina got married in 1984, six months after her high school graduation. Over a decade later, she gradually became ill with ME/CFS and went from a well person to someone very ill, visiting many medical specialists to find an accurate diagnosis and treatment.

After giving up the small-market newspaper that she had started, she became a freelance writer. When she can, she manages websites, writes letters and speeches for clients, and writes feature articles for a magazine. She won first-place awards for her work in the 2012 and 2014 Alabama Media Professionals Communications Contest. She has testified at CFSAC meetings on behalf of PANDORA Org, a patient advocacy organization. Tina also provides communication services for research organizations.

As a very active person with church, volunteer work, and a job that kept me connected to the public, I occasionally met someone who had that drained look. They seemed to struggle to just walk and talk. They complained of fatigue, pain, and other problems that no doctor could figure out. I used to say, "That would be the worst thing that could happen to me."

I loved to hike and canoe, and zipping here to there made me feel alive. So I thought that losing that ability would be the worst thing that could happen to me. I was wrong.

THE GRADUAL ONSET

Aside from a blood pressure and fainting problem that I developed as a child and that hardly bothered me in adulthood, my overall health had been very good until my thirties. In early 2004, at the age of thirty-six, I was running a small-market newspaper in my local city. I was the owner, editor, and publisher. Looking back on the previous year, I realized I had lost a total of about five months of work due to illness or brief periods of depression. I never was one to go to the doctor, especially for colds or flus, but I seemed to have caught a lot of them that year. I figured my immune system was overtaxed by the stress and responsibilities of my job. So I decided to discontinue my volunteer work.

Both the viral infection symptoms and brief bouts of depression lessened after I cut back my responsibilities. However, in 2004, I developed extreme fatigue, extreme headaches, and hot flashes that coincided with my menstrual cycle. I tested negative for menopause, and I didn't think the previous recurring infections could be connected, so I didn't say anything to the gynecologist about them. He changed my birth control pills, but the symptoms continued, and I started arranging my work according to the times that I could function.

Over the following three years, the severe menstrual symptoms gradually went from one day a month to two days a month, to three, etc. I also felt so tired that I would spend my weekends folding clothes instead of walking my 100-pound dog. I occasionally wondered if I was developing one of those mystery illnesses that I had seen in others, but I also thought that maybe this is what age thirty-nine feels like.

As 2006 started, the fatigue on weekends stopped me from going to church. I would also get sudden extreme fatigue at about 4:00 p.m. on many days. It was as though someone pulled a plug out of the bottom of my feet, and all my energy flowed out all at once.

My hot flashes eventually became a daily experience (even though my gynecologist tried two other hormone treatments), and I started to make mistakes in my news reporting: inverting figures, leaving out important words, and throwing away important papers. I was unable to keep a phone number in my head long enough to dial it and was not remembering phone calls I had received the day before. But I had no way of knowing whether these symptoms were within the normal range of someone my age: Everyone gets tired, forgets things, and makes mistakes. And my doctor told me many women in their mid-thirties experience headaches and hot flashes due to hormonal changes.

By the summer of 2006, I was forty and not making any appointments before 1:00 p.m. because I couldn't get out of bed before 11:00 a.m. I felt just as exhausted when I woke up as I did the night before. Transitioning from asleep to awake took hours. I was often in a mental fog, as though I had a hangover every morning.

THE PLUMMET

Then, on July 16 of 2006 around midnight, I was on my recliner, typing away, trying to get the newspaper off to the printer by the deadline. My menstrual cycle was also about to start. But that night, a new and severe pain started. It was sharp and moved around to different parts of my body. This is what I refer to as the day my health plummeted.

That's when I knew for sure that I was sick and not just overworked or just feeling the effects of age.

Since I didn't have a primary doctor, I made an appointment to see my gynecologist. The night before my appointment, I stumbled upon a description of chronic fatigue syndrome on a website, which seemed to fit what I was experiencing. When I read that there was no cure and that all my activity would have to be greatly reduced, I cried.

The worst thing that I thought could happen to me had happened. I would likely never hike or canoe again. It was my first big loss from the disease.

When I saw the gynecologist, he took one look at me and said: "This is more than hormones; I think you have chronic fatigue syndrome or fibromyalgia, but I don't treat it. You need to see a rheumatologist."

I was told by the rheumatologist's receptionist that it would be three months before he could see me. Later, I discovered many rheumatologists don't treat CFS. After researching online, I found that CFS is diagnosed by eliminating other conditions that can cause the symptoms. So I decided to see a local internist. I figured he could run the tests to exclude other diseases. However, before the tests were even ordered, he diagnosed me with depression—a "different kind of depression." I asked him if he believed chronic fatigue syndrome and fibromyalgia were organic diseases, meaning they are caused by a defect in a body organ. He said, "No."

Knowing that he would not treat an illness he didn't believe in, I told him I would take his anti-depressants if he would run tests for rheumatoid arthritis, lupus, and multiple sclerosis. In my view, seeing if the antidepressants made me better or not was part of the process for eliminating other conditions. He agreed to do the tests.

A week later, he told me a test he did showed I had hypothyroidism, so I stopped taking the anti-depressants. This new diagnosis was a surprise: I was thin, and in his exam, he did not feel anything abnormal in my thyroid. I started treatment and made arrangements to see an endocrinologist. By the time I got in to see the endocrinologist, I had waited three months for the appointment and was experiencing about four hours of normal energy each day because of the thyroid treatments.

The endocrinologist increased my dosage of thyroid medicine to hopefully give me more energy. Unfortunately, the fatigue became more debilitating, and the pain became much worse. When I told him how bad I felt, the endocrinologist said: "Well, from the tests, it looks like I overmedicated you. I'll put you back on the lower dosage, and if that gave you only four hours of energy, then you likely have something more like chronic fatigue syndrome or fibromyalgia, and I don't treat those. You need to see a rheumatologist."

"That's another three months to wait," I told him, as I cried in his office.

The doctors seemed to be just fine with the system that was passing me on to the next guy with three more months of waiting every time. Yet, this was the time of my greatest suffering with this illness. I needed to know what I had and whether it was treatable. I needed to know whether to close my business. By this time, I had been severely debilitated for seven months with no firm answers. I was frustrated and miserable. I never imagined modern medicine could fail at something I thought was easy and done by doctors every day – make a diagnosis and send me to a specialist.

I eventually saw the rheumatologist. She determined I did not have fibromyalgia, said she did not treat CFS, and suggested I see a neurologist.

That was when I realized that no standard medical specialty is responsible for diagnosing or treating chronic fatigue syndrome, despite the large number of people who have it. Even my health insurance company didn't know who to send me to. At this point, I had seen a gynecologist, an internist, an endocrinologist, and a rheumatologist. All of them either misdiagnosed me or suggested I might have chronic fatigue syndrome, but didn't treat it. So I didn't expect the neurologist would either.

I called support groups in my state, looking for a local doctor who treated chronic fatigue syndrome because fatigue was my main symptom. Unfortunately, there were none. All the group leaders said they go out of state for treatments, except one who sees a retired neurologist who does not see other patients.

THE DIAGNOSIS AND TREATMENT

I ultimately found an integrative clinic that focused on both chronic fatigue syndrome and fibromyalgia in Atlanta, Georgia, where my parents lived. The clinic was expensive, and I had to file to get reimbursement from my insurance company after I paid up front for their services. But I liked their holistic approach of lifestyle, diet, Western medicine, supplements, and alternative therapies. If I was going to have to go outside my insurance network, at least these people claimed to know the disease that I likely had.

So I got an appointment at the clinic and traveled to Atlanta by a shuttle van service, lying down in the back seat during the whole three-hour trip.

At the integrative clinic, the doctor ran extensive blood tests. He also confirmed, through a different type of touch/pressure test than the other doctor had done, that I had fibromyalgia. Most importantly, he officially diagnosed me with chronic fatigue syndrome.

He gave me prescriptions, showed me lots of supplements I could buy, gave me a restrictive diet, told me to start getting massages, and advised me to get a sleep study. I was to also see a gastroenterologist to make sure I didn't have intestinal cancer. Ironically, when I was sick with cognitive and physical limitations, this doctor was giving me more to keep up with and a lot more to do.

The tests at the clinic in the spring of 2007, nine months after my plummet, revealed many biological abnormalities, including low-functioning natural killer cells (a first-line defense of the immune system); reactivated parvovirus; high fibrins (a blood clotting factor); low cortisol (a hormone produced by the adrenal gland); and the highest homocysteine[210] the doctor had seen in many months.

Around this time, I read a book about CFS that said treatments have a better chance of working early in the illness. So I gave treatments my main focus. I rationalized that I could either spend lots of money and reduce my workload for a short time now, or lose my abilities for many decades.

I hired more help for the business. My husband helped with cooking, cleaning, and grocery shopping; and my mother helped with filing the insurance claims. I saved up energy for two days at home, working from my bed and laptop at only an hour at a time so that I could have one day with four hours of energy for doing things outside the house.

---

210 Homocysteine is an amino acid. Elevated levels of homocysteine are associated with greater risks of blood clots, stroke, and heart disease.

I was using all my mental and physical energy to keep the business going and to follow the treatment plan.

Thankfully, neither my husband nor any of my friends and family ever doubted that I was really sick with something. They saw the drastic change in me. My husband never complained because he had to do more, and he warned me when he thought I was doing too much.

After speaking with other patients, I realized how fortunate I was, and still am, that my family and friends believed me and made an effort to understand my disease. Their attitudes and assistance relieved me of an unnecessary stress so that I could adapt to the illness limitations and focus on healing.

In 2007, I discovered a study by Harvard Medical School's Dr. Anthony Komaroff that showed a large percentage of people with chronic fatigue syndrome also have low or suddenly dropping blood pressure, especially upon standing. It was then that I knew for sure that I had the right diagnosis.

I had a problem since I was seven of fainting occasionally (once every couple of years) from suddenly dropping blood pressure. I told all my doctors about it and insisted that all blood draws be taken while I am reclining to prevent a fainting episode.

If my gynecologist or any of the other doctors I saw knew of the study connecting the blood pressure problem to chronic fatigue syndrome, I would have been diagnosed much earlier. I was particularly angry with the internist who said I had "a different kind of depression" but didn't know of the connection between the blood pressure problem I told him about and chronic fatigue syndrome, basically dismissing both conditions because of ignorance.

THE IMPROVEMENT

I stopped going to the integrative clinic in Atlanta: The financial strain and the demands on my time and energy caused me to look for other options. The monthly expensive trips to Atlanta turned into phone visits with the doctor and my going to a local hospital for lab work. After improving over a couple of years, I felt I had plateaued and that I could get supplements with the same ingredients cheaper elsewhere.

I found an integrative doctor in my city who knew a lot about hormones, metabolism, and alternative treatments. Although she did not specialize in my disease, she was willing to learn. I already knew what supplements I needed, and started seeing her in 2009.

Between 2007 and 2009, I saw enough improvements in my health that I believed I could take a job working thirty hours a week, as long as I could rest lying down for forty-five minutes in the middle of each day. Many ask me whether the Atlanta clinic's treatments were responsible for my improvement. The improvement could have been just a natural stage of the disease – a sudden plummet and then some improvement. I just don't know. I attribute much of the progress to pacing, which I did simultaneously with the treatments from the Atlanta clinic. Pacing is the practice of alternating rest periods in a dark and quiet room with short periods of mental or physical activity throughout the day.

In 2009, I closed the newspaper, thinking I had another job offer that would be less demanding. When I didn't get that job, I started doing freelance writing work. I was told I was not eligible for Social Security disability benefits because I had not been paying into it, so I had to continue to work.

THE RELAPSE

In the beginning of 2010, I took on a challenging project with more work and stress. As a result, I started to go into a relapse. In the latter part of 2010, I caught the flu twice, which caused my CFS symptoms to get even worse. I had to stay home for two days in order to get out of the house the next day. Earlier, I had hoped to eventually recover, but I then came to realize this chronic illness would likely be with me for the rest of my life.

By the spring of 2011, I weighed only eighty-eight pounds (I am 5'4"). During this time, I'd wake up at 10:00 a.m., prepare breakfast and take it downstairs to eat it while lying on my recliner. After eating breakfast, I would start computer work. By lunchtime, I was too fatigued to go upstairs to prepare lunch, so I just kept typing or stayed curled up on the recliner. The fatigue was stronger than the hunger. After finding out how much weight I had lost, and with the help of a scale my husband bought for me, I put forth a concerted effort to eat more food, more often. I gained my weight back over time.

THE STABILIZATION

Since then, my energy levels have increased to about sixty percent of what a healthy person can do, and the pain is now almost completely gone. The pain comes back when I have extra physical demand, of course, but I try to pace my activities and avoid stress. Aside from the low dose of naltrexone and the birth control pill that I take to even out my sex hormones, and the thyroid hormone I take, I have no idea if all the other medicine or supplements help. I can only do what makes sense and what I can afford.

Due to the lack of knowledge among the medical professionals and very little research on treatments, ME/CFS patients become their own physicians, researchers, and guinea pigs; and they have to pay for all the experimentation themselves while their ability to earn money is greatly diminished.

I still have some days when I am not able to do anything but watch TV, curled into a fetal position on my recliner. However, in 2012, I had a small garden and even did some leaf raking for short periods of time. Any exertion means the next day must be a day of rest. The nausea, headaches, hot flashes, and chills come only when I've pushed past my limit or my hormone levels are off. Light sensitivity and sound sensitivity are still with me, but much less. The vertigo and bruises seem to be completely gone. I cannot stand in one place for longer than ten minutes or sit upright for more than two hours without getting extreme fatigue or dizziness, likely due to the blood pressure drop. And every day is ruled by some level of fatigue – mild or severe.

THE APPRECIATIVE ATTITUDE

I thought having a disease that took away my energy and my fun and exciting life would be the worst thing that could happen to me.

However, I learned by this experience that I was wrong. I could have ended up with some disease that took away everything, like someone I grew up with, who recently had a stroke at age forty-five and is now permanently bedridden; or I could have ended up with a severe case of chronic fatigue syndrome, which leaves people completely homebound or bedridden. Every human alive has to deal with some limitations: financial, family, health or other.

So while I wait for news of better treatments or a cure, I focus on what I can do instead of what I can't do. I accepted my limitations early in the journey and have adjusted my life accordingly. I have the support of my family and am not financially destitute. If I am having a "bad day," I stay in bed. On "good days," I am still able to do some writing on my laptop in my bed, which gives my life purpose. I am able to leave the house and go to meetings or run errands once or twice a week. I sit in my small garden, pull the weeds, and check the progress on my vegetables almost every day. I spend a lot of time in my lounger on my back deck, watching the birds at my feeder. I find comfort in my "rest buddy," my cat, who keeps me company no matter what I am doing or not doing. I have not been able to bring myself to sell my canoe. It is a tangible representation of the hope that one day I will get that life back. I may not have the life I planned, but – on most days – I still have an enjoyable and fulfilling life.

CHAPTER 2

CFS Kids – Unique Challenges and Considerations

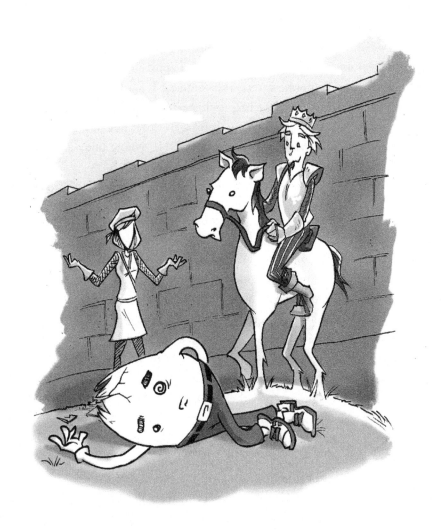

Sidelined: Growing Up with
Chronic Fatigue Syndrome [211]

Peter Madden | March 2012 | U.S.

Matthew Lopez-Majano wakes up feeling warm and safe. And why not? The nineteen-year-old's bed rests in a comfortable room on the second floor of a house in Chester Springs, Pennsylvania, a wealthy bedroom community an hour west of Philadelphia. His twenty-year-old brother and closest friend, Alexander, is still in bed down the hall. Their mother, Denise, probably has breakfast waiting on the kitchen table. In those brief moments of dreamy semi-consciousness, Matthew is happy.

It takes a few minutes before he detects the coldness. It starts in his fingers and toes, then spreads to his hands and feet, traveling up his extremities and throughout his body. He wraps his blankets tighter and wills himself back to sleep, but he cannot regain that feeling. The warmth is gone; Matthew is tired, weak. His young body always seems to grow old within the first few minutes of the morning.

Matthew has chronic fatigue syndrome.

In 2005, he developed pneumonia as an energetic twelve-year-old swimmer in Kansas. Six months later, the pneumonia was gone, but many symptoms remained: headaches, muscle pains, weakness. Suddenly, he was hypersensitive to light, sound, and smell. Physical and mental exertion, even expending the energy for a quick jog or the concentration required to study, left him exhausted and disoriented. He developed a kind of vertigo that prevented him from sitting or standing up straight for any length of time. Matthew disappeared from school and from swimming.

Soon after Matthew's diagnosis, his father accepted a new job and moved the family from Kansas to Pennsylvania. Since the move, Matthew has scarcely left the house, except for medical treatment. His arms and legs have grown thin, his skin pale. He completely missed high school.

"Swimming miles on end became laboring up the stairs," Matthew said. "Doing six-figure multiplication became trying to maintain a coherent train of thought. I just existed on a day-to-day basis without any larger vision for myself."

---

211 This piece was excerpted and adapted from Peter Madden's journalism thesis, which you can find in full at Columbia University Library: library.columbia.edu/locations/journalism/masters/2012MP.html (accessed May 28, 2016).

On the surface, Matthew lives a teenager's dream – no alarm clock, no school, no need to fill out college applications. But he said, "The average teenager's life is my dream."

Matthew's typical day: He wakes up around 11:00 a.m. and lies in bed until noon, when his mother helps him down the stairs for a meal. She lays out his meds. He takes twenty-one pills per day, each of them differing in size, color, and function. Turmeric is an anti-inflammatory. MigreLief holds off migraines. Spirulina combats mental fog. Cymbalta is an antidepressant. Propranolol is a beta-blocker that slows his heart rate. Matthew also pops a plethora of vitamin supplements that span the alphabet.

Mom makes the beds, does the laundry, drives to doctors' appointments, and remains on standby for emergencies. "It's not intensive care," she said, "but there has to be someone around. You don't know when something might happen." Her life is complicated by the fact that her husband is now working in Ohio and only visits the family in Pennsylvania every other week.

Denise performs many roles – nurse, cook, chauffeur – but that of liaison to the outside world might be the most important. Once the family realized that life with chronic fatigue syndrome was their new normal, as Matthew's older brother was diagnosed with a less debilitating case of chronic fatigue syndrome about a year after Matthew,[212] Denise began home schooling her sons, adapting her lessons to their limitations.

Their schooldays with Denise were brief, no more than an hour with a full day off in between, but with enough repetition, she found the material sinking in. "I would try something and back off, try it another way and back off, and try again," she said. "You just have to go at their pace."

Although she dispensed with formal home schooling when Matthew reached adulthood, Denise still collects articles on politics and current events and stacks them neatly in a pile on the kitchen counter for her sons to read when they can, an evolving encyclopedia of the world they barely know. "I hope it gives him a connection," she said of Matthew. "I hope it's to prepare him for the day he gets back out there again."

Denise is encouraging Matthew to pursue his GED, and they have applied for special accommodations from the Pennsylvania Department of Education. Denise estimates that the test, a seven-hour, bubble-filling marathon, would take Matthew about two weeks, accounting for time to crash and recover. They are awaiting the board's decision.

Denise estimates the cost per year to her family, with two sons afflicted, to be approximately $4,000.[213] It's impossible, however, to put a dollar amount on the time lost in growth and experience, she said. "No matter how flexible and accommodating I can be, at a certain point, I just wish they were out there making their way in the real world."

---

212 Fifteen months after Matthew became ill, in 2007, Alexander's gradual fall into moderate-severe CFS began. He was 14 years old. This required him to leave his schooling and activities as well. Mr. Madden focused on Matthew's story to be able to give the most detailed chronology of one young person with the illness.

213 This is over and above health care coverage, and Denise says it is an underestimate.

Through photography, book clubs, and the support of family and friends who "comprehend" her sons' condition, Denise copes, though she remains on high alert to "over-explain" the illness to disbelievers. "There is such a stigma attached to it," she said, "and they [Alexander and Matthew] don't have the energy to defend what they're enduring. The knowledge helps me help as much as I can."

❦

After breakfast, Matthew retires to the computer room, where he and Alexander play computer games and surf the Internet, side by side, for the remainder of the day. The conversation between them is sparse; there isn't much to talk about. No school. No homework. No social obligations. Matthew might watch some television, or perhaps try to read, but for the most part, the images and plots are foreign to him.

"People talk about friends and about dating and about jobs and about emotions, but it's hard to respond to stimuli I haven't had," he says. "It feels so far away from me that I automatically dismiss it. It's not personally relevant, though I know it should be. Even reading about issues in those articles – starvation, disaster, war," he adds. "I feel like I'm contributing to a failure to act by living a life that's not really helping anyone. I sit at a $1,000 computer and play my games while all these terrible things are going on."

Matthew says that asking him what he would do if he woke up one morning completely cured is "like asking what I would do if I had a million dollars." It's a seductive daydream, a guilty pleasure, something to be enjoyed on occasion but never fully embraced as a legitimate possibility. Nevertheless, he said, "I would run as fast as I could in whatever direction I was facing, and then run back twice as fast, and then I would sit down and start thinking as hard as I could about all the things I wanted to do. I would want to see how much I was different."

In a standing letter dated April 18, 2011, explaining Matthew's condition, Peter Rowe, Professor of Pediatrics at Johns Hopkins University and Director of the Chronic Fatigue Clinic, wrote that Matthew suffers from a "moderately severe category" of chronic fatigue syndrome that leaves him with "very little ability to perform normal activities outside the house without days to weeks of post-exertional increases in symptoms" and estimates a general wellness score of 35 to 40 out of a possible 100.

Rowe noted that Matthew is prone to post-exertional malaise, or a "crash," commonly described as a "muscle wilting meltdown," after periods of activity, and his symptoms, of which there are many, are generally unrelieved by Matthew's diligence in attending physical therapy twice a week and taking a host of daily medications. The orthostatic intolerance, or sudden vertigo, is perhaps the most vexing.

"We do not have a clear understanding of the etiology…but both he and his brother are affected, suggesting a genetic component and perhaps a shared infection," said Rowe.

Absent a major new discovery or treatment option, and given low rates (less than five percent) of spontaneous improvement among patients whose symptoms have persisted for three or more years, Rowe anticipated "that he [Matthew] will remain…unable to attend college or work at least for the foreseeable future.

"One of the great frustrations for me is that here's a guy who embraces the challenges and wants to do everything he can, but he's hit a wall," Rowe said in an interview. "Matthew is appropriately frustrated because of his desire to get on with things despite the limitations that have been imposed upon him."

∞

One recent evening was interrupted by an unfamiliar sound in the Lopez-Majano household – the ringing of the doorbell. Denise greeted her guests as they filed in, directing the younger crowd to the kitchen, where they found workstations equipped with gingerbread houses and all the colorful tools of candy carpentry. Most teenagers don't spend their Saturday nights doing arts and crafts with their parents. But with so few opportunities for pediatric patients to be social, Denise hosts regional gatherings of families with children affected by chronic fatigue syndrome.

Matthew and Alexander were the eldest in the room but had the least social experience. Children with chronic fatigue syndrome who are unable to attend school miss out on important developmental opportunities and milestones.

The group was equal parts children and parents, social gathering and support group. Guests came from Connecticut, New York, Delaware, and Pennsylvania. The snow deterred many more. With their sons and daughters pasting solid sugar to miniature mansions, parents compared notes and found their anxieties and complaints echoed in one another.

"These people get it," said Ken Jackson, a chemical engineer from Delaware, whose two sons, Jamie, seventeen, and Craig, fourteen, both have chronic fatigue syndrome. "We don't have to explain anything to each other."

Older patients arrived to help out as well: Joseph Landson, forty-three, traveled from Virginia, where he lives with his mother in Fairfax County. He was an information technology specialist for a government defense contractor until 2006, when he left to pursue a master's degree at James Madison University. Landson was diagnosed with chronic fatigue syndrome about halfway through the program and, though he is still enrolled, he has yet to receive his degree. Only his thesis (a history of chronic fatigue syndrome) stands between him and the cap and gown, but he must work within the limitations imposed by his illness.

"I slow down, but the world keeps going," Landson said of his three-year-old project. "As bad as the physical symptoms are, I think the mental symptoms are worse. The more I talk, the more I walk, the more I do, the more likely I am to crash."

Landson and the other adults brought each other up to speed on the latest research and shared tips on coaxing school administrations to shatter the traditional definition of special accommodations.

"You can't deal with this teacher by teacher," said Susan Jackson. "You have to get the administration on board."

But the knowledge of a childhood lost strikes a nerve for the parents.

"Watching them miss out is the hardest thing," said Jackson. "Parents are supposed to make things go away. You feel helpless. You can only help them manage."

While the parents talked, the kids played. They laughed. There was little mention of the illness that brought them together, except to poke fun at it. Matthew was slow to join the circle, but eventually he did, if only at the periphery.

In jest, Jamie Jackson, Ken and Susan's son, performed the strange greeting that he receives from his high school classmates whenever he returns to school following a long absence due to ME/CFS: "JAMIE! WE THOUGHT YOU WERE DEAD!"

They went at their own pace. If someone got tired, he or she just stopped talking and lay down – no questions asked. The shared understanding borne from an extraordinary illness allowed them, if only for one night, to be normal.

About the Author of *"Sidelined: Growing Up with Chronic Fatigue Syndrome,"* Peter Madden

Peter Madden | CFSAC Testimony [214] | March 2012 | New York, U.S.

"I am a twenty-five-year-old journalist from New York City and recent graduate of the Columbia Journalism School. Every student there must produce a master's thesis to graduate; 4,000 words on any subject worthy of such lengthy treatment. I chose to write about ME/ CFS." P. Madden – CFSAC public comment, March 2012.

My father was diagnosed with chronic fatigue syndrome when I was young. He left work on disability and later retired. I remember him, so angry with those who thought him a liar, so desperate for relief from a revolving door of doctors and specialists and so-called healers, so addled by the pain he perceived and the painkillers he was prescribed that I barely recognized him by the time he left our family.

My master's thesis began as an investigation of my father's illness. I started with very basic questions. What is it? How do you get it? Can it be cured? I suppose I should be disappointed that I'm still searching for answers to these questions (along with ME/ CFS patients, advocates, and researchers, unfortunately), but that quest brought me to Laura Hillenbrand, who supports the CFIDS Association, and who introduced me to the Lopez-Majano family.

During my investigation, I read about this woman [Laura Hillenbrand] who overcame crippling fatigue to publish two epic histories of courageous victory that parallel her own; I spoke to advocates and researchers[215] who overcame the stigma of an invisible illness to support a patient community desperate for vindication; I met the Lopez-Majano family... who overcame the loss of the happy trappings of a normal life just to love one another.

In a way, what I found, in the face of so much doubt and disappointment and anguish, was a story of triumph, one that repeats itself every time Hillenbrand pens a sentence or researchers make a breakthrough or Denise helps Matthew down the stairs. With all the new questions I've discovered about his illness, I know perhaps less about my father than when I started. But I found the Lopez-Majano story; one of a struggle shared by millions of Americans – and thousands of children – that needs to be shared. I should have been looking for them all along.

---

214 This comment was excerpted from P. Madden's CFSAC public presentation (given by telephone) in 2012. Find it in full at www.hhs.gov/advcomcfs/meetings/presentations/madden_061312.pdf (accessed May 27, 2016).

215 Including Dr. Peter Rowe, Drs. Alan and Kathleen Light, and Staci Stevens.

A Child's CFS, Misdiagnosed as
Munchausen's by Proxy

David S. Bell, MD, FAAP | U.S.
Introduction by Valerie Free

This CFS patient case history is excerpted and adapted from "Faces of CFS: Case Histories of Chronic Fatigue Syndrome" by Dr. David S. Bell, August 2000.[216]

Karl Friedrich Hieronymus Baron von Munchausen was a German "soldier, adventurer, and a teller of tales," according to one description, who lived from 1720 to 1797. His fantastic lies about his daring and his conquests were so notorious that their memory survives to this day as German lore.

Medical science has borrowed from this ancient character's name to categorize the patient who engages in equivalently tall tales, all having to do with physical illness. When a parent or caretaker makes up bizarre tales concerning the health of their child, doctors call it *Munchausen's syndrome by proxy.*[217]

Sometimes the parent intentionally harms their child, by poisoning for example, to create the symptoms. Experts suggest the parent is motivated by a need for attention, which they eventually get one way or another.

Women are more vulnerable than men to being suspected of Munchausen's syndrome. This is because women typically take the dominant role in helping children through the maze of doctors' visits, hospitalizations, and treatments when children fall chronically ill. Every year, parents in this country and abroad face court hearings before judges and juries in which they are subsequently found guilty or innocent of intentionally harming their child due to Munchausen's syndrome by proxy.

---

216 This CFS patient case history is excerpted and adapted from "Faces of CFS: Case Histories of Chronic Fatigue Syndrome" by Dr. David S. Bell. MZR Publishing. August 2000. It can be found at web.archive.org/web/20140213014605/www.mecfs-vic.org.au/sites/www.mecfs-vic.org.au/files/Resource-BellFacesOfCFS.pdf (accessed May 27, 2016). Arnie's full story can also be found at www.prohealth.com/library/showarticle.cfm?libid=16108&dupeVote=yes (accessed June 23, 2016).

217 The diagnosis of Munchausen's by proxy (or as it is more currently known "Factitious Disorder imposed on another") is all too common for parents of children with ME/CFS – often because of a failure to diagnose or recognize the illness. "Factitious Disorder imposed on another" is the current terminology in the DSM-5 and can be found under the category Somatic Symptoms and Related Disorders. The diagnosis was formerly known by other names – including Munchausen's syndrome by proxy (MSBP), Factitious Disorder by proxy (FDP) or Pediatric Condition Falsification (PCF). At the October 29, 2009 CFSAC meeting, Dr. Bell gave a slide presentation "Factitious Disorder and CFS in Adolescents." www.hhs.gov/advcomcfs/meetings/presentations/091029.html (accessed May 27, 2016).

The notion of a mother deliberately hurting her child is difficult for most of us to comprehend. Nevertheless Munchausen's syndrome by proxy has been accepted by the medical profession as bona fide, if somewhat baffling. And there is no question that it occurs. Hidden videotapes in hospital rooms show parents either injuring their children, or doing things that make it appear that a child is ill.

Because this does occur, physicians have grown suspicious, particularly when confused by symptoms in the patient they treat.

So imagine what might happen when a mother becomes the advocate of her child suffering from an extremely complex, misunderstood – even overlooked – chronic disease.

Imagine the situation from the perspective of the sick child, who can barely articulate to his friends, much less to an attorney or a psychiatrist, what ails him. Imagine how, over time, these quiet struggles can escalate, thrusting mother and child into a firestorm of accusations by authorities of all stripes, as they attempt to salvage their dignity and even their right to remain a family.

A chronic disease robs children of many things, but it should never destroy the life-affirming refuge children find in their home, as it did with a boy named Arnie.

Arnie was ten when he experienced the onset of CFS, but for much of his brief life he had suffered a seemingly endless succession of colds, allergies, sore throats, stomach aches, and headaches.

The doctors that his parents took him to somehow failed to notice a pattern of minor infections that, in retrospect, strongly suggested Arnie may have had a medical problem for some time before the symptoms suddenly escalated. Instead, it was attributed to an over-anxious parent worried about trivial illnesses.

In July 1990, Arnie's heightened level of exhaustion, hitting him hard after an intestinal flu, heralded the onset of full-blown CFS. By the time school began that September, Arnie was too weak to stand and was confined to bed. His mother took him to see a pediatrician numerous times, but the doctor was unable to explain Arnie's profound fatigue.

By law, school systems are required to provide home tutoring to students who are too sick to come to school, but they also require that the child carry a diagnosis before they hire a private tutor using state dollars. Arnie had no diagnosis. The school year ended, and another began. Arnie failed to receive either a diagnosis or an education.

Arnie was still housebound because of the exhaustion.

He suffered from sore throats, headaches, sensitivity to light and blurred vision, pain in his muscles, joints, and lymph nodes. His ability to learn was diminished because of difficulties with memory and attention. He could not remember what he had read. His attempts to physically exert himself uniformly resulted in relapse or worsening of his fatigue.

Aside from ruling out thyroid disease, lupus, multiple sclerosis, rheumatoid arthritis, HIV disease, and hepatitis, doctors found immune abnormalities that suggested that Arnie was suffering from an ongoing viral infection.

But they believed that the abnormalities failed to fit a pattern associated with any particular disease – at least, any disease with which they happened to be familiar. Neurological tests revealed that Arnie suffered from vertigo and lacked the kind of fine motor control in his hands that might be expected of a boy his age. Other tests of intellectual capability demonstrated that Arnie's short-term memory and concentration skills were impaired.

All in all, everything about Arnie – his long history of illness, his physical exam, his laboratory tests – was typical of CFS, a disease his doctor did not believe existed. It was just eight months after Arnie had become severely ill that his parents began arguing about whether or not he was really sick. Arnie's father sided with the child's pediatrician and other specialists who had suggested that there was nothing medically wrong with the boy. Arnie's father was particularly tired of paying for medical exams that failed to provide definitive answers. He believed his son needed psychiatric care.

Arnie's mother felt differently. She did not believe the doctors. Instead, she began to explore unconventional treatments for her son, embracing, for a time, the "fringe" medicine offered by "ecologists," naturopaths and acupuncturists, each of whom seemed confident that they understood Arnie's problems, yet each of whom had a different explanation for them.

Whatever the explanation, Arnie's father thought of these alternative healers as shams. Large conflicts and petty complaints that had smoldered for years between the two parents erupted in a war centered on their son. Naturally, the boy tried hard to feel better in order to bring an end to the war. When his illness continued, in spite of his best efforts, he became withdrawn. And when Arnie's father moved out of the house, Arnie assumed he had caused the breakup.

Arnie's parents were unable to separate their private conflicts from their son's illness, leaving him caught in the crossfire. What followed was probably inevitable: a kind of chain reaction in which a sick child became a battleground, fought over not only by his parents, but by the local school system, and, eventually, the state of New York.

As far as Arnie's pediatrician and his teachers were concerned, the issues were clear: Arnie was suffering a kind of psychiatric meltdown because of his parents' acrimony.

The principal of his school made several visits to the boy's house during the first year he was absent, acutely aware that neither his parents nor his doctors had been able to offer the school a diagnosis. Each time she visited, Arnie was in the living room, seated, and watching television. He did not look sick to her.

The principal assigned a truant officer to the case.

The officer saw Arnie in his backyard one spring day, resting in a lawn chair, sipping lemonade. Finally, the school filed a truancy petition with the local court in order to force

Arnie to return to classes. In addition, the local social services department launched an investigation of Arnie's parents to determine if they were guilty of child abuse.

At the court hearing on the matter of truancy, the judge listened to the attorney representing the school argue that Arnie had been absent without good cause. Arnie's mother, representing herself, told the judge about her son's medical condition. She called it *chronic fatigue syndrome*. In turn, the judge inquired about the impending divorce, as well as the custody hearing.

Not surprisingly, the judge, who knew of CFS only as the rather flaky sounding "yuppie flu," concluded the hearing by ordering a psychiatric evaluation of Arnie. He also ordered Arnie to return to school.

After only three days at school, Arnie found himself confined to his bed, once again.

Despite the mother's attempt to explain chronic fatigue syndrome and the alternative treatments she'd explore to help her son, the court-mandated psychiatrist seemed to remain unimpressed and skeptical and eventually called Arnie's father, who said the sick one was his wife, not his boy.

A week later, the psychiatrist submitted his report to the court. His diagnosis: Munchausen's syndrome by proxy.

In his report, he pointed to evidence that Arnie wasn't medically ill, that he was at the center of a custody battle between divorcing parents. More critically, the psychiatrist noted there existed an unusual degree of "enmeshment" between mother and son.

The judge ordered that Arnie be removed from his mother's custody and placed in a foster home. He ruled that the final determination of Arnie's fate would be decided in the custody hearing. He also demanded, for a second time, that Arnie return to school and receive twice-weekly psychiatric counseling. In a small concession to the boy's claim of illness, the judge ruled that Arnie could be excused from gym class.

One week later, Arnie was admitted to a psychiatric hospital after he swallowed a handful of aspirin and several sleeping pills he found in his foster mother's medicine chest. Though it had never been Arnie's specific intent, his suicide attempt had confirmed beyond all doubt the diagnosis of the court's psychiatrist, school officials, and the judge who had presided over his truancy hearing: He suffered from a serious psychiatric illness.

During his incarceration, Arnie was unable to see his mom and was given a large daily dose of tricyclic antidepressant medications, which made him feel much worse. Hospital staff demanded that he participate in all the ward activities, which he did dragging himself from activity to activity all the while feeling he was dying a slow death.

He would remain incarcerated and drugged until he was successfully "rehabilitated," which chiefly meant renouncing his absurd belief that he was sick.

ᏏᎧ

Doctors like to solve problems. They like to make people well. Nothing makes them happier. Sadly, when they fail, their universal fallback position amounts to blaming the patient for his or her own disease. Even when the evidence points in the opposite direction, doctors frequently come up with psychological diagnoses in the absence of clear answers.

Children may be the most vulnerable of all to such treatment. It's hard for them to fight for their rights, or make the case for their own sanity. Pediatricians, when flummoxed by their small patients' complaints, tend to cast a suspicious eye at the child's home environment: If the parents are in distress, pediatricians are provided with a convenient explanation for mysterious symptoms in the child.

As a pediatrician, I know that a child's home can play a big part in his or her health. But I do not automatically exclude the possibility of medical illness in a child because his parents are on the verge of a divorce, or if a grandmother died.

Just as it is possible to have a child with diabetes living within a family in turmoil, it is possible to have a child with CFS living within a family in turmoil. Family dysfunction has its own signature; it creates its own particular pattern of difficulties in children, and these problems are very different from the problems of CFS.

Demanding that a diagnosis of CFS may be made only in perfect families makes no sense at all.

In my view, psychological diagnoses need to be made with the same specificity and accuracy as medical diagnoses. It is not enough to pull a psychological diagnosis out of your hat if you are stumped. Autism is a severe neurologic disease of childhood, but for many years doctors ascribed autism to family dysfunction. We now understand that autism has nothing to do with poor parenting; it is an organic disease.

I am not going to debate the legitimacy of Munchausen's syndrome by proxy. It exists – a sad commentary on modern society. But the diagnosis should be made after obtaining absolute proof of a parent inflicting conscious and active harm on their child.

In Arnie's case, neither the court nor school officials bothered to offer proof of his mother's intent to cause harm, or even actual harm, no doubt because they had no proof.

Their actions were based on conjecture.

❧

Unfortunately, these events are becoming increasingly common, as more and more children and adolescents fall ill with CFS.

The medical establishment and our federal health agencies are digging in their heels, so to speak, hewing with vigor to the mistaken belief that CFS is psychiatric in origin. As a result, more and more children who suffer from CFS are being diagnosed with Munchausen's syndrome by proxy, and the courts are remanding them to foster homes.

Arnie's suicide attempt under such conditions is hardly uncommon either. Too often, children with CFS, who have been taken from their homes, told they are imagining their illness, and sent to live in strange homes with adults who refuse to acknowledge their symptoms and disability, find death to be a better option.

Like Arnie, these sick children frequently end up in psychiatric institutions, deprived of the comfort of their parents, who may be the only people who understand they are ill.

Failure to diagnose a condition is, in some circumstances, malpractice. Failure to properly diagnose Arnie resulted in a forced separation from his mother – his only advocate – and his subsequent suicide attempt and incarceration. For Arnie, failure to diagnose had serious consequences.

∾

The existence of CFS has been confirmed by the National Institutes of Health and the Centers for Disease Control. There continues to be legitimate debate as to what causes the illness, but to deny its existence because of a collective failure to understand its cause is inexcusable.

The American Academy of Pediatrics has stated that at least one part of its mission is to act as advocate for children. Yet on the contentious matter of CFS, the Academy has remained silent, which I see as equivalent to child abuse. Our court systems have an obligation to protect the young and the helpless. Our courts, however, take their advice from the medical profession.

There are many forms of child abuse: neglect, physical abuse, sexual abuse ... I would like to suggest that the term "medical abuse" be used when children are directly hurt by apathy or ignorance of health care providers – not the ignorance expected prior to scientific discovery, but ignorance defined as refusal of accepted fact. We are not talking about a new religion here. CFS has been recognized and studied in this country for nearly twenty years.

Arnie is nineteen years old now and remains disabled by CFS. His incarceration in the psychiatric institution lasted six months, after which he lived in foster care for another several years. He has reunited with his mother and is at last receiving basic symptomatic care for his illness.

CHAPTER 3

Severity

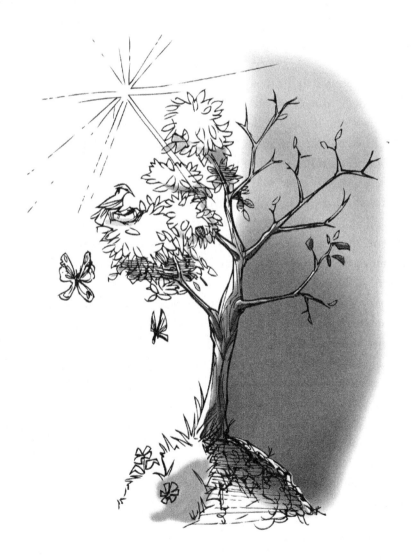

From Life to Darkness

A New Year's Never to Be Forgotten

Laurel [218] [219] | May 25, 2009 | Arizona, U.S.

I remember the moment I became ill. It was December 31, 1996 around three o'clock in the afternoon. I was twenty-four years old. Walking down the hallway of my cheerful two-bedroom apartment, I was about to shower and get ready to go out with friends to celebrate the New Year. As I got about halfway down the hall, I literally felt like I had been hit by a ton of bricks. I stopped in my tracks and leaned my hand against the wall to hold myself up. "What is happening?" I murmured out loud, astounded by how abruptly ill I felt.

Dizzy, I made a beeline to the living room to lie down on the couch and rest, hoping that would be enough to make whatever this was go away. What bad timing, I thought, to have come down with the flu on New Year's Eve. I turned on the TV to distract myself from how sick I felt, but the images on the screen seemed so dizzying that I could barely tolerate two minutes of it. I had to turn it off.

My roommate walked in and I told her I might have the flu and didn't think I'd be able to go out that night. I distinctly remember thinking (and perhaps intuitively knowing) that this was something much more significant than your average virus.

However, not one to be deterred by a silly bug (I virtually never called in sick to work), it didn't take much for my roommate to convince me to go out anyway. I told myself I'd feel better after I showered. I didn't.

We took the city bus to a club in Boston to meet up with friends. As I sat in my seat, eyes closed from lights that felt too bright, I remember everyone's voices seemed simultaneously too loud and yet somehow distant and muffled, as though we were all traveling underwater. I felt myself sweating from fever, though it was below freezing outside. My temperature that night, I later learned, was well over 104.

I honestly am not sure how I got through the evening except to continuously tell myself all would be better in a few days. I remember laughing and drinking and even dancing on the dance floor. With the exception of my roommate, my friends remained clueless to the fact that I felt at all unwell. As midnight approached, I counted down the seconds with a room full of people as we all shouted out loud: "Ten ... Nine ... Eight ..." Little did I know that I was not just counting down the last few moments of 1996, but the last few moments of my life as I had known it.

---

218 To learn more about Laurel from her CFSAC public comment dated September 2009, go to www.youtube.com/watch?v=LvweCk44WHs (accessed June 29, 2016).

219 Originally posted on www.dreamsatstake.com, Laurel's blog.

The next morning, I woke up in a pool of sweat with swollen glands and a terrible cough. I got out of bed and clung to the walls as I made my way to the shower. Moments after turning the water on, I collapsed onto my knees with dizzying exhaustion. Something was dreadfully wrong. I fumbled my way back to bed and called my doctor.

Two days later, the nurse phoned to tell me that I had mononucleosis. "You'll need to stay home for at least two weeks," she said.

"Two weeks?" I replied in dismay. "I'm going to feel like this for at least two whole weeks?"

It's now been thirteen years, and I am still counting.

When months went by and I did not seem to fully recover, I went through a myriad of tests and skeptical doctors (which took two years) before I had an official diagnosis: CFS. I remember the first time a doctor suggested it to me. "You might have chronic fatigue syndrome," he said. "Some people develop that after severe cases of mononucleosis."

The funny thing was, I didn't realize at the time that he was actually diagnosing me with anything. I thought he was just telling me what I already knew: that, following mono, I had become chronically ill and exhausted. It wasn't until another doctor brought it up again that I realized chronic fatigue syndrome was actually a name for an illness. "I feel way too sick to have something called chronic fatigue syndrome," I told her.

I have always been a very determined person, often to a fault. I went back to work the very morning I woke with a temperature below 100 degrees (three weeks after that fateful New Year's Eve onset), though I otherwise was not much improved. Clearly, it was too soon. Within a month, my 104-degree fever was back, and I was off of work for another three weeks.

Following that setback, I was able to push myself to continue working full time for the next few years; however, not without great difficulty. I often had to rest in my car during my lunch hour, and went straight to bed upon getting home. I was running my body to the ground, and though I knew this, I did it anyway. I thought that I could push through anything and with enough determination, I would eventually overcome.

Not so.

❧

I learned the hard way that CFS does not reward that kind of forced perseverance. After years of pushing my body beyond its capacity, I had a setback (known in the CFS community as a "crash") so severe that I ended up housebound and had to quit my job. Not long after that, I had another crash that left me bedridden and unable to speak above a whisper. That was nine years ago. I have spent what was supposed to be the most vibrant time of my life sick, barely able to speak, and confined to my bedroom.

As with many who are stricken with this illness, I was previously a healthy, energetic, ambitious, and well-educated young woman. I graduated magna cum laude with a BS in psychology from Tufts University. I worked in human resources, first at an internationally known publishing company in Boston, then at a state university. I traveled extensively, including a year abroad in London, during which time I backpacked through Europe for a month at spring break. After college, my friend and I spent nearly two months driving 6,000 miles across the United States.

I love to travel, read and spend time with friends and family. I love dancing, taking photos, and exploring the great outdoors. It's not that I no longer want to do these things. It's that I can't.

Despite my situation and isolation, I was fortunate several years ago to find a friend and companion who can relate to my struggles and who brings me hope and laughter every day. We met online, and we write daily. His friendship and sense of humor are my strength. He, too, has a severe case of CFS and is wheelchair bound. And he, too, became ill at a young age after a severe case of mononucleosis. He has been ill for nearly twenty-five years now.

Somewhere in the midst of writing each other, we became best friends and fell in love. He's the most extraordinary person I know. Last spring, he found the strength to fly out to surprise me and propose, and I enthusiastically said yes. We are thrilled to be engaged, and can't wait to be well enough to get married someday. We dream of having children, of successful careers, volunteer work, travel, adventure, and much more. A former athlete in high school and college, my fiancé hopes, one day, to run again. He has a PhD in mechanical engineering from Carnegie Mellon and might like to teach someday.

I hope to get my master's in speech pathology and work with deaf or special needs children. I also have aspirations of starting my own business.

I dream of the little things too, such as being able to walk down the hallway or outside to stroll in the yard, or spending time with my friends and family to catch up on so many years lost. I dream of walking, running, and dancing. Most of all, I dream of the vibrant, glorious feeling of good health, and I strive for it every day.

But instead, I remain forced to continue watching through my bedroom window as time slips by, and the battle goes on.

Update | January 2015 | Note from Valerie

Laurel remains very ill and bedridden with severe ME/CFS. Her relationship with her fiancé continues to be long distance due to their health. Laurel maintains a blog called Dreams at Stake where she writes about her experiences of living with the disease.

Four Red Hearts for My Son

Barbara | June 2014 | California, U.S.

All is ready. I knock on his door. He is silent, not moving. My heart skips a beat and flutters. I hold my breath, trying not to think of losing him. No response, but I hear a sigh. I quietly wait. At last I hear a groan as he rises to his elbow. I hear him drink water from his straw. I then hear him pick up a urinal. Yes…one more day.

୭

Right now at thirty years old, Mark can't communicate with us by speaking, listening, or texting. He can barely manage to push his call button, which rings a bell we can hear from everywhere in our home. I have made a lot of small cards for him to communicate: "open door," "more," "less," "close door," "rub feet," "back rub," "apple juice," "yogurt," "need help," and so forth. If and when he wants something, I've also placed numbered dice for him to indicate how much of it he wants (e.g. how many minutes he would like me to rub his back, how much apple juice he would like…)

We've also come up with a color system for him to use, whereby a red post-it arrow means "no" or "not now," a green one means "more," a yellow one means "not working," a purple one means "move," and a blue one means "needs attention." Even so, quite often, I cannot figure out what Mark means by the arrows and cards he has placed, which frustrates him, making his symptoms worsen. It's so stressful. He then puts out his "sorry" card, one that he drew himself when he was a bit better – the one with a big heart on it.

We write to him, too: His dad updates him with his thoughts about the science of CFS, research he has read, possible treatments, or supplements that might help. I write to him about my conversations with his doctors and what has been happening outside his room. Our notes have to be short, and not too many.

୭

Mark spends his days just lying in bed. Sometimes he's able to watch a TV show on his iPod. Other times he listens to music. But mostly, it's just silence. He can't tolerate anyone other than his dad or me going into his room. He's usually calm and detached, but occasionally gets panic attacks. His breathing becomes shallow and fast. He moans, and I calm him down as best as I can with a back rub; or I just sit outside his door when he can't tolerate my presence. Anything he doesn't expect makes him crash. So I follow the same routine every time I am in his room, with the same order and the same movements.

Mark only gets out of bed every two or three days to go the bathroom, but it's not usually long enough for me to change his bottom sheet, which hasn't been changed in months. I can tell when it's time to straighten up his covers, and I do so while he lies there with his eyes closed. Other cleaning is done one small bit at a time, quickly and silently – no vacuum.

❧

He now has dark circles under his eyes, but that doesn't change the fact that I find him so beautiful – inside and out. I pull down the covers to massage his stomach ... He is so thin, his ribs are sticking out.

In the hope he will get an appetite and to help get his digestive tract moving, I massage his stomach before he eats – sometimes four times a day, sometimes more. I then get up quietly, gaze at him to try and send him love and energy, and pull his covers back up to his chin.

Mark can't eat much anymore. Most foods make him nauseous or cause stomach pain. He mostly eats yogurt and apple juice. I once considered giving him IV nourishment, but a nurse advised against it and suggested medical marijuana. After getting a card request from him, I got edible things for him to try, in vain...He never touched them and eventually put a red arrow on them. He finds some relief in acupuncture, which, with the help of my daily massages, enables him to eat 2000 calories of yogurt and apple juice a day.

❧

Our routine goes on day after day – his trays of yogurts, a hot wet towel for his dry eyes, his meds, vitamins and supplements, ginger tincture, his apple juice (which I have to open since he can't do it himself), three liters of warm water (he's always cold), gum to help digestion.

We've developed a schedule for bringing him food, emptying urinals, opening his door, and more: We get everything ready and knock on his door. Then we wait – sometimes for fifteen minutes or more. If he knocks back, we can go in. If not, we knock again thirty minutes later. Some days, we spend all afternoon waiting for his response, which puts a knot in my stomach. What if he's dead? We have set times for the knocks, too: at 3:00 p.m., 7:00 p.m., 9:00 p.m., and again at midnight.

His sleep is so disturbed that he often can't manage it until early in the morning. I often stay up until 2:00 a.m. myself so that I can be there with him, sitting quietly outside his door, until sleep comes. His dad works all day, and we are now using our retirement money to get some help because I can never seem to get anything done.

Mark can't really tell us what he needs, so any little mistake on our part (like putting something on the wrong side of the bed or out of his reach) can make him crash, which is both stressful and devastating.

When we are not in his room helping, his dad goes back to reading the ME/CFS literature or doing work-related tasks, while I go back to talking with doctors, ordering things we need, keeping things organized, and so forth. I spend hours trying to get meds or procedures covered by Medicare or Blue Shield. For the most part, they either don't cover it or have requirements that are impossible to meet, like in-person meetings with doctors, tests that Mark is unable to tolerate, or unbelievable paperwork. I've cut back on my own professional life significantly, which puts more of a burden on our finances.

❦

Our house seems to be overrun by Mark's stuff: the bottles (which seem to multiply); towels, eye drops, toothbrush, breathe-right nose stickers… Everything he uses is outside his room so we can take it in when he needs it. He can't do anything for himself.

We have four different specialists now, and they all come to him.

Mark's dad and I can't leave town together anymore. For our annual two-week trip to participate in a spiritual ceremony, Mark's dad will go alone while I remain and care for him. When his dad travels for business, I am also alone caring for him. Our daughter, who's pursuing her own career, helped for months last year, but she became so emotionally wrought that she couldn't function.

A couple of months ago, Mark had a spurt of energy and held out his arms to me for a hug. We held each other and sobbed together. At another time, he got to hug his father, his sister, and his cousin, whom he hadn't seen for months.

Throughout this journey, we've felt like Mark's losses have been so tragic. He was once a very successful, prize-winning artist, traveled all over the world, and (even though his health was already compromising his ability to work full time) he ran a campaign office for a candidate in the 2008 election. He is very creative and wants to make a difference in the world.

People suggest that CFS is psychogenic or is depression, and it makes me angry. Mark was a vital, independent, active young man who was excited about his life and pursuing his ideas. This is not depression, and it is not psychiatric.

His gradual decline started with a bad case of mono in high school in about 2000. He has been bedridden for four years and his health keeps declining. Now I long for the time when he could talk, even for only five minutes. Or look up at me and smile. Or spend a few minutes a day on his art projects.

❦

It's 2:15 a.m. I'm so tired. But I ask myself, "What would I rather do than help him feel a bit better?" I sink into the music he now has playing, gently rubbing my son's back; caressing each bone, each rib, his hips, shoulders, up and down, deep and soft. He sinks into relaxation, and I tiptoe out.

I text to him four red hearts. Tears run down my cheeks, and I ache for his life.

Update | January 2015 | Barbara

Mark is now unable to eat at all. He receives his nutrition through a PICC line. He recently had three life-threatening infections with high fevers, which were successfully treated with antibiotics. Occasionally, he is able to write a card expressing how much he wishes he could get better, be able to communicate, eat, or spend time with his family and friends. On Thanksgiving, he wrote his dad and me cards with a heart and "Thank you." Recently he wrote: "I want cookies." Yes, and a life.

Down the Rabbit Hole: Reality or Dream?

Bradshaw | December 2014[220] | Alberta, Canada

Like Alice after tumbling into Wonderland, I feel like I've fallen down a rabbit hole and am in a universe where normal rules don't apply. Unfortunately, for me this is not a fantasy but reality. I don't ask "Why me?" That is something I have never done. Stuff happens, and sometimes it happens to me.

I slowly roll over, trying to mitigate the pain as much as possible. Turning on the light, I note and enter the time in my medical journal, journal number 46 – over 300 pages each, more than 12,500 pages total – which cover the last nine years of my thirteen years ill.

Checking the last time I took a painkiller and calculating the total so far for the day, I realize I have taken two. I have tried over thirty different medications of varying dosages to arrive at a combination with the fewest adverse effects and the most positive ones. They have included antidepressants and painkillers, as well as medications for sleep, high blood pressure, thyroid, and digestive problems. Charting these things, along with my sleep quality and duration, is imperative so my doctor and I can make the best decisions. Sadly, none of these combinations have helped me recover any quality of life, but do help with some symptoms I cannot bear.

My life consists of sixteen to twenty-four hours a day in bed, in severe and continuous pain, which even creeps into the majority of my dreams. For years, my dreaming was better than my times awake. I usually dreamt of work or pleasant things from my past, but now even my dreams make no sense. When I do have a rare one that is happy and fun and I begin to realize it is a dream, I try my damnedest not to wake up. No success. I am trapped in a hidden world worse than any I could have ever imagined, and the ways out are extreme. ME/CFS is a piece of reality I want no part of.

What happened? How did I get here?

Nearing fifty years of age, I had a great career going nowhere but up. I was working as a specialist in the demanding field of high tech communication systems. The company I worked for supplied support to military, police, public service, and large industrial corporations. My life had been fun, active, and happy.

My daughters, now young adults, had just left home to be on their own. My job as a single parent could now change its focus from them to me. I was and always will be a

---

220 This story was updated in March 2015.

very proud father, and I looked forward to enjoying my independent children and the grandchildren that would soon be part of our lives. Life couldn't have been better from my point of view, and the future looked bright.

I planned to learn to ski and return to white water rafting, canoeing, camping, hiking, and rollerblading. My financial plans for the next fifteen years, until official retirement at age sixty-five, would leave me a nice house barely an hour from the Canadian Rockies. I would have a worry-free retirement. I knew I wouldn't completely quit working – maybe consulting or part-time work as needed. I wouldn't live in a mansion and drive a foreign sports car, but I would be comfortable and never have to worry about where my next meal was coming from.

All this shattered shortly before I turned fifty.

❧

Now, at age sixty-three, life looks a whole lot different.

In the fall of 2000 at age forty-eight, I caught a bug that came and went and came again. It seemed I was always stuffed up and feeling like I had the flu. That November, I attended a week-long course for my job, just one of many I had taken over the years. The first day, I could hardly get out of bed. Class was a blur, and as I sat looking at my dinner in the restaurant that night, I couldn't eat. All I wanted to do was sleep.

The whole week went by like that. Focusing on the material was difficult, and for the first time in my life, I failed a test.

The flu cleared up the next week, and I had no other medical problems for a while. My job was going very well. I was working the usual sixty-plus hour weeks that I thrived on, and I enjoyed flying back and forth to work sites all over Canada.

In April, I had my annual physical. All the tests came back normal.

In July, I bought a top-of-the-line set of rollerblades. During my second outing on my favorite freshly paved trails, I was going down a hill with a T-intersection at the bottom. Left or right? At over twenty-five miles per hour, I decided on turning left. At that moment, an elderly couple appeared out of the trees, not two feet from where I was going to be within seconds. I called out a warning. Missing them was my priority. Hitting someone at that speed would surely cause significant damage. I had to somehow get around them.

Barely missing the couple, I was looking at my feet as I rounded the corner and realized my right skate was going to hit the edge of the grass. Thank God I was wearing a BMX racing helmet, and not the cheap plastic bicycle kind. Wearing only wrist guards, I knew I had to land with my wrists first. These thoughts took only a millisecond. Then blackness.

I landed in the brush about twelve feet from the trail, later finding out that I had been unconscious for almost two minutes. Lying on my back, I awoke on the lap of the man I had just avoided crashing into. "Breathe, breathe, please breathe," he was saying. I could barely pull air into my lungs, as I watched his wife locate my cell and prepare to call 911. "I'm fine," I croaked, "no ambulance." In shock and too proud to ask for help, I dragged myself up. Against their objections, I managed to skate the mile back to my car. As I drove home, it hurt to breathe. It hurt everywhere.

At the insistence of my daughter, I let her take me to the nearest emergency room. The X-rays showed several cracked and a few broken ribs. No big deal. It would heal, and I would go on as before.

❧

Three weeks later at work, I fell asleep at my desk – yet another thing that had never happened before. It scared the hell out of me.

I was at my doctor's the next morning, then off to the lab, and back to my doctor the next day to find out what was going on. The results were shocking: My liver had failed.

Off to the hospital, where the specialists said they would be very aggressive in helping me. After about three weeks, I was put on the transplant list. All the forms were filled out, and the preparations were made so that if my temperature ever went above 103 degrees, I was to call the hospital. They would then send an ambulance to take me to the airport to be transported to a different city where an expert liver transplant hospital was located.

I rested at home, and in the following weeks, I was so sick that all I could do was drink liquid meal replacements for food as well as pray when my temperature hit 104 to 104.5 degrees, which it did several times. By this time, what started as a yellow color in the corner of the whites of my eyes had spread to the rest of my eyes and skin. One of my daughters insisted I wear sunglasses so she did not have to see my eyes that sickly. My skin looked like I had been spray tanned with bright yellow dye, which was not very flattering. Even my hair and fingernails were discolored.

I did not want a transplant. I would not, and did not, call for the ambulance. I convinced myself that I was going to get better! The lab took blood by the pint twice a week, but the tests never revealed what had caused the liver failure. They wrote it off as hepatitis, which really means "swollen liver."

After three months of testing, by the grace of God, my liver function tests indicated that it was healing. The good news was that no transplant was required! I was off the danger list and recovering, chomping at the bit to get back to work.

My skin and eye color were turning back to normal, but I wondered why I didn't have the energy to get out of bed and why I had trouble walking any distance when I did get up. I couldn't understand why my mind, usually sharp as a scalpel, was so slow and dysfunctional.

Thank God I had an excellent doctor who was, and remains, very supportive. He ran every imaginable test on me. This took three more months, which I spent lying in bed, exhausted and weak. Though I was itching to return to work, my overall health never improved.

When I went for the final results and asked him what I had and how we were going to fix it, I got the shock of my life: "You have chronic fatigue syndrome, also known as myalgic encephalomyelitis. There is no cure. There is no treatment. The best we can do is to try to alleviate your symptoms." He wrote prescriptions for what was the beginning of a long battle to find the most effective combination.

My world collapsed into a tiny space, consisting of shock, horror, and disbelief.

∽

We tried every treatment available in this country. No luck. Now what? Just the spring before this, my life was grand. Instead of time filled with enjoyment, work, laughter, and activity, my life became one of sleep, pain, confusion, and a feeling of having woken up one day trapped in a different universe. I felt alone and lost in a world gone terribly awry – my rabbit hole.

It was only a few months after my fiftieth birthday, and I had to end my career prematurely and apply for long-term disability. While still reeling from the fact that I was now chronically ill, I had to jump through hoops to fill in form after form that the insurance company required. Why didn't they send all the forms at once? It took almost four months for the insurance company to grant me long-term disability, and that was only with my doctor and employer pushing them!

My world shrank to my house and my two cats. Eventually, friends, co-workers, and family got on with their lives. I was left behind. They had jobs, kids, and lives that I could no longer participate in. Nobody wants to put their life on hold and listen to the same things over and over again. Pain, confusion, boredom, and loneliness don't make for good conversation.

"How are you feeling today?" I heard again and again.

If I lied and said, "Fine," and the insurance company heard of it, there went my income. If I told the truth and said, "Like a pile of shit run over by a steamroller," nobody wanted to hear it. My standard answer became, "As good as I get, thank you! Yourself?" The only in-person conversations I had were with my daughters, my one neighbor, and my doctor. Luckily I also had a couple of close relationships by phone.

The next six years were a jumble, and I had a real problem adjusting. After that, I think I started accepting my situation and my brain seemed to function a bit better – the key word being "seemed." In reality, I spend ninety percent of my time in bed or in front of the TV.

I wouldn't have made it without my cats. They have kept me constant company and are just happy to be with me. That has maintained my sanity more than anything else in the last thirteen years. It is only when I am with them that I know for sure I am awake and not dreaming. Otherwise, it is hard to tell reality from a dream.

꩜

One of the main problems with this illness is the lack of knowledge and acceptance of it by the health care system. I have friends who have waited years for a diagnosis and/or for a doctor that would take their case. A great many are told they are depressed, crazy, lazy, or misfits. I'd give anything to be able to do advanced aerobics and go to the gym several days a week. How dare anyone suggest we're just unmotivated or depressed?

Are we depressed? It doesn't take a rocket scientist to figure out that a life-destroying chronic illness will likely cause depression. Unfortunately, if that were the cause or an important piece in my illness, I would have responded positively to the many antidepressants I have tried.

Research is now proving our intolerance to exercise and activity of any kind and shows that our brains are negatively affected by this illness. However, this knowledge is not reaching mainstream yet. Due to these systemic failures, we are left to learn about our disease from the Internet, fellow patients, advocacy organizations, and from reading research papers.

꩜

I have a close friend who has celiac disease along with ME/CFS. Celiac disease is a genetic autoimmune disease that is triggered by certain gluten proteins found in food (rye, wheat, barley and sometimes oats). It has a prevalence of one in 100 people in North America, and many remain undiagnosed. Finding out that celiac disease is more common among chronic medical conditions, I started doing research into it.

After nine years of ME/CFS, I asked my doctor to send me for a blood test, and I tested positive for celiac disease. The normal range of antibodies for people without celiac disease is zero to twenty. Mine in the year of 2010 was 156. Celiac disease can be very serious and does not always create only digestive problems. It affects all systems of the body and has a high rate of certain cancers, if left untreated.

Nine months of eating gluten-free, and my antibody level dropped to ten, but my symptoms and overall health had not improved. Could discovering the celiac disease immediately upon my diagnosis with liver failure in the year 2001 have saved me from this Satan's curse? I'll never know.

꩜

From what I have read, the main causes of death for those with ME/CFS are, various organ and system failures due to the illness, thirty percent; heart disease, twenty percent;

cancer, twenty percent; suicide, twenty percent. Depending on the person's age and their severity, the chance of getting their pre-illness health back is at a minuscule seven percent or less.

The average life span, according to one study, is fifty-seven. I'm now six years past that expiry date. Yikes! Remember, these numbers are only as accurate as the information I have obtained from the Internet and knowledgeable friends. I'm pretty confident in them personally – as sure as I can be after years of researching.

I have to live at least as long as my cats. We are a team: We have been together 24/7 since they were kittens, and they do not tolerate change of any kind. My heart breaks when I think how abandoned they would feel if I were suddenly gone. I can't and won't do that to them. But when they are gone ...

❧

Sleep comes.

I'm walking through a small city. I am sure it is a place I once lived, familiar but somehow slightly different. I am looking for something, someone, somewhere. I'm not sure which, but I keep on looking. Maybe I'm just trying to go home. It's winter. I'm dressed for the cold and am enjoying wandering my old haunts. I notice that it is very quiet.

Things get a bit stranger, and I don't feel quite right. My muscles ache as if I'd just overdone it at the gym or like the day after the first baseball practice of the year, when my body reminds me of muscles I forgot I had.

The pain and the dream are entangled. It's like feeling I have the flu, a massive hangover, and have been beaten all over with a two-by-four simultaneously. I am neither in a deep sleep nor completely awake – a middle zone that I can't escape. The pain, noticeably more intense, is unfortunately not part of the dream – a pain that the most powerful medicines available cannot stop entirely – a pain that is physical, mental, and emotional.

As I become more conscious, the quiet winter setting of my dream blurs into a familiar rectangle – the rectangular doorway that I have been looking at from my bed for most of the last thirteen years.

❧

This afternoon, I had the rare energy to go out. I stopped for a soft ice cream cone, drove slowly into a beautiful nearby park, ate the ice cream and listened to 1960s music very, very loud. I stopped to throw the cone in the garbage: I can't even eat it because it contains grains of some type that will flare my celiac symptoms. Some symptoms have worsened now when I consume gluten by choice or by mistake ... but I have to hold the ice cream somehow. It is just one more inconvenience.

I start the car, crank the music, and drive around slowly, thinking of the best period of my life. I grew up in the 'sixties, and there is no way to explain how much better life was for me back then. You had to have lived it.

Time to return home. That was hard, sad, and fun. I realized that I had made a decision. If I can't be one of those who get well or improve to a decent quality of life within the next five years or so, I will become a *"butterfly."* I think of our time here as only a stage of our journey similar to a caterpillar before transformation. I will not spend the next ten, twenty, thirty years in this alternate universe that I have become a part of. I will be healthy or I will be free.

CHAPTER 4

Those Who Have Died

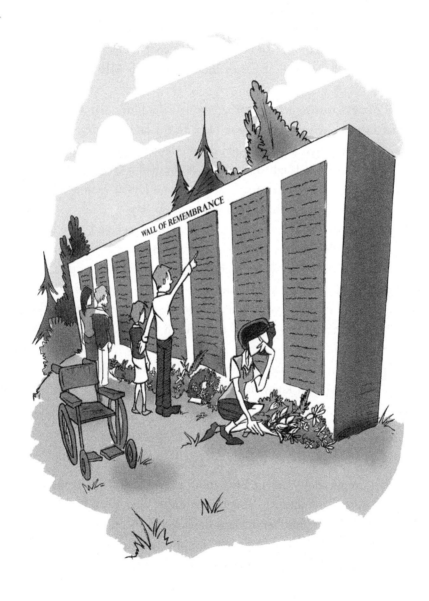

Missing Lisa

Valerie Free | March 21, 2015 | Alberta, Canada

By chance or destiny, through a common illness – ME/CFS – I made a lifetime friend. Her name was Lisa.

Lisa heard of my plight a few years after I became ill and contacted me. On our first phone call, we instantly connected. I learned she was a hairdresser and was married with three children before this illness "happened" to her. Over our many conversations, she shared some of the complications that being very sick contributed to: a divorce, financial and legal struggles, and the medical fiascos those of us with ME/CFS all seem to find ourselves in.

It is rare to come across someone nearby who has the illness, let alone someone like Lisa. After that first phone call, which took place in the late 'nineties, we spoke at least twice a week. We chitchatted about normal day-to-day living and about our lives with ME/CFS. We told jokes and laughed regularly, as she had a great sense of humor. We confided our struggles, disappointments, frustrations and joys as we fought to regain our health and to maintain a place within our families and society.

We had so much in common. We were about the same age and were each raising a daughter. They are also close in age. Lisa's sons were already teens and were not living with her most of the years I knew her. We both enjoyed our homes and our pets. Our level of functioning was also approximately the same over the years – between twenty and fifty percent on the Karnofsky scale,[221] which meant we were not permanently bedbound, nor were we very highly functioning – both of us living in what I called "the middle zone"; the one between here and there.

It was a surprise when, years after we met, we realized that one of Lisa's brothers lived in my original hometown and knew my parents, family, and friends. Our worlds were so connected.

However, the complications I mentioned above affected her life over the years – as if having ME/CFS wasn't complicated enough. She didn't have disability income; lacked help from outside the home; and her medical providers in the more recent years did not include an expert in ME/CFS. Unfortunately, she also had to deal with the fallout that can come from divorce, split parenting, and having three children going through different stages of life.

---

221 For more information on the Karnofsky scale, refer to Appendix H.

In the midst of this, an angel did eventually appear in the form of a loving partner, Tray, who took her illness seriously and was extraordinarily compassionate and helpful. Despite the constant limitations the disease imposed, Lisa and Tray both felt blessed by their loving relationship.

⁊∾

Lisa would always try to tend to her family's needs. She would tell me that she had been on the roof fixing something, that she had caulked her bathtub, or that she made a meal that she could stretch over two suppers to conserve her energy. She enjoyed that type of work. Lisa was so sensible and practical that I always felt more grounded after our conversations.

We mothered our girls in a similar way and often shared our stories by phone while lying down. I could hear the patience, love, and tolerance that she exercised – she was a good and loving mother.

In 2014, alongside our two grown daughters, Lisa and I sported matching T-shirts and hosted the May 12 International Awareness Day at a local health food store. As I looked at her that day, I realized that her blond hair and bright blue eyes, as well as her enthusiastic demeanor, made it hard for me to remember how sick she was, and this reminded me that it is hard for everyone to spot invisible illness, even when you have it yourself. It was this day that our daughters (also dressed in the ME Awareness tops) finally met, and they shared with each other and the passers-by what it is like to live with a neuro-immune illness in the family.

⁊∾

In the early days of my illness, I only knew three people as friends who had been diagnosed with CFS: Lisa was one of them. They lived locally and made up most of my illness community for years. Many years later, through writing and researching for my book project, I got to know others in the global community. Although Lisa did not have the time or energy to make these connections herself, she was exposed to some of the people, organizations, and the research through me. She enjoyed that and found it comforting.

⁊∾

Over the last months, Lisa expressed some concern about new symptoms such as dizziness and vision problems along with a worsening of others, such as muscle weakness, increased pain, and memory and concentration loss. She was very frustrated about the constant post-exertion relapses and felt very sick every day. Although she went to her family doctor to explore these regularly, they remained unresolved. We had a standard reply to each other when relapse would rear its ugly head, and that was: Go lie down, relax, drink water with salt, and eat something! We will try again tomorrow.

Sometimes we would call our conversations "taking a walk around the block." We would try and solve one of the problems revolving around CFS, like health care, only to find ourselves back where we started. Other times, the overwhelming symptoms created confusion and fear within us, which made us wish for an illness more definable and treatable. One would calm the other in response: "We have a serious and complex disease that not many understand yet. It is important we not beat ourselves up, keep our expectations realistic, and be gentle – with ourselves and with each other."

On March 5, 2015, Lisa took her life. She was fifty years old.

Although I have been writing about my own illness experience – as well as that of others – for five and half years, I cannot grasp that I am writing about one of my best friends in the section of "Those Who Have Died" due to ME/CFS. It is shocking to me that I am telling you this story. As one of my friends reminded me after this tragedy: "ME/CFS is a vampire of a disease and can test people to their core – and more."

Now, when my symptoms flare because of a local weather change and I pick up the phone to compare symptoms with Lisa, she is not there. When I go to email her the latest exciting news from the ME/CFS scientific and research world, I realize she won't be on the receiving end. Never again can I read aloud to her some of the cool stuff in my book as she puts her earphones on, sits down and puts her legs up to rest. May 12th will be coming soon… Who could replace Lisa's help and encouragement on this important day?

I will always remember her closing words on our final call. We had diverted our conversation because of my dog, Cotton, who was barking about something. So I said, "Cotton, you should go play with Lisa today – she is having a rough one." Lisa very quietly laughed and said, "You are so sweet – you are so sweet."

My heart goes out to her loved ones.

My beautiful and devoted friend, Marlisa Wolfe: December 14, 1964 – March 5, 2015. May she rest in peace.

Emily's Appeal: Give Us Reason to Hope

Emily Collingridge | March 22, 2012 | U.K.
Introduction by Valerie Free

On March 18, 2012, Emily Collingridge died in hospital at the age of thirty. Approximately a year before she died, Emily wrote a direct appeal for more understanding, support, and research for ME. Her family released it after her death. It was posted at a number of sites including the ME Association [222] on March 22, 2012. Her appeal "Give Us Reason to Hope" ended with the following paragraphs:

❧

My entire future, and the greatly improved health I so long for…currently hinges on luck alone. This is wrong.

As I lie here, wishing and hoping, and simply trying to survive, I (and the thousands like me – severe ME is not rare) should at least have the comfort of knowing that there are many, many well-funded scientists and doctors who are pulling out all the stops in the quest to find a treatment which may restore my health and that the NHS is doing everything possible to care for me as I need to be cared for – but I don't.

This wretched, ugly disease is made all the more so through the scandalous lack of research into its most severe form and the lack of necessary, appropriate support for those suffering from it. This is something that must change.

And that is why I tell my story; why I fight my painfully debilitated body to type this out on a smartphone, one difficult sentence at a time and to make my appeal to governments, funders, medical experts and others.

Please put an end to the abandonment of people with severe ME and give us all real reason to hope.

Emily Collingridge, 1981-2012.

❧

Update | August 6, 2016 | Note from Valerie

In Remembrance of Emily, her mother Jane Collingridge acknowledged the 4th Annual Day for Understanding & Remembrance, August 8, 2016, with some of Emily's other writings. The 25% M.E. Group – www.25megroup.org

---

222 Excerpted. Published on March 22, 2012.www.meassociation.org.uk/2012/03/emily-collingridge-1981-2012-such-a-short-life-such-a-huge-legacy (accessed July 12, 2016).

From Six to Thirty: A Life with ME [223]

Emily Collingridge [224] | 2010 and 2011 | U.K.

Note: Here is Emily's story in her own words.

I was a very happy six-year-old. I loved school and my boyfriend; I could spend hours in a swimming pool and always wanted to climb everything in sight; I couldn't wait to have a proper bike without stabilisers. Life was out there, and I was going to live it to the full. Then mumps hit my class.

My peers continued to run around the playground, but I was in bed for weeks. In time, I went back to school, but gone was my childhood vigour. I would return home so desperate to sleep that sometimes I wouldn't make it past the downstairs floor where I would lie still for a couple of hours. I had mysterious pain migrating across my body and was driven crazy by an irritable bladder. I struggled to hold a pen, and my eyes wouldn't focus properly. My sharp brain became increasingly fuzzy – teachers were confused to hear their consistently competent and confident pupil repeat, "I can't do it, I really can't."

I was a shy, sensitive child, and these mysterious symptoms were so strange, inconsistent, and confusing that I was embarrassed – and even ashamed – of them. When doctors didn't show any significant concern, I began to hide everything that I was experiencing and struggled on alone. My mother knew that I was "different" from other children, but it was not until my symptoms became hard to conceal that anyone realised that something was very wrong with my health. By this point, I was nearly ready for secondary school.

It was now the early 'nineties, and ignorance about ME was still widespread. With no obvious cause to my constantly deteriorating condition and still no support from doctors, I was forced to pursue as normal a life as possible. For me normal meant being physically dragged from my bed in the mornings only to collapse at school and be sent home or worse, carted off to the hospital in an ambulance. It meant standing at the foot of the school stairs crying at the thought of having to climb them. It meant my best friend carrying my school bag because I was too weak to do so myself. It meant being bullied and ostracised for having an unlabelled illness. It meant painful self-doubt, which soon turned

---

223 This story has remained unedited.

224 Emily is the author of "Severe ME/CFS: A Guide to Living." www.severeme.info (accessed May 28, 2016).

into self-hate – if I wasn't ill, then clearly I was a defective human being. Most of all, it meant isolation and misery. Was I going to suffer like this for the rest of my life (alone)?

By the age of fourteen, both school and home tuitions were a physical impossibility. With little to no functioning in my legs, I was now in need of a wheelchair. At last my doctors paid attention; at last they realised what was wrong: ME, a chronic neurological condition triggered by a virus. In my case: mumps.

My relief was incredible. I wouldn't have to fight against my pain and ignore my disability daily any longer. And surely if it were an illness, it would one day go away. It's hard to imagine how I would have felt if I'd known that, fifteen years later, I would not only still be waiting for that elusive recovery, but would be far sicker.

The decline continued, and at the age of sixteen, I found myself housebound. But I was now absolutely determined that ME would not ruin my life. The Association of Young People with ME (known as AYME) was looking for volunteers, and I embraced the opportunity. My career aspirations had long been charity PR, and I was amazed to find myself fulfilling them despite my circumstances. And I was not disappointed in my choice of occupation.

The next five years were extremely rewarding, and I felt honoured that my achievements were twice recognised by the Whitbread Volunteer Action Awards.

But my disability was now profound. I needed someone to bathe me and at times to dress me, feed me, and help me to the toilet. I worked from bed. At the end of each day, I lost the ability to speak, and the pain was so bad at night that my mother had to get up to provide additional care. This was not going to stop me from moving on into the wider world though. At twenty-one, I commenced what would be three satisfying years working (still from bed) as a project adviser for various charities, including the U.K.'s leading family support organisation Home-Start.

But in 2005, when I was twenty-four, life took a very cruel turn.

For some time, my doctors had not known how to manage my extreme pain, and I was once again pushing myself too hard; I then found myself spiralling into a level of illness that was both shocking and overpowering in its severity. I had no idea that modern medicine could allow such suffering. I knew that my family and doctors felt as helpless, desperate, and afraid as I did. I lost the ability to swallow, speak, see, and move. I was doubly incontinent, often paralysed, tube-fed and in unbelievable pain, only partially relieved by high doses of morphine. My nausea was so extreme that it had to be treated with drugs normally reserved for patients undergoing chemotherapy.

I could bear no stimulation – even though I couldn't open my eyes and was in a blacked-out bedroom, my eyes had to be covered at all times. I wore earplugs twenty-three hours per day, and someone's mere presence in my room was like an assault. At times, I didn't recognise my own mother and was confused about where I was.

In 2006, there were rare complications that almost cost my life. For much of 2007, as the misery dragged on, I regretted the life-saving treatment and yearned to be released from the hell that was my life. But I was incredibly fortunate. By the end of 2007, when I truly felt I could keep going no longer, my body rallied.

The improvement came slowly. The first major milestone was washing my own face. Eventually, I progressed to having my curtains open. Then I was able to prop up in bed and later sit on the edge of the bed – my family and I could not stop beaming with excitement at my managing to place my feet on the ground without agonising pain or blacking out. In time, I started taking a few wobbly steps with a walking frame, having a bath thanks to an electric reclining bath lift, going downstairs with the aid of a stair lift and even managing to go outside in the sunshine for a few minutes using a super duper reclining wheelchair. At last I could spend time with my loved ones.

My parents and I began to have weekly family film nights, which, though difficult physically, were an almost unbelievable joy. I also got into a routine, which allowed one phone call to a treasured friend each week. I even – and I do not know how I managed this as I was still so very ill – wrote my first book, *Severe ME/CFS: A Guide to Living*, which was well received by my fellow sufferers, carers, and professionals. Orders flooded in from around the world within days of publication. My dreams seemed to be coming true. Finally I felt I could dare to imagine one day having a life that was not dominated by a crippling illness. I was so full of hope and love for life. But such happiness was not long lived.

A difficult and unavoidable hospital admission in 2009 brought with it a crushing blow; devastating relapse. There are no words for the disappointment I felt. I was thrown back into the indescribable hell that is ME at its worst, and I did not know how I would stand it. I was once again trapped in a body that was torturing me twenty-four hours a day, and there was no way of escaping.

In the first six months of 2010, I was hospitalised four times as my body struggled to survive the intense symptoms. I spent a total of nine weeks as an inpatient; it should have been longer, but the hospital failed to meet my needs during the last admission, and I was forced to discharge myself before irreparable damage was done.

Some of my days in hospital were amongst the most frightening of my life, and all because the hospital did not provide a care environment appropriate for someone with severe ME. My condition was thus magnified a hundred times over. (It was so bad that I don't know how I stopped myself from screaming – I certainly could not hold back the sobbing.) I was given a central line for long-term intravenous nutrition and medication, but it had to be removed when I developed a serious infection. This in itself was another significant blow as other methods of delivering the symptom relief so vital to me are not so effective, and complications had made feeding tubes dangerous for me. All I wanted was to be able to turn the clock back a year. The old cliché that the simplest things in life are the best is true. I yearned to feel fresh air on my skin, to eat a meal, to enjoy the sensation of clean hair ... but most of all, to feel less ill. Of course, nobody could make this happen for me. Somehow, I had to find the strength to accept the nightmare I was stuck in and to have faith that, in time, my health would start to improve again.

❦

So what is my life like now?

Thanks to the strong drugs delivered round the clock by syringe driver and injection that currently keep certain symptoms reasonably stable, I am managing to stay out of the hospital. However, it would take very little to change this. So my family and I constantly live worrying about when my next health crisis will strike.

It is impossible to describe how ill I feel every minute of every day – many people would find this hard to believe, but it is becoming worse than when I was in a High Dependency Unit, my body in shock and my organs failing. It really does seem incredible that I am not actually dying. I sleep for up to twenty hours a day, and the only people ever to enter my darkened room are my mother (who is my twenty-four-hour carer and as such is virtually housebound herself) and the community nurses who support us.

I have no direct contact with anyone else, not even my father – despite living in the same house – as I'm simply not well enough. I am mostly cared for in silence, as I myself can only whisper. Hearing other people talk can make me feel even more horrendous. But when my mother comes in the room, my head fills with all the thoughts, feelings and ideas that I would like to share with her, and not being able to do so is beyond hard.

Even worse is having to spend so much time lying here alone because just having her company can intensify my symptoms to an unbearable degree. I desperately miss communicating with friends – I keep hoping to send them messages, but I never find the strength.

❦

I have not been washed properly for months. It's just not feasible.

We've had to make the very emotional decision to cut off all my hair, as my inability to cope with having it brushed meant that it had tangled itself into a huge, tight lump, which was horribly uncomfortable. I have to wear nighties that button up at the front so that my mother can roll me into them, but I still have to leave a couple of weeks between changing as it is such a strenuous task (despite the fact that they are frequently soaking wet due to the sweats I have on an almost daily basis).

The sheet on my bed is often left unchanged for weeks because my body's reaction is extreme: seizures, breathing difficulties, tremors, spasms, pain, and nausea. I struggle to cope whenever my mother changes my incontinence pads and find myself dreading those times. I always have to lie flat and have pillows surrounding my body to support it. Just lifting my head up for a few seconds, if possible at all, can leave me on the verge of losing consciousness. For hours each day, my body is so hypersensitive that contact with bed covers can send me demented with pain.

I require a drug that is one hundred times the strength of morphine just to be able to manage some ice cream, and even then the swallowing exacerbates my pain and many of my other symptoms. Having once been dangerously underweight, I can now do nothing to stop my ongoing weight gain caused by a restricted diet, medication side effects, and the illness itself. I worry constantly about my teeth, as brushing them isn't possible – it would make me dramatically ill and could send me back into the hospital.

The basic necessities of daily life are so far past my physical capabilities that my overall condition is steadily declining through the accumulative effect of chronic over-exertion. It always seems hard to see how I could get any worse, and yet I do.

It is impossible not to be frightened by this. The highlight of my day – my only real distraction – is going through the lovely post that kind and thoughtful friends keep sending me; some days, I just can't manage reading them though, and often, when I do, the effort results in a fever.

Mine is a tough life filled with constant physical pain and almost unbearable suffering, but I try not to dwell on it. Amazingly, I am not currently depressed, though I inevitably have my low days, and I do get angry when I think of the huge negative impact that doctor ignorance and mistreatment has had on my body. I still have the intense passion for life that I had when I was that healthy little girl, and I can't wait for the day when I can get out of bed, walk out of my room, and embrace every opportunity that comes my way. Sadly, I cannot see this happening before my thirtieth birthday, in the spring of 2011. It's hard to believe that I am approaching such a landmark date. Everyone questions where their twenties have gone as life flies by so fast. But I really feel that mine have been stolen from me. And not just my twenties, but also a large chunk of my childhood and teenage years.

ME has taken so much from me and inflicted so much pain. After twenty-three years, there is still no end in sight. It truly is a hideous illness.

Much of this was written prior to my relapse (in 2010). Recounting what has happened since my relapse has been a huge undertaking, which has taken fifteen weeks to write one sentence at a time and had a significant impact on my symptoms. However, I feel it to have been a very important task. ME is extremely underestimated. If there is a chance that describing my current life as well as my past experiences will help people to understand the enormity of this largely hidden illness, inspire health professionals to improve the care offered to sufferers, or provide the small comfort of knowing one is not alone to others who are struggling with severe ME, I am pleased to do so no matter how difficult.

∽

My Symptoms

> **Pain:** muscle, joint, bone, neuropathic, vein (anywhere and everywhere in body), headache/migraine, abdominal, pelvic, toothache, earache (and itching inside ears).

> **Muscle:** pain, weakness (despite natural strength remaining evident at times), fatigue, tightness, stiffness, spasm (inc. dystonias), twitching, tremors, rigidity, hand/foot clawing, transient paralysis, inability to open eyes, extreme problems with sustained muscle use.

> **Joint:** pain, stiffness flu-like: malaise, exhaustion, aches, (post-exertional), low grade fever (approx. 37.5-38.0 deg), sore throat, tender/swollen glands.

> **Sensory:** light/sound/touch/smell/chemical/taste/vibration/movement/medication (e.g. antibiotics)/weather hypersensitivity, extreme reaction to sudden noises/movements (e.g. doorbell or door opening), extreme pain response to only slightly painful stimuli, extreme pain response to painless stimuli, sudden sensory overload, inability to filter unnecessary sensory information (leading to significant restriction of cognitive abilities and increase of ill feelings), strange sensations (e.g. pins and needles), loss of sensation, inability to judge position of limbs.

> **Gastrointestinal:** nausea/vomiting, acid reflux, increase or decrease in appetite, severely impaired motility leading to constipation, paradoxical diarrhoea, bowel cramping/pain, flatulence, digestion difficulties, faecal incontinence.

> **Urological:** difficulty emptying bladder (leading to frequency and leaks), painful spasms, pain during urination, bladder ache, incontinence.

Cognitive: impaired memory (including temporary loss of significant information from the past, forgetting things I've been told recently and stopping speech mid-sentence as a result of being unable to remember what I'm saying), (occasionally) inability to recognise familiar people, poor concentration, brain fatigue, impaired intellect, confusion/ disorientation, sense of disconnection from environment, brain "freezing", cognitive slowing, difficulties normally associated with dyslexia/ dyscalculia/dysgraphia/dyspraxia, difficulty learning entirely new information, difficulty or inability to understand speech, reading difficulties (including word blindness), using wrong word in writing or speech, difficulty/inability to make decisions (trying to make decisions can cause overwhelming ill feeling and brain paralysis, sometimes leading to panicky feelings), difficulty multi-tasking (despite natural ability!) loss of meaning of time, difficulty with telephone conversations.

Eye: blurred vision, "floaters," other visual disturbance, pain, twitching, inability to open, watering.

Sleep: hypersomnia (up to twenty hours sleep in a day), insomnia (up to about sixty hours without sleep), frequent waking, disruption of circadian rhythm, difficulty getting to sleep, light/unrefreshing sleep, dream changes.

Temperature: extreme temperature fluctuations (largely unrelated to environment), cold hands and feet/poor circulation, (post exertional), low grade fever, (often (approx. 37.5-38.0 degrees), sweats sudden onset).

Other: excessive thirst, salt cravings, dizziness, vertigo, orthostatic intolerance/difficulty standing still, fainting, myoclonic jerks, clonic seizures, absence seizures, hallucinations, palpitations, raised resting heart rate/ tachycardia, swollen feet/ankles, extreme pallor, cyanosis, tinnitus, panicky feelings (associated with degree of illness rather than thoughts/ circumstances), difficulties with speech, difficulties with chewing/swallowing, allergies, poor fine motor skills, difficulty with physical tasks requiring a sequence of movements/actions, clumsiness/poor coordination, problems with balance, episodes of feeling high/hyperactive thoughts/behaviour, weight gain independent of calorie intake, hypoglycaemia-like symptoms, breathing problems, mouth ulcers, bacterial or fungal skin infections, menstruation changes, painful menstruation.

My Brother By Choice – A Goodbye to Tom Hennessy

Cort Johnson[225] | September 28, 2013 | U.S.

Of all people, I thought, "Not Tom Hennessy." Tom was such a fighter. It was true he had the most painful case of ME/CFS I ever encountered. A couple of years ago, ironically on his way to see a doctor, he'd fallen asleep and slammed into the back of an eighteen-wheeler, severely injuring himself. I don't know how he kept going after that, but he'd been dealing with horrific pain for decades.

Finally it got to be too much, and he took his life.

One of his last emails to me started off, "Hey Cort, LONG time no speak! How are you doing, my brother by choice?"

"My brother by choice." Who says stuff like that? It makes me want to cry.

I met Tom some years back at the *HHV6 Symposium of Viruses in ME/CFS* in Maryland. He was alternately alarming and charming; alarming some people as he buttonholed them on issues – sometimes a bit obsessively – but absolutely charming when he let those issues drop.

I drove him back home, and he started popping Fentanyl – "the strongest pain drug possible," he told me – as I watched the sweat starting to trickle down his face and the pain starting to hit. He'd been at the symposium for most of the day – probably the longest time he'd been out in years.

When I think of Tom, though, I don't think of his death, but of what he got robbed of in his life. I felt Tom had a touch of genius. He was a born leader. A former salesman, he could enroll you with a word. A former executive, he was an organizer with vision. A former PR man, he knew what the press wanted. Package all this together in someone who's utterly fearless, and you've got a formidable force.

He always went right for the jugular – not just in his advocacy, but also in his thinking. He tried unsuccessfully to get the advocates for other CFS-like illnesses, such as fibromyalgia and Gulf War Illness, to work together. He was on *Larry King Live* several times and other media outlets many times.

As a former PR man, he immediately recognized what a terrible cost the name would bring: "I explained to that audience back in April 1989 that IF they didn't change the

---

225 Cort Johnson, founder of both Phoenix Rising and Health Rising, posted this tribute to Tom Hennessy on Health Rising the day before Tom's memorial service. The full title of Cort's article was "My Brother by Choice: A Goodbye to Tom Hennessy – Fierce Advocate," and the article can be found at /www.healthrising.org/blog/2013/09/28/my-brother-by-choice-goodbye-tom-hennessy-fierce-advocate-memorial-tomorrow (accessed June 24, 2016). This has been excerpted and adapted for this book.

name that very day, and nip this problem in the bud, it would cause a mess for decades, and it has."

If Tom had been healthier, I think he would have created an *Act-Up*-like advocacy organization that would have become the perfect foil to the CFIDS Association. They needed him to rock the boat, and he needed them to be the ultimate dealmakers.

If he had been just thirty percent better, I think he could have changed the history of chronic fatigue syndrome.

That Tom I've been describing was mostly gone, though, by the time I got to know him. He was simply too sick, too racked with pain, too injured to really use his talents anymore. He was yet another example – a glaring one – of the tragic loss of talent and skill this disorder is too often associated with.

I think of Mary Dimmock's son who was trekking across Asia by himself pre-CFS and is now mostly confined to his house. I think of Mike Munoz with his grand vision for ME/CFS, who is just barely hanging on. I think of Bob Miller, the most vigorous and bold person I've ever met, who spends much of his time in bed. It makes me want to cry.

Tom had so much. He was so gifted, and yet much of it disappeared. That loss is what I think of most when I think of him now.

Here are Tom's own words describing what he was doing before he got sick:

> *Sales and advertising was my job for two decades. I did a national campaign for Subaru that inspired their "official car of the US ski team" that ran for seventeen years. I did a program for Marriott Hotels that used a Gold Gambits card to use for discounted rooms and upgrades for frequent guests that is still running twenty-five years later. I was working on a program for BMW to upgrade their customer service when I got sick. I had seen how the Japanese work up close and personal while living in Japan from 1968 to 1972. My BMW friends laughed at me but the Japanese ate BMWs and Mercedes lunch for the next fifteen years.*
>
> *I was a BMW sales manager in Marin County, California, just over the Golden Gate Bridge. I was making six figures, and I had a new BMW company car, and I was planning to start a computerized database for people to buy and sell cars, boats, motor homes, and motorcycles – sort of like a dating service for yuppies involving anything with a motor. I had possible investment bankers, several hundred clients – life was great!*

But then ME/CFS hit in classic style; a depleted system almost completely folding under one last insult, and almost everything changed. To think it all probably came down to eating some raw oysters (he'd had a bad experience with oysters before):

> *I had constant sore throats, chronic mono, and I just didn't feel well. I couldn't get restful sleep. Then one day, a fellow salesman offered to pay off a*

*loan to me by taking me out to dinner. We drank a bunch of margaritas and
ate ceviche and raw oysters. I went home to sleep it off – the next morning
I couldn't move. I felt like I had been given a Rodney King style beating the
night before.*

*I have hardly gotten out of bed again for the past twenty years. The crippling,
burning, searing nerve pain is still my worst symptom, but with the exception of raccoon eyes (very black deep circles in my eye sockets) and totally
atrophied muscles, I don't look quite as sick as I claim to be.*

Tom's career as an advocate began way back in 1989, when he gave a speech before
600 people at the first *International Meeting on ME/CFS* in San Francisco. He was almost
prescient in his grasp of how widespread this disorder was, stating that almost one million
people in the U.S. had it, and that five to six million people were "one viral, bacterial, or
physical insult away from complete and crushing disability."

Tom was bold like no one else. At one point he called ME/CFS patients "the n...rs of
the medical world" because of the second-class treatment they'd received. At one point,
they even called the meeting's security guards in when Tom got too confrontational.

Tom explained his first speech at the San Francisco meeting:

*I gave an in-your-face speech saying that we are SICK, often deathly ill and
we are NOT fatigued!" I said. "If you do NOTHING else today, then lock
the doors, get together and knock heads and come up with an ACCURATE
definition and CHANGE THE GOD DAMN NAME!" This got a HUGE
response, and all the major media ended up interviewing myself and
Melinda Paras, a gay, Latino woman who gave an equally moving and rip-
roaring speech.*

Tom knew how to push buttons and generate buzz better than anyone. He was a
natural – we've never seen his like since. About one of his *Larry King* appearances, he said:

*That show got pretty heated when I claimed that "many of our brave veterans
are returning with very similar symptoms as all these 'alleged whiney white
women' who can NOT handle stress! I went on to say that "if these highly
educated, mostly male, stunningly victorious soldiers who only fought for
four days could come down with this terrible illness, then maybe the NIH
and the CDC will be forced to stop telling lies about it." I got TONS of mail
from all over the world.*

But then in 1994, he relapsed badly, and that was really it for our most gifted advocate
ever. The website and the organization RESCIND survived, but mostly in name only. He
was in incredible pain, taking Fentanyl patches almost daily at times and finally resorting
to morphine. As always, he described the pain in his own evocative way: "The doctors told

me that I was taking MORE pain medicine than a dying cancer patient whose tumors were crushing his very bones."

Tom was one of the most aggressive advocates I've ever met, but it wasn't personal. At one point he compared me and other advocates to "lobsters sitting in a pot of lukewarm water" that was slowly coming to a boil. It was framed in such an evocative way that you just had to smile. It meant nothing regarding our friendship. Tom would show up from time to time with his long emails of unpunctuated, run-on sentences with capitalized phrases, which were both difficult and oddly thrilling to read. The genius, the pain, and the loss that was Tom Hennessy were embodied in each one of them. I feel honored to have been Tom's "brother by choice."

Tom died on September 9, 2013 after a twenty-five year battle with CFS. He was fifty-nine years old.

Thomas M. Hennessy Jr. 1954 – 2013.

CHAPTER 5

Speaking Out to Government

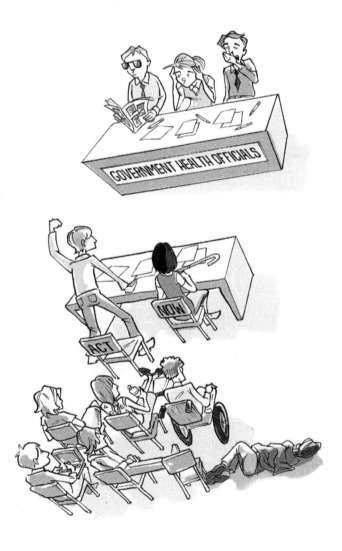

U.S. Government Agencies Hear From the ME/CFS Community

Valerie Free | January 2015 | Canada

I remained unaware of the political importance of the research, funding, and care of chronic illness for most of the years I have been ill. I was very busy surviving/navigating the ME/CFS experience and raising a family until, many years later, I had the opportunity to meet people in Canada and the United States who introduced me to the politics of this disease.

One of the first things I learned was that in Canada, this particular illness community does not have the attention of our Health Minister and associated agencies. This unconscionable neglect exists despite attempts by Canadian organizations to provide them with statistics and information about ME/CFS, fibromyalgia and multiple-chemical sensitivity.

So I became hopeful when I learned there were opportunities for people in the U.S. to present their illness experiences to government officials – figures who have the influence to trigger change for all of us.

I became familiar with two primary opportunities for the ME/CFS community (patients and professionals) to advocate with their stories and presentations:

1. The Chronic Fatigue Syndrome Advisory Committee
    (CFSAC) meetings.

    CFSAC meetings have taken place in Washington D.C. two times
    per year for more than a decade! These meetings provide the public,
    patients, caregivers, and professionals the opportunity to give presenta-
    tions that then become part of public record. This committee is made
    up of board members from many different areas such as medicine,
    research, law, and patient advocacy; and it makes recommendations
    to the U.S. Secretary of Health and Human Services on issues related
    to ME/CFS.

    There are hundreds of powerful, moving testimonies and presentations
    covering all the concerning aspects of care, cure, and prevention for

ME/CFS posted on the CFSAC website.[226] The recommendations made to the Secretary of Health by CFSAC and the results, or lack thereof, are listed at the same site and are available to the public. There is also a separate chart under "Recommendations" which sorts them by focus area, agency, and progress.

Unfortunately, CFSAC meetings have not yet moved the powers-that-be to implement all of their recommendations – many of which would improve the quality of life for people who suffer from the illness. Despite this, CFSAC is an informative structure and process that is in place, and there have been some positive results.

෨෴෨

2. The Workshop on Drug Development for CFS and ME, organized by the U.S. Federal Drug and Food Administration (FDA).

Whereas CFSAC meetings are ongoing, the FDA Workshop on Drug Development for CFS and ME was a one-time opportunity. The workshop took place on April 25-26, 2013. Patients and medical professionals conversed about the symptoms of ME/CFS, and patients offered their experiences with various treatment trials. They also discussed ways to measure the efficacy of these treatments and other medical interventions.

These outcome measures are a necessary requirement for drug development to progress. In addition to comments made at the meeting, there were more than 220 comments submitted to the public docket.[227]

A twenty-three page report was generated as a result of these meetings. "The Voice of the Patient, Chronic Fatigue Syndrome, and Myalgic Encephalomyelitis"[228] revealed that the patients had been heard in a way they hadn't been before. The report concludes:

---

226 The comments and transcripts from these meetings become part of the public record and are available for everyone. The testimonies made at these structured public meetings target a specific audience such as the Secretary of Health and other influential forces. People are directly fighting for advances: for example, more funding for research, an illness name change, or training for the medical profession on ME/CFS. The issues addressed are endless and they are all very important. You can find all recommendations and presentations at www.hhs.gov/advcomcfs/meetings/index.html (accessed July 2016).

227 To view the Webinar archive, the transcript, and the summary of the Workshop, go to www.fda.gov/Drugs/NewsEvents/ucm369563.htm (accessed July 2016).

228 "The Voice of the Patient" report is at www.fda.gov/downloads/ForIndustry/UserFees/PrescriptionDrugUserFee/UCM368806.pdf (accessed July 2016).

"This meeting was the first of the Patient-Focused Drug Development initiative meetings. It allowed FDA to obtain patients' point of view, in a systematic way, on the severity of CFS and ME, its impact on daily life, and available treatment options. FDA recognizes that patients have a very unique ability to contribute to our understanding of this broader context of the disease, which is important to our role, and that of others, in the drug development process. We share the patient community's commitment to facilitate the development of safe and effective drug therapies for this disease."

The FDA later issued a Draft Guidance[229] document on March 10, 2014[230] for the pharmaceutical industry to utilize. It is intended to assist sponsors in the development of drug products for the treatment of chronic fatigue syndrome/myalgic encephalomyelitis (CFS/ME).

Although some people choose to give comments by phone, many others make the trip to DC to participate and offer testimonies in person. Their efforts are remarkable considering what traveling can cost them, both financially and physically.

Thanks to the Internet, I was able to virtually attend these meetings, which allowed me to learn more about the role of government health agencies.

Furthermore, these testimonies changed my perspective: Not only do I now understand that many others are facing the same challenges as I am, I also see how active the illness community is becoming. In spite of all the suffering that is clearly portrayed in the public comments, as well as that from medical professionals who care for the people living with ME/CFS, I began to feel a sense of empowerment.

Here are excerpts of three meaningful testimonies out of many – one from the FDA meeting and two from the CFS Advisory Committee meetings. In addition, the CFSAC testimony of P. Madden is in Chapter 2 and that of M. Fairman is in Chapter 11.

---

229 Draft "Guidance for Industry" at www.fda.gov/downloads/Drugs/GuidanceComplianceRegulatoryInformation/Guidances/UCM388568.pdf (accessed July 2016).

230 As of May 2016, the "Guidance for Industry" remains a draft document but does provide useful information for drug developers.

Help Those of Us Still Able to Work

Jon Kaiser, MD.
Comments at the FDA meeting [231] | April 25, 2013

Good afternoon. It's going to be a challenge to condense my experience with this condition into just a few minutes, but I'll do my best. My name is Dr. Jon Kaiser, and I practice medicine in the San Francisco Bay Area.

In 1987, after many stressful years of pre-med, medical school, residency training, and working as a solo doc in a busy emergency room, I developed ME/CFS. I had severe fatigue, recurrent sore throats, chronic pain, and unrefreshing sleep. If I exercised just a modest amount, I would experience a devastating crash with an exacerbation of all my symptoms, and I never knew how long a crash would last. Sometimes it would last only a few days, and other times it would last several weeks.

My ME/CFS had a significant effect on my work and my personal life. I had to cut down my work hours. I remember lying down on the couch frequently between patients. And if I was able to socialize, I never knew how long it would be before I went up to my wife and said, "We need to leave now." It's like you just hit a wall and you become dizzy and lightheaded and your brain clouds over.

Fortunately, after five or six years of working really hard to rebuild my health, including taking a job with much less stress and leaving emergency medicine, I was able to recover to a significant degree; however, I still experience relapses of these symptoms that significantly impact my life. When a relapse occurs I cannot participate fully as a father or a spouse, I need to lie in bed for hours at a time, and I experience total body pain during these relapses.

Now, there are a lot of people who are totally disabled from this condition, bedbound, or can't leave their homes, and they're a lot worse off than I am, but I'm not here to speak for them. I'm here to speak for the thousands of people with CFS who are able to work but struggle to make it through each day and each week. People who are able to work with CFS struggle to get [their] minds clear enough to function and to be able to think well enough to perform. We struggle to make it into work by nine or ten in the morning and be as productive as everyone else, and we struggle to make it through an eight-hour workday without having to lie down and take a break.

The worst part about this condition, from my point of view as a person with CFS who is still able to work, is the toll this disease takes on my family. I don't know if I can

---

231 This testimony is from Page 37-41, FDA transcript, "Drug Development for Chronic Fatigue Syndrome and Myalgic Encephalomyelitis: Public Workshop, Day One," and can be found at www.fda.gov/downloads/Drugs/NewsEvents/ UCM354951.pdf (accessed July 13, 2016).

convey the psychological distress I feel when I'm unable to spend time with my daughters or participate in family activities because I'm in bed on the weekend recovering from all the energy I expended during the week. This, for me, is the worst part of this condition: the fact that during exacerbations I have no energy left to participate fully in my family and social life. And one other terrible thing, which I'm sure all of you are familiar with, is that family members and friends just can't understand how I can feel so sick when I'm at home, if I'm still able to work and hold a job.

So I want to thank the FDA for holding this meeting and for getting input from patients themselves. I hope they will work to identify treatments that not only help those that are bedbound get out of the house, but also help those of us still able to work be able to think more clearly and function at a higher level. And I look forward to hearing other people's perspectives and having a productive sharing of ideas. Thank you.

People Are Dying

Billie Moore | Testimony at the CFSAC meeting[232] | October 4, 2012

My name is Billie Moore. I am the Advocacy Chair of the New Jersey Chronic Fatigue Syndrome Association and, in this statement, am speaking for myself, my son, and a man who wishes to remain anonymous.

The following are this man's comments to you:

I would like to share with you something that we ME/CFS patients all think about and know, but do not discuss, because we are afraid that revealing the full horror of our disease will leave us vulnerable to ignorant, facile attacks. I have come to understand the meaning of suicide. I am loath to admit it, lest you dismiss me as simply depressed, rather than as tortured and utterly, hellishly hemmed in. But I share myself hoping that if you can see how horrific, how hopeless and forlorn our lives are, you will take action to rectify the monstrous situation that you and your peers have helped to create...

In my life now, I taste only rarely and fleetingly the small pleasures that once made my life so rich. Music was once the great small pleasure of my life, but listening to music now is too physically painful for it to light up my days as it once did. Reading was another great small pleasure of my life. I can no longer read for pleasure, because the mere act of reading confuses me and otherwise exacerbates the symptoms of my disease so quickly that I can barely follow the plot, never mind find joy in the endeavor. Reading is now punishment. Even listening to crickets on a summer night or lying in the grass on a sunny day cannot bring me the joy it once did; I am just too sick.

When a layer of horrible pain, suffering, and debility permeates every moment of your life, you find that you cannot appreciate even the simplest moments that you once treasured. To understand what this is like, imagine for a moment the simplest pleasure that you cherish. Now imagine that every time you experience it, you are zoned out and dizzy; sensitive to light, sound, and touch; your head hurts; your muscles are sore and your joints ache; your eyes burn; and you are exhausted beyond compare. If you felt this daily, you would find life's little pleasures rapidly receding into memory.

---

232 Excerpted from the public comment given at the CFSAC meeting, Fall 2012, by Billie Moore. The full comment is available at www.hhs.gov/advcomcfs/meetings/presentations/moore_billie_100412.pdf (accessed August 6, 2016).

Loss of these little pleasures is torture, because the small things make difficult lives bearable. But ME/CFS also steals life's greatest pleasures, laying waste to our dreams. Like you, I hoped to one day raise a family, develop great friendships, and build a career. Heartbreakingly, those dreams have vanished...

Until our government begins to take this disease seriously, I will live every relentless, soul-crushing day knowing that my life will never improve. I will be the "living dead," until I am dead. And because I am so sick, because we are all so sick, we cannot even advocate for our own futures. To the extent that we do, we sacrifice what pitifully little quality of life we have.

It is in this respect that suicide becomes a positive, life-affirming option. When your dreams are foreclosed, when your ability to appreciate life's small moments is nearly eliminated, when all you know is pain, and you have no hope of recovery and no way of bettering your life, suicide ceases to be an attempt to escape reality, but becomes a conscious choice for a better future, even if that future is the deep black unknown.

This is the unimaginable reality of ME/CFS. We struggle every moment of every day to face pain that knows no end and to cope with the loss of nearly everything meaningful and real in life, and we have absolutely no reason to hope that our future will be any better than our present, because our government has ignored our plight for the last twenty-five years and continues to do so, prioritizing protection of the twisted and broken status quo over creation of a framework capable of providing for our health and our dignity.

That is the end of the man's statement. He is not alone. Countless sufferers of ME/CFS have found in suicide their only relief from indescribable total-body pain, loss of any quality of life, complete lack of hope of a treatment that works, and the disrespect shown by the medical profession and the U.S. government agencies. My own son was severely disabled with ME/CFS for twenty years. He had been to multiple doctors, tried multiple drugs – none of which helped much. His words are as follows:

Since very early on in my illness, when it truly sank in that I was "incurable," I knew that I felt so bad that without the "realistic hope" that I would get better, I could not live indefinitely in this state. That was over nineteen years ago, and I haven't experienced a day yet in which I would be willing to spend decades living life knowing the next day would be the same forever, that's how unpleasant it's been ... I have needed to have REALISTIC hope (the suffering I serve demands this as non-negotiable). I've done extensive research recently, and hope seems to possibly be gone for good for me.

My son committed suicide in June 2011, at age forty-six. He had lost his entire young adult life, and finally life itself, to this disease.

CFSAC members, people are dying. Do not go back to your offices and ignore these desperately sick patients. PLEASE, push for change in your departments and throughout the DHHS [Department of Health and Human Services] regarding ME/CFS.

I Am Having Déjà Vu

Terri Wilder | Testimony at the CFSAC meeting | May 18, 2016
Introduction by Valerie Free

Terri has been a social worker since 1989. Motivated by social justice, she took an interest in the people living with HIV/AIDS and in the illness itself. She has been advocating for the HIV community for over 25 years. In 1996, Terri became very ill, leaving her bedbound at times. Despite thorough medical investigation, including testing for HIV, she did not receive a diagnosis. Since then, her health has been undermined to varying degrees. Only ten weeks ago, March 2016, she was diagnosed with ME by a leading expert in the field. Here she begins to advocate for her own health to U.S. health agencies.

๛

Good Afternoon. My name is Terri Wilder and I'm a person living with ME.

I should tell you that I was only diagnosed about ten weeks ago so it feels strange for me to introduce myself to you this way as I typically introduce myself *this way:*

"Good Afternoon, I'm Terri Wilder and I'm an AIDS Activist and a member of ACT UP/NY."

Yes, that ACT UP – the AIDS Coalition To Unleash Power – the infamous activist organization that shut down the FDA, demanded that the CDC change the definition of AIDS to include women specific illnesses, and stormed the NIH. If you worked in government for any length of time, I'm fairly certain you have heard of ACT UP.

While I have only been diagnosed with ME for ten weeks, I can tell you that it didn't take me very long to figure out that we are repeating history with ME. I have told multiple people that I'm have déjà vu. You see, I have been working in HIV since 1989.

One of the reasons ACT UP was founded was because health officials, government researchers, medical bureaucrats, medical providers and pharmaceutical company executives believed they were the "AIDS experts" when in fact the experts were the people living with AIDS. The persons with AIDS points-of-view were made invisible and their real-world knowledge about the changes that needed to be made to end the crisis were ignored.

I need to be honest with you and tell you that people told me that nothing would happen today if I gave public comment – nothing would change – and that the government would continue neglecting people like me with ME as they have for the past 30 years by throwing us a few crumbs.

For the past ten weeks, I have had two things on my mind – how long am I going to be able to hold on to my job so I don't lose my health insurance, and how could government institutions like the NIH, CDC, HRSA, and FDA repeat history by doing nothing for the millions of people who have this disease?

If I end up really sick in the next few months or years, it will not be because the disease or its complications made me sick.

If I'm getting sicker from anything, I will be getting sicker from the sexism and psychogenic views that are so deeply entrenched in this disease; I'll be getting sicker from the CDC for pushing unexplained fatigue definitions and putting incorrect information on their website about ME; I'll be getting sicker from the neglect and disdain that has driven away researchers and pharmaceutical companies that could discover a treatment for my disease; and I'll be getting sicker from government committees that won't allow people like me (with ME) to sit at that table and help inform policies and programs that might actually save my life. We have a model allowing people like me at the table – people just refuse to use it. I know this because my friends with HIV have a seat at the table.

So how many people are dead either directly or indirectly from this disease who might be alive today if research had been done to develop drugs for ME?

Would they be here today if the government took this disease more seriously and established ME Centers of Excellence around the country? Would they be here if the government invested funding to the tune of $250 million vs. 5-7 million? Would they be here if the designated federal official for this advisory committee actually had something in her bio on the womenshealth.gov website that gave me a clue that she actually had some commitment to ME? (The name of the disease can't be found anywhere in her bio.)

So – how many lives?

Someday, this will be over. Remember that. And when that day comes, there will be people alive on this earth who will hear the story that once there was a terrible disease in this country and that a brave group of people stood up and fought, and in some cases gave their lives, so that other people might live and be free.

I'm having déjà vu...and I don't want history to repeat itself.

If you work for HHS, the CDC, NIH, the FDA or any other government agency – write down my name.

My name is Terri Wilder and I don't want my tombstone to say I died of government neglect.

❧

Originally posted on Occupy CFS, www.occupycfs.com, May 18, 2016

CHAPTER 6

Policy and Funding

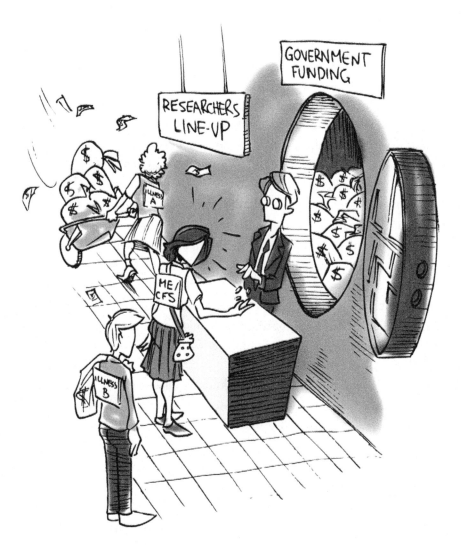

The Shame of Biomedical Research in the U.S.

Llewellyn King[233] | January 19, 2014 | U.S.

When the dark shadow of incurable disease settles across a life, it is brightened only by the hope that science is on the job: The cavalry will come.

Horribly, the cavalry – researchers in the big pharmaceutical companies and the government-run National Institutes of Health and the Centers for Disease Control – may not even have mounted. New drug development is a murky business governed by huge risks, inertia, bureaucracy, and politics.

I've been looking at the role of biomedical research and the development of new therapies and drugs through the lens of one disease, chronic fatigue syndrome (CFS). But it is symptomatic of the whole struggle for cures, which means funds. It is a peephole into a system in chaos; where good intentions, economic reality, public pressure, politics, and bureaucratic apathy play a role in where the research dollars go.

I've been writing about CFS for several years now, so I understand the dilemmas those who are in charge of biomedical research in government and private industry face. It is a disease of the immune system, like AIDS, but it is mostly a medical enigma. It is hard to diagnose because there are no normal markers in blood or urine. It prostrates its victims essentially for life. In its severest form, patients lie in bed in darkened rooms, often feeling that their bones are going to explode. It cries out for more research, as do many other little-understood diseases.

A very small coterie of physicians – not many more than fifty in the United States – specialize in CFS and have developed private clinics for research into alleviating therapies. None of them are set up to do major drug research in the way that pharmaceutical companies do.

Big Pharma – as the drug behemoths are known collectively – is at the heart of new drug development, aided by preceding biomedical research that takes place through government grants to researchers in universities, teaching hospitals, and private clinics. It is a complex matrix.

A new drug can cost over $1.2 billion to develop. It is a very high-risk undertaking – maybe the riskiest investment decision made in the private sector is developing a new drug. It is also a tortuous undertaking.

First, a target has to be selected where there is a large enough patient cohort to establish a market. Then the science begins. Diseases that are straightforward, in medical terms,

---

233 Llewellyn King, journalist and co-creator of the video series ME/CFS Alert, originally published this article for the Hearst-New York Times Syndicate, http://whchronicle.com/?p=1971 (accessed August 6, 2016). It has been excerpted and adapted for this book.

edge out those where the causes may be multiple and the resolution may require a cocktail of drugs. Understandably, a rifle shot is more appealing than a shotgun blast. Eight out of ten drugs fail and are abandoned at some point. The winners have to pay for the losers.

If, after years of research, a compound that may work is discovered, the laborious business of testing it on animals must precede human trials with control groups and years of analysis. Finally the drug must be approved by the Food and Drug Administration, which looks for efficacy, safety, risk benefit, and manufacturing stability.

Into this already difficult world of new drug development, enter the politicians.

Some believe private enterprise will shoulder all the risks and is the right place for research. Others don't understand the vital role that government research grants – administered by NIH and CDC – play in the development of biomedical knowledge [which is] the essential precursor to new drugs and therapies. Its funding is on a seesaw: it was down under sequestration, and [now] funding is restored but not boosted under the new budget deals. It tops out at $29.9 billion, a decline of twenty-five percent since 2003, according to *The Atlantic* magazine.

Chronic fatigue syndrome gets about $6 million a year from NIH. What's wrong with that largesse? Well, remember, it costs $1.2 billion to develop a new drug once the biomedical case is made. As they say, you do the math – and don't expect the cavalry to ride to the rescue anytime soon.

Obama Responds on Chronic Illness [234]

Llewellyn King | August 18, 2012 | U.S.

On April 21, 2011, at a town hall meeting in Reno, Nevada, local resident Courtney Miller asked President Obama for help. Specifically, she asked the president what the administration was doing to fund research into the debilitating, lifelong illness, chronic fatigue syndrome (also called Myalgic Encephalomyelitis). Miller's husband, Robert, is a sufferer.

The president has now responded extensively. [See President Obama's letter next].

Obama has designated his deputy chief of staff for policy, Nancy-Ann DeParle, as his point person for dealing with the disease and to work with the National Institutes of Health. She has been in contact with Miller by email and phone.

The president has asked DeParle to convey a sense of urgency about CFS and to raise its standing. In a two-page letter to Miller, he said: "I have asked Nancy-Ann to stay in touch with Dr. [Francis] Collins at NIH and Dr. [Howard] Koh at HHS [Health and Human Services] about my interest in their efforts on CFS. And I have asked her to update you from time to time. She reports that you are extremely knowledgeable about developments in the research on CFS, so I hope you will keep in touch with us as well." In his letter, Obama said he had asked Collins for a report on NIH funding of CFS research, and he was told that last year the NIH spent $6.1 million on CFS research, which represented a thirty-one percent increase over the level of spending when he took office.

The CFS community – an estimated one million people with the disease in the United States – has long felt slighted by government and ignored in the media.

The community notes that spending to this point in time has been minimal by Washington and NIH standards. Multiple Sclerosis (MS), a disease with half the sufferers, gets about $100 million in research funding.

The politics of disease are like all politics: size matters. Money is important, media access counts, and it helps to have a celebrity to front your cause. AIDS had Elizabeth Taylor, and [MD] had Jerry Lewis. On all these fronts, CFS comes up short.

Also it does not have a national voice, as cancer, diabetes, heart, lung, and many other afflictions do.

The name itself, chronic fatigue syndrome, sticks in the craw of the sufferers. Patient advocates – a dedicated but scattered band of sufferers and victims' family members, like Courtney Miller – hate the name. It was conferred on the disease by the CDC and is the official name in the United States. In the rest of the world it is called by its old name,

---

234 Excerpted from the original post in the Indiana Gazette written by journalist L. King. www.indianagazette.com/news/
    opinions/llewellyn-king-obama-responds-on-chronic-illness,140245 (accessed July 15, 2016).

Myalgic Encephalomyelitis, and the community much prefers that name. Obama used both names in his letter to Miller.

The complaint, which I have heard without exception from patients and their families, is that the name CFS trivializes a terrible disease and brings with it an undeserved stigma: a suggestion that the victims are not really sick, but malingering.

Another deeply felt anger among patients worldwide has been a consistent attempt by psychiatrists to claim the disease as psychosomatic, despite palpable physical debilitation. In fact, it is a disease of the immune system, according to doctors who have made a career of treating it.

Miller told me she was ecstatic about the president's letter and her communication with DeParle. "It is all that I had hoped for," she said.

Obama has some new friends.

President Obama's letter to C. Miller | President Obama | July 26, 2012

THE WHITE HOUSE

WASHINGTON

July 26, 2012

Mrs. Courtney Miller
Reno, Nevada

Dear Mrs. Miller,

At a town hall meeting in Reno, Nevada last April, you asked me about the level of funding for research at the National Institutes of Health (NIH) devoted to Chronic Fatigue Syndrome (CFS). I told you I would ask NIH for a report on what they are doing to address CFS. I understand that my Deputy Chief of Staff for Policy, Nancy-Ann DeParle, spoke with you last week about this, and I wanted to follow-up with you personally.

I asked Dr. Francis S. Collins, M.D., Ph.D., the Director of NIH, for a status report on what NIH is doing to find a cure for CFS. He reports that NIH has spent $6.3 million on research on CFS in FY 2011, which is an increase of $1.5 million (31 percent) from the level of spending on this disease when I took office. This research, he explained, is promoted and facilitated through the coordinated efforts of the Trans-NIH Myalgic Encephalomyelitis/Chronic Fatigue Syndrome (ME/CFS) Working Group.

The National Institute of Allergy and Infectious Diseases (NIAID); the National Cancer Institute (NCI); the National Heart, Lung, and Blood Institute (NHLBI); and the National Institute of Neurological Disorders and Stroke (NINDS) supported 36 research projects on CFS in FY 2011. As part of these projects, NIAID is supporting a multisite study of unprecedented scale designed to address whether a murine retrovirus is associated with CFS. NCI supports intramural and extramural research on viruses linked to both cancer and CFS. NHLBI supports research projects examining circulatory dysfunction, orthostatic intolerance, and the autonomic nervous system as they relate to CFS and NINDS supports extramural research on the effects of CFS on the central nervous system.

In addition, Dr. Collins reports that NIH hosted a State of Knowledge Workshop on ME/CFS last April that Nancy-Ann told me your husband Robert attended. The workshop brought together a broad group of attendees and investigators from various scientific disciplines and identified gaps in knowledge and new opportunities for biomedical research on CFS.

I understand that NIH will continue to encourage research on CFS through two Program Announcements of the same title (Myalgic Encephalomyelitis/Chronic Fatigue Syndrome: Etiology, Diagnosis, Pathophysiology, and Treatment). NIH expects these research programs will enhance our knowledge of the disease process and provide evidence-based solutions to improve the diagnosis, treatment, and quality of life of all persons with ME/CFS. Dr. Collins also advises that the Department of Health and Human Services (HHS) has launched an Ad Hoc Workgroup on CFS and is working to develop a Department-wide strategy to address the disease. This effort is being led by Howard Koh, M.D., Assistant Secretary for Health at HHS.

Finally, I should also note that – as I am sure you know – we are engaged in a debate in Washington about the appropriate level of funding for research at NIH and other important government services such as funding for education and clean energy. If the House Republican budget were to be enacted, the Office of Management and Budget (OMB) estimates that the number of new grants from NIH for promising research projects would shrink by more than 1,600 in 2014 and by over 16,000 over a decade, potentially curtailing or slowing research to find a cure for Alzheimer's disease, cancer, and CFS. I will continue to fight to cut the deficit and build a stronger economy through balanced deficit reduction that asks all Americans to shoulder their responsibility and pay their fair share of taxes, cuts spending, and invests in areas critical to job creation, innovation, and growth. But you should know that this is an area of considerable disagreement between my Administration and many Republicans in Congress.

I have asked Nancy-Ann to stay in touch with Dr. Collins at NIH and Dr. Koh at HHS about my interest in their efforts on CFS. And I have asked her to update you from time to time. She reports that you are extremely knowledgeable about developments in the research on CFS, so I hope you will keep in touch with us as well.

Sincerely,

Unfulfilled Commitments/Broken Promises: The NIH and Chronic Fatigue Syndrome After Twenty-Five Years[235]

Cort Johnson | December 22, 2013 | U.S.

National Institutes of Health (NIH)

The NIH, with its 30 billion dollar budget, is easily the biggest medical research funder in the world. Buoyed by powerful supporters on the Hill, the NIH has had a remarkable ride over the past 20 years, with its budget (not accounting for inflation) tripling over the past 15 years.

NIH Total Funding

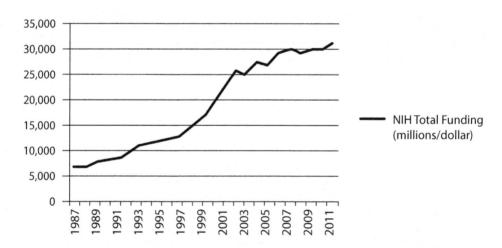

Funding for the NIH has increased nearly fivefold since it began funding ME/CFS in 1987. The NIH, to put it plainly, has been rather flush. The last twenty years have been a good time to be a medical researcher.

---

235 Excerpted and adapted from the original article written by Cort Johnson, www.cortjohnson.org/blog/2013/12/22/
unfulfilled-commitments-broken-promises-nih-chronic-fatigue-syndrome-twenty-five-years (accessed June 20, 2016).
All the NIH information is derived from report.nih.gov/categorical_spending.aspx (accessed March 1, 2016).

NIH Funding Goes Up/Chronic Fatigue Syndrome Funding Goes Down

From 1987 to 1995, the rate of growth in research funding for CFS equaled or exceeded the rate of growth in NIH funding. Around 1995, however, something happened: From 1995 to 2002, ME/CFS funding remained flat, which meant that, accounting for inflation, it declined. Ironically, the plateau in ME/CFS funding roughly coincides with an enormous increase in the NIH's budget that began around 1997.

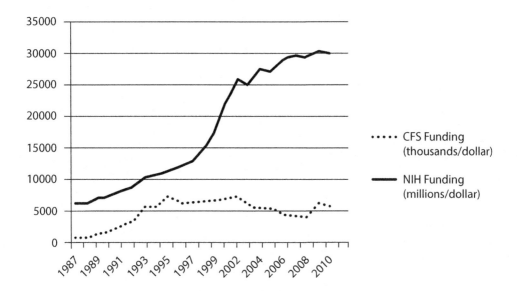

As NIH funding levels explode, funding declines for chronic fatigue syndrome[236] [This translates to over $30 billion total for NIH funding at its peak and $6 million for CFS funding in the same timeframe.]

Ill-Fated Move

One particularly ill-fated move at the end of this period cemented chronic fatigue syndrome's position as little more than an afterthought at the NIH. The transfer of the CFS research program from the powerful National Institutes of Allergy and Infectious Diseases (NIAID) to the small Office of Research on Women's Health (ORWH) in the early 2000s began a decline in its funding, from which it has not recovered.

---

236 The chart has two scales in order to get the CFS figures on it; NIH funding is in millions of dollars, and the CFS funding is in thousands of dollars.

Not only was the ORWH not given any direct funding for CFS, but the funding mechanism instituted (a consortium of institutes tasked with funding a disorder they had no direct responsibility for) heralded a dramatic decline in funding as could have been predicted.

Over the next five years, NIH funding increased 20 percent while funding for chronic fatigue syndrome funding fell almost 50 percent, hitting its nadir in 2008. In 2009/2010, the NIH halted the slide by returning funding (not accounting for inflation) to 2003 levels.

Chronic Fatigue Syndrome Gets Lost

From 1997 to 2002, the NIH underwent the most rapid budget growth in its history, almost doubling its budget in five years.

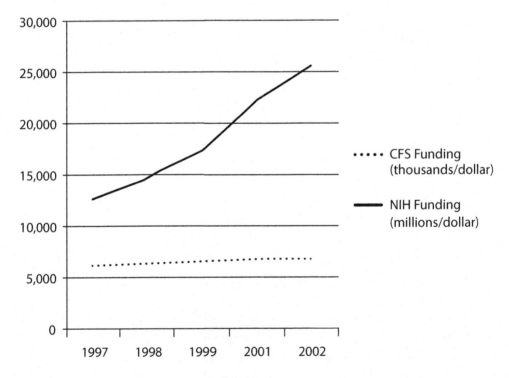

Chronic fatigue syndrome loses ground as the NIH coffers fill.[237]

---

237 The chart has two scales in order to get the CFS figures on it; NIH funding is in millions of dollars, and the CFS funding is in thousands of dollars.

Adjusting for Inflation Reveals Large Drop in Funding Over Time

Adjusting for inflation using the U.S. consumer price index relative to 1987 (the year the NIH program on ME/CFS started), we see that, in real terms, the NIH is currently [2013] spending about as much money on ME/CFS as it did back in 1992, only five years after it began funding CFS research.

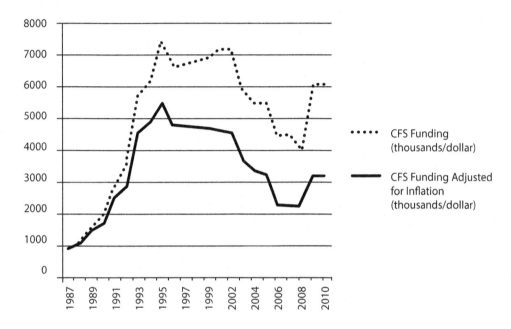

Adjusting for Inflation Reveals Large Drop in Funding over Time

Similar Pattern in Chronic Fatigue Syndrome Studies

The pattern of studies funded is similar. The number of NIH-funded ME/CFS studies peaked in 2001 and underwent a steep decline as the ORWH fumbled its commitment to this disorder.

The increased number of NIH-funded studies from 1996 to 2001 was almost certainly due to the CFS research centers.[238] Their closure around the year 2000 forced ME/CFS researchers to submit their grants to the Chronic Fatigue Syndrome Special Emphasis Panel, which ironically has few, if any, ME/CFS experts on it. Without the insulation of the special CFS research centers, ME/CFS grant approvals fell precipitously.

Without spikes from the neuro-immune grant in 2006 and several XMRV studies in 2011, the trend in studies would have remained flat. [XMRV studies investigated a possible retrovirus as a factor in ME/CFS.]

NIH Funded ME/CFS Studies
(1988-2011)

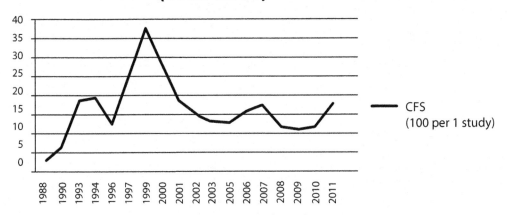

A similar pattern prevails with chronic fatigue syndrome studies.

---

238 The NIAID (National Institute of Allergy and Infectious Diseases) chose to fund three CFS Cooperative Research Centers from 1998-2002. Each center proposed a different model for CFS. A University of Washington center, led by Dr. Dedra Buchwald, adhered to a psychiatric, perception-based model. A New Jersey clinic, headed by Dr. Ben Natelson, researched neurological, autonomic nervous system dysfunction. A Miami center, headed by Dr. Nancy Klimas, favored a system and organic model, focusing on immunology, circulatory dysfunction, and coping strategies. In concert, the three models provided the NIAID with a multidisciplinary approach to CFS. Yet by 2002, the NIAID decided to not renew the funding for the three centers. That money was sent back into the NIAID budget to be spent on other issues. www.cfidsreport.com/Articles/NIH/NIH_CFS_2.htm (accessed Dec 2015).

Looking Back at 1992

What was happening in 1992, the last year, adjusted for inflation, in which the NIH was spending similar amounts of money on ME/CFS as it is today?

In 1992, federal estimates suggested chronic fatigue syndrome was a rare disease, and "yuppie flu" was not necessarily considered to be a misnomer. None of the supposed building blocks for ME/CFS – including the Fukuda definition; the federal advisory committee (CFSAC); the special review panel for CFS grants (CFS SEP) – that were designed to foster further development in this field, had occurred.

The field was almost wholly unformed in 1992. Of the 6160 citations PubMed pulled up for a chronic fatigue syndrome search on Dec 8th, 2013, only 500 (about 8 percent) had been produced by 1992.

In 1992, Manu's overview of all of thirty-two studies[239] indicated that most people with ME/CFS were white middle-aged women with abnormal personality traits and high rates of somatoform disorder. Higgins called CFS a depressive disorder,[240] Simon Wessely was trying to measure fatigue, and Bill Reeves published his first paper on CFS.

Epstein-Barr Virus was a hot topic. One author asked if CFS was an "epidemic," and another study indicated CFS was "rare"[241] (only 1 of 13,538 people examined had it). The following year, the CDC estimated that two to seven people out of 100,000 had chronic fatigue syndrome: ME/CFS was considered a rare disease.

Flash Forward Twenty Years

It wasn't until Jason's 1999 paper[242] indicated that approximately 800,000 Americans had chronic fatigue syndrome that researchers began to be aware of its impact. A CDC prevalence paper in 2003 concluded CFS was "a major public health problem."[243] A 2004 CDC paper indicated that productivity losses caused by CFS ran to the tune of 9.1 billion dollars a year.[244] A 2008 Jason paper[245] estimated both direct and indirect costs to the U.S. from ME/CFS at about 20 billion dollars.

---

239 www.ncbi.nlm.nih.gov/pubmed/1338059 (accessed July 11, 2016).

240 www.ncbi.nlm.nih.gov/pubmed/1548851 (accessed July 11, 2016).

241 www.ncbi.nlm.nih.gov/pubmed/1329134 (accessed July 11, 2016).

242 Jason LA, Richman JA, Rademaker AW, Jordan KM, Plioplys AV, Taylor RR, McCready W, Huang CF, and Plioplys S. 1999. "A community-based study of chronic fatigue syndrome." Archives of Internal Medicine 159(18):2129-2137.

243 Reyes M, Nisenbaum R, Hoaglin DC, Unger ER, Emmons C, Randall B, Stewart JA, Abbey S, Jones JF, Gantz N, Minden S, and Reeves WC. 2003. "Prevalence and incidence of chronic fatigue syndrome in Wichita, Kansas." Archives of Internal Medicine 163(13):1530-1536.

244 Reynolds KJ, Vernon SD, Bouchery E, and Reeves WC. 2004. "The economic impact of chronic fatigue syndrome. Cost Effectiveness and Resource Allocation." 2(4).

245 Jason LA, Benton MC, Valentine L, Johnson A, and Torres-Harding, S. 2008. "The economic impact of ME/CFS: Individual and societal costs." Dynamic Medicine 7(6).

It appears that none of this made any difference to the NIH. Studies demonstrating dramatically increased incidence of a disorder should, one would think, attract more resources, but that was not to be. In the most real terms of all – money spent – chronic fatigue syndrome remains the same, small, poorly funded illness it was in 1992. It might as well still be the "yuppie flu" many considered it to be in 1992.

The NIH has funded one grant package (request for applications) for chronic fatigue syndrome in the last twenty years.

❧

A Commitment to What?

The NIH's "commitment" to "enhancing the health" of people with chronic fatigue syndrome has declined dramatically over time.

Funding for chronic fatigue syndrome made up less than .04 percent of the NIH's budget in 1992. By 2012, the NIH was devoting less than half of that, or less than .02 percent of its budget, to ME/CFS. If the condition had just maintained its meager share of the NIH's budget from 1992, the NIH would be spending 10-12 million dollars annually on this disorder today.

The NIH was providing about $400 in funding per patient in 1993. It's now providing about $6 a patient. (If the NIH currently provided the same funding per patient in 2013 as it did in 1993, the ME/CFS research budget would be around $400,000,000).

NIH Does Not Consider Need in Its Funding Decisions

One might think that "need" should play a role in the funding decisions of an agency tasked with enhancing the health of Americans, and at times it may. But not with chronic fatigue syndrome.

In 1993, when the NIH was spending 6 million dollars on ME/CFS, the CDC estimated that out of every 100,000 people, somewhere between two and seven people had chronic fatigue syndrome. Studies now indicate ME/CFS affects about 60 times as many people as was believed in 1993. (That would be one of every 300 people in the US). But the 985,000 more people believed to have ME/CFS might as well not exist. The NIH is still providing funding commensurate with the 15,000-person disorder ME/CFS was thought to be in 1993.

Conclusion

Some progress was made recently. The fact that a million dollars was allocated to produce a clinical definition of ME/CFS suggests the NIH may be starting to unclench its tight hold on its purse. With the FDA taking up chronic fatigue syndrome as well as the numerous advocacy efforts over the past couple of years, the NIH may be getting enough pressure to improve its commitment to ME/CFS.

Compared to the needs present (demonstrated by NIH and CDC funded studies[246]), this is a baby step, however. The NIH still has twenty years of ignoring the health needs of a significant part of the population to answer for.

At some point, someone or some group of people at the agency may decide that people with chronic fatigue syndrome are worth it and that need does count for something in their funding decisions. They may take a stand that the NIH is committed to improving the health of everybody under its watch, not just the disorders it wants to study, but everyone – no matter how difficult or confusing or poorly named a disorder they may be suffering.

---

246 A list of publications by the CDC CFS Public Health Research Program from 2009 to 2013 is at www.cdc.gov/cfs/publications/index.html.

Advocate Jennie Spotila has written a number of articles on yearly NIH funding. A recent one analyzed NIH funding for 2015 with links to the articles she wrote for 2011 to 2014. www.occupycfs.com/2016/02/17/2015-nih-spending-on-mecfs-studies (accessed July 11, 2016).

CHAPTER 7

The Good Fight

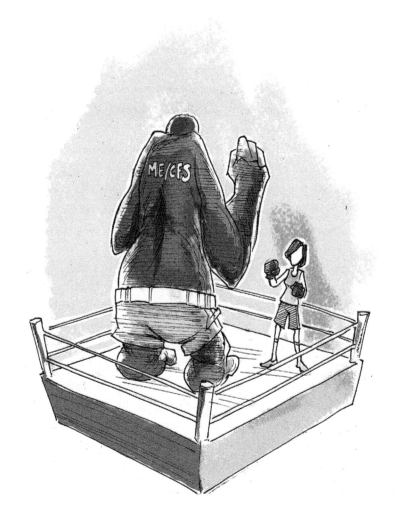

Claudia's Story: A Race to Action and The Unpredictable Journey

Claudia Goodell | September 2013 | New Mexico, U.S.

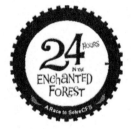

A Race to Solve CFS

My hope is that by telling my story to healthy people like you, the world will begin to understand that ME/CFS can strike anyone at any time – men and women; adults and children; and it can forever strip away the life and people you love.

ME/CFS is a thief of time that reduces a full functional day to a fraction of a healthy person's. It is an energy crisis that forces us to sacrifice the things that bring us joy; things we often take for granted when well. ME/CFS has relegated approximately one million Americans and millions worldwide to be partial-participants in life. It has undermined our ability to contribute and forces us to be a cost to society because of the lack of effective treatments or cure.

The financial cost to societies created by these failures is exorbitant, and ME/CFS affects everyone in some way.

This is why I wanted to engage the public in an exciting fundraising event, which I'll tell you about later. Things are slowly improving, and there are many opportunities to contribute to the ME/CFS cause, ensuring the bright future we envision around the globe.

My name is Claudia Goodell, and I was diagnosed with chronic fatigue syndrome and fibromyalgia in 2005 by a rheumatologist. Although my doctors and I suspected CFS and fibromyalgia beginning in 2003, these diagnoses were not confirmed for two more years: I received the final diagnosis only after we had ruled out every other possible cause. Following this, the rheumatologist said she didn't need to see me again because there was nothing more she could do for me. I was forty-five years old at that time.

Mine was not the sudden onset you may hear about more often, but a slow and gradual one into serious dysfunction. My diagnosis took nearly twenty years and was complicated by a history of thyroid dysfunction, periodontal disease, two viral infections in 1985 at age twenty-five, and endometriosis leading to a hysterectomy in my thirties.

During all of those years, I was shuffled from one specialist to another so they could assess me and offer treatment within their specialty. If I had followed all the different medical advice I received, I would have taken a dozen various hardcore medications, in a feeble attempt to mitigate the underlying symptoms. As I have seen in many other ME/CFS patients, doing this can further complicate an already bad situation.

Although I am learning to accept my existence with a very restricting chronic illness, I still wage war against the total lack of control I have over my own life. I am a keen person trapped in a dysfunctional mind/body. I am treading in a society, government, and healthcare system that remains mostly unaware of, or misinformed about, ME/CFS and the scope of its violation.

❧

I have a bachelor's degree in psychology with a minor in American Sign Language, and a master's degree in audiology. In wellness, I enjoyed many athletic accomplishments, but now I have found a new love and skill as an artist, which I find therapeutic. My health and family remain my priorities, and as an artist, I can work with my experiences and project them onto a canvas. I am inspired by nature and music and paint in a newly developed style called Curvismo, which transforms real objects into abstract movement.

I have always considered myself a pioneer of change and have applied my influence to situations that require forward thinking. Bringing something new to the table was a challenge I enjoyed. I co-authored a publication in my undergraduate program in psychology and initiated a new course in counseling for the audiology program curriculum.

My only child was born shortly after my eighteenth birthday, and her father and I were married for eight years. It was the year after our divorce that I became ill with viral infections, later diagnosed as Epstein Barr and Herpes Simplex.

At age twenty-six, I met my current husband, and we began to enjoy an active and athletic lifestyle together.

I began to notice a significant decline in my energy level and general wellbeing despite our healthy ways. Because of my youth, I attributed my periodic exhaustion to being a single mom, dating, working, attending college, and then graduate school. Although, as I look back to try and understand what happened to my good health, I question my exposure to the odor and powder residue of hearing aid plastic that I was exposed to while working as a technical audiologist in an open-format hearing aid factory. Two others out of the hundred workers there also became chronically ill – one of those diagnosed with CFS.

My work, family, love for travel, and volunteering for other causes had kept me happy and busy, but as time went on, my symptoms became more pervasive, and I slowly lost my ability to continue this life I loved so much.

❧

ME/CFS reduced me from the rewarding position of a professional to the unfamiliar territory of being largely dependent on my husband for income and health insurance. My only means of contribution was the tedious, and for me, unrewarding duties of cooking and light housekeeping (which even now, I am sometimes unable to complete due to my level of function).

Pacing and conserving my energy have become a daily and life-long practice. Relapse from using more energy will bring on some of these symptoms and aggravate others. At times, the onset or worsening of them can even be caused by simple reading and/ or conversation.

My major symptoms and overlapping conditions include:

- Pain

- Fever

- Exhaustion

- Dehydration

- Chronic infections

- Swollen lymph nodes

- Food and environmental sensitivities

- Cognitive and/or memory problems

- Liver function and blood abnormalities

- Light headedness

- Sleep disorder

- Chronic migraines

- Thyroid dysfunction

- Heavy metal toxicity

- Vitamin D insufficiency

- Irritable bowel syndrome (IBS)

- Temporomandibular disorders (TMD)

- Post-exertional malaise (PEM) (a period of intense exhaustion and other symptoms lasting more than 24 hours following physical/ mental exertion)

- Postural Orthostatic Tachycardia (POTS) (a sudden drop in blood pressure and increase in heart rate when in an upright position)

In addition to over-the-counter pain relievers and a few supplements, I rely on only two prescription drugs: one to treat my migraines, the other for thyroid function. Western medicine has had little else to offer me as a solution.

At my worst, I was barely functional – bedbound or housebound much of the time; twenty percent on the Karnofsky Scale (as adapted for ME/CFS). Over the years, I improved to about forty percent, which felt like a great deal. I accomplished this by not working, staying at home most of the time, doing only minimal household chores, and trying alternative care. By living in this way and sacrificing other activities, I have been able to continue to develop as an artist and occasionally ride a bike and do other athletic things – even though I rarely escape without some consequences of a flare-up complete with exhaustion, fever, swollen lymph nodes, pain, and migraine.

❧

In 2012, I received the additional clinical diagnosis of Lyme disease, which has created complication and confusion. Because of the controversial nature surrounding chronic Lyme, CFS, and fibromyalgia, a clear diagnosis remains uncertain. According to certain CFS diagnostic criteria, people can be diagnosed with Lyme disease and CFS if the Lyme disease does not resolve after traditional treatment. Of course, what matters most is finding appropriate therapy and feeling better.

I can happily say today that after following the treatments recommended by a holistic neurosurgeon in my hometown, I am about sixty percent functioning on that Karnofsky Scale, and the treatments seem to have a cumulative effect. My improvement is gaining momentum. I still have to pace myself, and I have limited my activities to do what I consider worthwhile.

However, each stage of this chronic illness brings different challenges. The one that is most difficult for me is the separateness it creates in my relationships, including the most important one to me – my relationship with my husband. He has always had a very active lifestyle and continues on as an endurance athlete. I am unable to participate in that part of his life, which is very hard on both of us.

Although this illness has stripped away much of what I can do, I try to remember that I am so much more than what I do or how I do it. The beliefs I hold about how to value myself within society now are in conflict because our culture generally defines people by their careers and accomplishments.

It is difficult to remember that the illness is only part of my experience, and that it does not define who I am. Working in advocacy makes this especially challenging because of the constant focus on the topic, but the overall intention is to create a better future for us all.

❧

With public recognition and support of complex chronic illnesses like these, progress is accelerated for treatment, cure, and prevention.

That is why in late 2009, I partnered with a bike race director (who also has this illness) to organize a fundraiser for it. Together with several volunteers, we created "24 Hours in the Enchanted Forest: A Race to Solve CFS." It is a 24-hour mountain bike race for healthy competitors and a weekend festival held in the New Mexico Zuni Mountains.

It was a challenge for some fellow patients to understand why a mountain bike race was a perfect venue for creating awareness about the illness, when most were unable to even attend. The event required travel and was held in a primitive, rugged location. Others commented that they appreciated the optimism and hope that it provided.

Throughout the weekend event, a patient advocate from The CFIDS Association of America[247] and I educated 300 captive racers, as well as 200 of their family members and friends about myalgic encephalomyelitis/chronic fatigue syndrome (ME/CFS). We were elated that these healthy people really had a sincere interest in helping the initiative and in learning about this disease that has remained off society's radar for decades.

Unbelievably in 2010, this was the first grassroots fundraiser to benefit the CFIDS Association in their twenty-two-year history. Over the next three years, the event raised a total of $17,500 for research, which was donated to the association. Creating, organizing and running this event was the most empowering thing I had done since becoming ill.

Unfortunately, after each year's event, as patient coordinators, we endured predictable but lengthy relapses. They would only subside in time for us to begin planning the next year's festival. Sadly, one patient volunteer fell into a regression from which he has yet to recover two years later. This is one of the reasons we need healthy individuals to become involved in fundraisers for our cause.

Although my role with the bike race concluded after three years, I continued to partner with the CFIDS Association on various projects with a common goal of advocacy and fundraising. Currently, I manage the Facebook page "Race to Solve CFS." Its goal is to increase knowledge and understanding about this illness and to engage the public.

We have proven it can be an exciting, unpredictable and challenging ride.

❧

Update | January 2016 | Note from Valerie

Claudia has advised me that she now supports several national advocacy groups and has served on two working groups for the chronic fatigue syndrome advisory committee (CFSAC) to the CDC. She continues to manage her Facebook page and is working with others to address the current political obstacles.

---

247 Now known as Solve ME/CFS Initiative.

Chronic Fatigue Syndrome:
A Celebrated Author's Untold Tale [248]

Aaron Gell | Laura Hillenbrand Interview
December 2010 | Washington D.C., U.S.

*Laura Hillenbrand spins irresistible accounts of heroic figures undaunted by
long odds. But she's frequently so unwell that she scarcely leaves home.*

❦

On a recent night, Laura Hillenbrand lay in bed dreaming of somersaults in the powder-blue bedroom she shares with her husband, Borden Flanagan, in their modest, yellow row house in Upper Northwest Washington, D.C. Dozing in REM sleep, the author of the acclaimed horse-racing history *Seabiscuit* (2001) imagined herself tucking her head to her chest, tipping forward, and letting her hips and legs pull her all the way over. A playful-seeming reverie, conjured out of the mists of an athletic childhood.

But then she didn't stop turning. She couldn't stop, flipping and flipping in a torment of constant motion.

Most of Hillenbrand's dreams are like this now, strange, panicked scenarios cobbled together somewhere inside her head – plummeting airplanes and storm-tossed ships are other recurring motifs – to help her process the strange and excruciating physical sensations that she lives with more or less all the time.

Hillenbrand has chronic fatigue syndrome (CFS), a cruel medical condition with an unfortunate name that fails utterly to do justice to an often debilitating array of so-far unexplained symptoms, including muscle pain, unrelenting exhaustion, digestive problems, environmental hypersensitivity, occasional fevers, and vertigo. "Laura is on the more severe end of the spectrum," says Fred Gill, MD, a noted specialist in infectious disease at the National Institutes of Health, who treated her for many years. "It's very serious. It stops people's lives."

"It's so frightening and hellish and disorienting," Hillenbrand says, "and on top of that there's this layer of gripping fear, because I don't know what will happen next – if it will get worse." She's sitting at her dining room table, one foot folded under her knee, looking like the picture of health, pretty and cheerful, in a black blouse, metal-rimmed glasses, and hoop earrings.

It's early afternoon, her best time of day. Since she first came down with the disease in 1987, the severity of her symptoms has shifted without warning or explanation, and

---

248 Originally published on ELLE.COM – reprinted with permission.

the ferocious relapse that began three years ago, as she was deep into the research phase of her second book, seems gradually to be abating. Over the years, Hillenbrand has often gone for long stretches without so much as leaving her room, but she's feeling strong enough lately to receive a visitor. Aside from Flanagan, a soft-spoken professor of political philosophy, who passes through from time to time; her new doctor, who by necessity does house calls; and one social visit a few weeks back, I'm the only person she's seen in months.

"When I was really dizzy, I was almost screaming with fear because it's so thoroughly disorienting, but it's not too bad right now," she says, smiling. "Things are moving in a liquid kind of way, and the floor is slanting and it looks like a really bad computer-generated image. Nothing looks real."

It's only then that I realize Hillenbrand has remained perfectly still – keeping her hands folded in her lap – since we sat down an hour before. Suddenly imagining how my own gestures must look to her, I try not to make any abrupt movements.

Reviewers and fans of *Seabiscuit*, which was dubbed "a model of sports writing at its best" by *The New York Times* before going on to sell some three million copies and spawn an Oscar-nominated feature film, praised the book's descriptive immediacy and the author's spooky ability to put the reader right in the saddle with jockey Red Pollard atop the squat, famously graceless horse as they thundered around the far turn in the legendary race at Santa Anita in 1940.

Only when Hillenbrand began to talk openly about her affliction did it become apparent that her astonishing prose wasn't simply a stylistic choice or a literary flourish but a psychic imperative. "I think riding along with those jockeys, creating that sense of movement and exhilaration, might have been the product of her desire to experience that in her own life, because she was living such a constrained existence," notes Jonathan Karp, the book's editor, who is now publisher of Simon & Schuster.

"It was all about motion," agrees Hillenbrand, "all about what I can't do."

It was during her research for *Seabiscuit*, poring over reports of the horse's match races in yellowing old 1930s broadsheets she'd found on eBay, that Hillenbrand first took note of another preoccupation of the era's West Coast sports pages: the story of Louis Zamperini, an incorrigibly rebellious teenager who competed as a miler in the Berlin Olympics. Zamperini's exploits, she thought, might make a good subject for her next book. Only later did she learn of the subsequent twists his life had taken: After enlisting in the Army Air Corps, he became a bombardier and was shot down over the Pacific. Somehow he swam from the wrecked plane and wound up drifting on a small life raft 2,000 miles across shark-filled waters for forty-seven days. Eventually, he and a fellow airman were spotted and captured by the Japanese, who interned them in a series of horrific POW camps. Fourteen months after the U.S. government declared him dead, Zamperini returned home to a hero's welcome – followed by a traumatic, whiskey-soaked readjustment. When Hillenbrand reached out to him, he was eighty-seven and living in California.

Zamperini's amazing tale is at the center of *Unbroken*, which arrives in bookstores November 16, [2010]. In it, Hillenbrand demonstrates a dazzling ability – one *Seabiscuit* only hinted at – to make the tale leap off the page. "It's like she sees in color and the rest of us see in black and white," Flanagan marvels.

"When I read it, I felt like I was right back there," says Zamperini, now ninety-three. "She brought my buddies back to life. I believe she actually relived every moment I lived in the prison camp."

Part of the book's power is attributable to Hillenbrand's tenacity as a researcher, her eagerness to immerse herself in the minutiae of, say, the cockpit layout of a B-24 or the physical effects of dehydration. She scoured countless war-crime affidavits and conducted hundreds of interviews, including more than seventy with Louis himself, many while she lay in bed. "I loved her relentlessness," he says. "She has a sweet personality and a soft demeanor, and yet her questioning was very intense."

Indeed, the sheer depth of her research allowed her to unearth visceral details Zamperini himself had forgotten or blocked out. "At one point I asked him, 'Were your eyes hurting because of the glare off the ocean?' He said, 'Come to think of it, yeah, we had headaches all the time.'"

And this is where Hillenbrand's illness actually serves her work. Compared to her own situation, the deprivations of a lost raft or the brutality of a prison camp can seem like an escape. "I climb into these stories because I don't want to be here," she says. "I don't want to be in this body and I don't want to be in this place, so I'm on that raft. It takes a while to get my concentration to that level, and then I lose all track of time." Which, it seems, is exactly the point.

She also developed a deep kinship with Zamperini and his fellow POWs, much as she did with Seabiscuit – all of them indomitable characters facing incredibly long odds. "I can't compare my experience to theirs, but something I do understand is being in a situation of ultimate desperation, or suffering to the last point of your ability to tolerate it. I can understand how bad it felt, and I can draw strength from the fact that they got through those things. What you feel more than anything else in these situations of great extremity is an experience of terrible aloneness, when you get truly desperate and hopeless, and it's reassuring to see that other people have gone to those places and come back."

As a child growing up in Bethesda, Maryland – the daughter of a lobbyist father and child psychologist mother – Hillenbrand was a hardcore jock. She swam competitively, spent her weekends riding and grooming horses on her dad's farm in rural Maryland, and became such an avid tennis player that when she enrolled at Ohio's Kenyon College, she chose a dorm based on its proximity to the courts. She was nineteen when she became ill on a road trip back to school after spring break. Feverish, her glands and stomach swollen, she soon found herself unable to walk, much less attend class, and so withdrew from school and returned home to Maryland. Except for Flanagan, her boyfriend, who stuck by her, Hillenbrand's tight circle of college friends seemed to forget all about her, and her family offered a collective shrug.

The isolation was devastating. "It's like you go to another place, like you're not on this planet anymore," Hillenbrand says. "You reach a level of despair and suffering where you just don't feel like the rest of the world."

"She didn't get the family support she should have," says Hillenbrand's sister Susan Avallon, a script reader. "That's one thing I still feel bad about. It took years, unfortunately, to find out how bad it was. For a long time we just expected she'd get better and go back to college. Then it became clear she wasn't getting better."

Meanwhile, a parade of doctors diagnosed her with strep throat, stress, laziness, anorexia, or depression. One told her, "The only thing wrong with you is an attitude problem."

"I think when Laura was first sick, a lot of them just thought, 'What's this little blond girl doing here in my office claiming illness?'" recalls Flanagan, who moved to Washington soon after his graduation to help care for her. "It's a combination of the arrogance that is an occupational hazard of medicine and a certain degree of sexism."

"In the early years, a lot of very good doctors didn't believe it was a syndrome at all," acknowledges Gill, who over time became one of Hillenbrand's best friends. "Well-meaning people would say, 'You need psychiatric care.'"

Several years later, when she was finally diagnosed with a mysterious new ailment, it was one with a name that sounded to most people like a joke. "Jay Leno was on TV every night calling it the yuppie flu," she recalls. "To think of how much suffering it's caused, just that name, how many people have been alienated from their families or been unable to get disability – that's a source of a lot of anguish and a lot of anger."

In the intervening years, Hillenbrand has experimented with an array of treatments, including steroid hormones, daily vitamin B-12 shots, a gluten-free diet, acupuncture, and Chinese herbal remedies. "They didn't help," she says, "and in some cases made things much worse. So because of the way a seemingly small mistake can land me in bed for years, I've become very conservative. The most effective thing I've done is to learn, through trial and error, how best to manage my body – eating bland, easy-to-digest food, keeping the temperature in the house low, and always stopping myself the moment I feel myself sliding into fatigue."

When possible, she also practices yoga, not only to prevent her muscles from atrophying but to maintain her emotional balance as well. "It's not just the poses, but also the meditation," she says, "and learning and applying the philosophy behind it: acceptance, living in the moment, focusing on being peaceful, being alive to what is beautiful and good all around me."

One night in July 2003, Hillenbrand sat in a corridor of the White House, not far from the East Room, where she'd been invited for a special screening of the film adaptation of *Seabiscuit*. She can't actually watch a bright screen, so while the film unspooled in the forty-seat family theater to an audience that included George W. and Laura Bush, as well as Steven Spielberg, Jeffrey Katzenberg, Tobey Maguire, and director Gary Ross, the author sat gazing out a window onto the Rose Garden. "I was just letting it sink in, and I thought about the years that I was stuck in my mom's house, and how the vertigo was so bad, and how I really had to think of a reason to keep going. It was a wonderful moment, realizing, 'that time is over. I'm in a different place now.'"

Still, the success of *Seabiscuit* didn't change Hillenbrand's circumstances as much as one might expect. She purchased her first home, but it was next door – and more or less identical – to the one she and Flanagan had been renting for years. Financial security was nice; after years in which she often found herself choosing between paying her rent or covering the massive phone bills she racked up doing all those interviews, she no longer had to worry about money. But since there's still no treatment for CFS, once she was diagnosed, her medical bills became quite low. The usual luxuries (travel, clothes, fancy restaurants) hold no appeal, either. The disease complicates digestion, so Hillenbrand's diet is spare and unchanging: Wheatabix and skim milk for breakfast, toast with almond butter and blueberry spread for lunch, and baked chicken with baby-food vegetables for dinner. She spends hours at a time on a balcony just off her office, gazing out at the cemetery behind the house and watching the comings and goings of a variety of animals. "I never move, so they've decided I'm not dangerous," she says, smiling as she relates recent developments involving the Carolina wren Petey, the cardinals Stanley and Gladys, and the squirrels Barnacle, Nosy, and Tum-tum. "They're my buddies."

One of her tricks for staving off depression has been to forswear daytime TV; at night, though, favorites include *30 Rock, So You Think You Can Dance?* and shows about astrophysics on the Science Channel. Her sister Susan mentions another coping mechanism: "When Laura feels really sad, often she will get on the Internet and find a horse that's destined for slaughter and find it a home. To me that says a lot about who she is." She also teamed up with actor Gary Sinise to cofound a charity, Operation International Children, that distributes books and school supplies overseas.

Hillenbrand's only real splurge since what Jonathan Karp describes as publishing's equivalent of "winning the lottery": a chairlift that snakes upstairs from the living room, which she rarely uses because riding it can set off her vertigo as easily as walking downstairs can.

The more significant change *Seabiscuit* wrought involved her sense of self. "Learning I could reach out into the world from here, that was really beautiful," she says the following afternoon, sitting in her office, a small space where she's stowed all the necessary provisions (toaster, mini-fridge, electric kettle, hair dryer) so she can conserve every ounce of available energy for work. "It also brought about a great change in the way I thought about myself. For a long time I felt stuck at nineteen forever, stuck in the way people saw me. It was truly shattering. The book changed my relationship with the world. You can't say I'm lazy."

The experience also made it easier, when she suffered her most recent relapse, to keep fighting. "I'm so impressed with her," Flanagan says, beaming. "I mean, in the beginning, she was sick to the point where it wasn't clear how long she could keep breathing. It was really awful. She was just flat in bed. And as soon as she could sit at the desk, she'd read. But she still couldn't lift her arms to the keyboard. She wrote this book under such extraordinary circumstances. She finished the very first draft basically only being able to move from the bedroom to the desk."

Watching Flanagan and Hillenbrand interact together, it seems clear that since first falling for each other in the campus deli back in 1986 (they bonded over a shared love for the Smiths), they have forged an extraordinary relationship, united in a wearying struggle and leavened with large doses of ironic humor. I ask Flanagan how he's managed to handle the pressure.

"I'm just so awesome," he says jovially.

"He tells me that every day," Hillenbrand jokes.

Flanagan adds, more seriously, "I can't tell you how demoralizing it is to be helpless when somebody you love is suffering. It's tremendously emasculating because the biggest problem you want to solve, you can't, so every day is an experience of failure." It helps, Flanagan says, that even at her sickest, Hillenbrand can be wickedly funny. "One time I remember she had this infection and this awful fever, going up and up and up," he recalls. "And it was 104, I think, and you said, 'When I hit 107, sell.'" They both laugh, a bit darkly.

Despite that levity and the tremendous accomplishment of completing *Unbroken*, which like her debut seems destined for best-seller status and critical acclaim, Hillenbrand still lives a sort of twilight existence, shadowed at all times by fear of the future. Indeed, a few weeks after our interview, I e-mail her with a question. She replies a day later: "In the last few days, my health has taken a sudden, very sharp downturn, and I'm back to being trapped upstairs. I'm scared to death that I'm sliding into another relapse. If you happen upon a magic wand, wave it my way."

Notes Louis Zamperini, "I suffered for a short period of time – her suffering is for life."

exactly

Susan echoes the idea: "She's still on the raft."

"I'm dealing with things that frighten me and with moments that are really miserable," Hillenbrand said when we met. "But overall I feel happy in a way that can't be shaken. A great deal of that is him" – she flicked a smile toward Flanagan. "And a great deal is the writing, because it's the one way in which what I am in my essence can be realized. Everything else has been compromised, but I found a way to be who I really am on the page in a way I can't be in my living-life, and that has made me really, deeply happy."

Singing for a Cause: The Story of Jacqueline and Stephanie Ko

Valerie Free | August 2, 2014 | Canada

In 2013, I was searching for inspirational stories about those who've raised awareness and funding for ME/CFS when a beautiful young lady on a poster caught my attention. The poster announced a unique gala concert in support of the 2013 International ME/CFS & FM Awareness Day on May 12th.

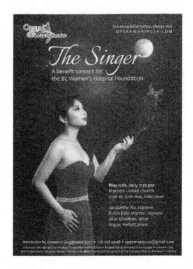

The show – simply titled *The Singer* – was presented by Opera Mariposa in British Columbia, Canada, and simultaneously broadcast live around the world. One hundred percent of ticket sales would go to support a new initiative, the Complex Chronic Diseases Program, located at BC Women's Hospital. This groundbreaking program (the first of its kind in Canada) is dedicated to helping men, women and children throughout BC with chronic, life-altering diseases like ME/CFS.

With my curiosity piqued, I wondered why anyone, especially an opera company, would be so committed and generous to a cause such as ours. To date, large ME/CFS events have been quite rare in Canada, even for International Awareness Day.

After the concert, I delved a little deeper, learning that it had been a great success and had raised $10,000 for the new specialty program. I began to get a more complete picture of the motivation and the hearts behind the event.

The picture-perfect young woman on the poster is Jacqueline Ko, at the time twenty-one years old. This Chinese-Canadian soprano is not only an award-winning opera singer, but she is also the founder and artistic director of Opera Mariposa. She had decided to hold a concert on Awareness Day for a very simple reason: She herself has had ME/CFS since the age of six.

With *The Singer*, Jacqueline wanted to use her passion for music to raise awareness for this devastating disease. "By holding a concert on International ME/CFS and FM Awareness Day, I hope to not only inform people about this illness, but support sorely needed treatment and research," she said in the concert media release. In blog posts on the Opera Mariposa website, Jacqueline explained that *The Singer* was a way for her to tell the story of her fight with ME/CFS. By choosing songs that were deeply meaningful to her, she took her audience on an emotional journey, conveying both her struggle with the disease and the deep love of music that had seen her through the darkest of times.

Initially, I contacted Opera Mariposa in the hopes of simply sharing the concert news release or a blog segment with my readers. I quickly received a response from the company's communications director, Stephanie Ko, Jacqueline's older sister by two years.

Stephanie, a lovely and articulate twenty-four-year-old, was kind enough to offer an interview. This quickly turned into a series of phone conversations and a personal connection, which we have maintained since. My first surprise in learning about this May 12 event was to discover that Stephanie also suffers from the illness.

୭୨

Stephanie and Jacqueline fell ill in 1998 when they were eight and six respectively, beginning with pneumonia and a diagnosis of mono. Both were academically advanced students and highly gifted learners. Stephanie had already skipped a grade, so she was in grade four, while Jacqueline was in grade one.

The girls never recovered their pre-illness health, Stephanie recalls, and eventually had a brutal relapse that robbed them of their remaining health. With no conclusive diagnosis in hand, doctors ultimately suggested depression and school avoidance. How could these little girls possibly be so sick if they could occasionally make appearances at school? Rumors that the sisters' excellent marks were due to parental pressure started to circulate. Maybe they were just acting out; maybe they were having a nervous breakdown – an all too familiar theme in children battling with ME/CFS – skepticism all around and lack of support.

Alone in her search, Stephanie and Jacqueline's mother came across myalgic encephalomyelitis/chronic fatigue syndrome, which seemed to fit her daughters' symptoms.

A few years later, Mrs. Ko found a reputable pediatrician who helped with a final diagnosis of CFS. He remained the girls' primary doctor until he retired, and he kept the maturing young ladies in his practice even when they advanced beyond the ages normally treated by a pediatrician. Due to the lack of knowledge among medical professionals about ME/CFS, there was simply nowhere to refer the girls.

This would eventually become one of the motivations for the benefit concert that started this story: Jacqueline and Stephanie had seen firsthand the need to increase awareness and education about their illness.

Sadly, a diagnosis didn't provide a solution for the sisters. By grade eight, the severity of their illness forced them to end their traditional schooling. In the struggle to continue their education, they had forced their bodies beyond their capacity and caused a total collapse from over-exertion. Years later, their attempts at home-schooling met with the same result, and today they still look forward to completing their high school diplomas when their health returns to a better status.

Despite all this, something wonderful was unfolding.

Jacqueline had just started singing lessons before her relapse. It turned out she had a natural gift for music and singing – particularly opera. As her proud sister was happy to share with me, Jacqueline Ko is actually something of a prodigy: With brief singing lessons as seldom as once every few months, she was able to advance her skill and technique with unusual speed, and her teacher identified her vocal range as almost double the standard size for a fully trained opera singer. Jacqueline could learn complex music just by listening to it a few times, and during a single lesson – punctuated by frequent rests – she could leap ahead without even practicing.

Why could Jacqueline sing like this and not be able to go to school? This is actually a contradiction associated with many ME/CFS cases that very few, if any, healthy people can understand.

Science has revealed that the brains of people with ME/CFS work differently than those of healthy people. The illness affects cognition in many ways: impaired memory, difficulty multi-tasking, slowed mental processing, and the decreased ability to work with numbers, to name but a few. Some people have told me that they lost certain developed skills, such as the ability to speak a second language in which they used to be fluent. Depending on the severity of illness, learning new skills can be challenging, too. But for some, certain tasks may be much easier.

At their current ages of twenty-three and twenty-five, Jacqueline and Stephanie are mature beyond their years. With their extraordinary talents and determination, as well as a supportive environment, they have accomplished many things – all in spite of over sixteen years of serious chronic illness. They must still live within the constraints of ME/CFS, doing everything according to the rhythms set by their condition.

Despite all their lost years, Stephanie still won national awards for her writing while Jacqueline received multiple awards and scholarships for her singing talent. In 2012, Jacqueline formed Opera Mariposa to create performance opportunities for other young and emerging artists, and the company has gone on to earn rave reviews in local and national media.

Following the success of *The Singer*, Jacqueline decided to make her Awareness shows an annual event. In May 2014, she wrote, directed and performed *The Butterfly*, an original Broadway revue show in which she told her life story through music; it raised over $13,000 for treatment and research for ME/CFS, fibromyalgia and other chronic, complex conditions.

Jacqueline and Stephanie have missed out on many things their peers take for granted, including getting driver's licenses, moving away from home, and completing post-secondary education. However, they recognize that their struggles have had a hand in shaping who they are today. To many, they are bright, shining stars offering beauty and hope for those with ME/CFS who are still left in the dark.

The sisters remain determined to not only pursue their dreams, but to use their talents to help others. When I asked Stephanie about their hopes and aspirations for the future, she said that they dream of continued education, increased independence, and travel – so that Jacqueline can further her singing career. With fewer health constraints, they would love to expand the scope of Opera Mariposa and pursue their individual careers, as a performer and as a writer, without limits.[249]

---

249 To get updates on Jacqueline's and Stephanie's endeavors, visit operamariposa.com (accessed June 2016).

A Young Man, A Big Disease and A Big Idea[250]

Llewellyn King | June 2013 | U.S.

We expect big ideas in computers, social networking, and music to come from young people; in medicine, less so. That is, until Ryan Prior.

Prior, twenty-three, is from Atlanta, Ga. and suffers from CFS, a ghastly disease of the immune system…His story begins on Oct. 22, 2006. Like many victims, he knows exactly when he was felled; when normal life had to be abandoned. He entered a dark world where good times are marked in hours; where bad times are days, weeks, or months in darkened, silent rooms.

Prior was student president at Warner Robins High School in Warner Robins, Ga., captain of the cross-country team, and was taking three advanced placement courses. "My goal was to attend Duke University or West Point with the ultimate goal of becoming an Army Ranger," he said.

But by Nov. 15, 2006, Prior had to quit school. Under a Georgia plan for educating sick students, "My physics teacher taught me heat transfer while I was lying on the couch," he said. But he slept through calculus.

Ryan still hoped to make it as an athlete. During a brief respite, he was back on his soccer varsity squad. But it was a disaster. He had been put on a drug that provided a short energy boost. "I went to a practice and played for about five minutes. I did OK for the first minute. After five minutes, I realized I had to stagger off the field as soon as possible. If I didn't get off voluntarily, I knew I would have to be carried off soon after."

After seeing fifteen doctors who knew little or nothing about the disease, Prior found one who has helped him. Now, he says, he functions ninety percent of the time if he takes fifteen to twenty pills a day and avoids overdoing it. Ultimately, he graduated Phi Beta Kappa from the University of Georgia.

But it's the almost complete ignorance of CFS by most doctors that has set Prior on his big idea project. He is making a documentary film about the disease [*Forgotten Plague: M.E. and the Future of Medicine* – see next essay] with young filmmakers and with a $12,000 budget. He hopes the film will lead to $50,000 in funding to create "an eight-week summer fellowship program" for medical students, between their first and second years, to study with recognized experts in CFS. They would, according to Prior, provide each student with a stipend of $5,000 for the eight weeks.

---

250 Excerpted and adapted from journalist, L. King's article, "A Young Man, A Big Disease, and a Big Idea" originally published on The White House Chronicle, June 17, 2013. www.whchronicle.com/?p=1509 (accessed July 15, 2016).

Prior has compiled a list of nine doctors or clinics preeminent in the field who he believes would accept the fellows. The end result: a flow of young doctors with knowledge of CFS and new ideas…

If Prior's plan works, it may lead to a much larger training effort in the United States and across the world.

"The message is simple: American history has progressed in a logical line from women's rights, through civil rights, then to gay rights," Prior says, adding, "Medical history has a similar process of ridicule, repression, and ultimate acceptance: MS, AIDS, and now we want CFS to be the next step."

The Making of *Forgotten Plague:*
M.E. and the Future of Medicine

Ryan Prior | December 2013 | Georgia, U.S.
Introduction by Valerie Free

Ryan Prior explains why he and Nicole Castillo decided to make a movie about ME/CFS and why they have formed the Blue Ribbon Foundation.

೧৲

A year ago, I wrote a story for *USA Today* about my experience with ME/CFS that changed the trajectory of my life. The response to my story taught me just how neglected the ME/CFS patient population is. My plan after graduating from the University of Georgia had been to write about politics. I thought I would move back to Washington to work as a political journalist or as a speechwriter for a congressman or senator.

But my story on ME/CFS kept tugging at me. If I didn't become that political writer, there was still a long line of applicants behind me who could easily and eagerly take up that mantle. To me, it felt far more exhilarating to break new ground and make a documentary. It was exhilarating to feel this work would never get done unless I, and others, made a conscious decision to do it.

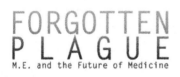
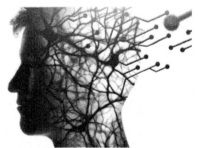

That's why Nicole Castillo and I set out six months ago on the journey of a lifetime. I was transforming from writing on politics to making a movie on microbiology. But Nicole was coming home. Her dream was to make documentaries on medical or social justice topics. And what better chance to fulfill her dream than to tell the great under-reported medical story of our time?

Making the movie[251]

So far, we've shot footage in California, Nevada, Alabama, Georgia, Florida, North Carolina, and the District of Columbia. We've filmed with bedbound patients, home-bound patients, and with many of the top experts in the ME/CFS and neuro-immune field: luminaries like Dan Peterson, Andy Kogelnik, Staci Stevens, Chris Snell, Mark Van Ness, Judy Mikovits, Charles Lapp, Nancy Klimas, and Gordon Broderick. We've also shot footage with an even longer list of brilliant researchers whom many patients don't know yet. For instance, there's Ron Davis, one of the men who very nearly invented the field of genomics, who is facilitating ME/CFS genetics research at Stanford. Then there's William Pridgen, who is leading a clinical trial on a new drug combo targeting herpes viruses with the University of Alabama.

We set out to make a film that would inspire people. And we think twenty-first century medicine is the best way to move the masses. As I look back at the footage, I like to think this is going to be the kind of a movie that a fifteen-year-old could watch and decide immediately to become a scientist. Throughout history, science has always made strides to improve human life, and this story is no different. As Dan Peterson said in his interview with us, "I'm a believer in the model, we just haven't gotten there yet."

Making the movie matter

But making the movie is only half the battle. Making the movie *matter* is the other half. To be sure, we still plan on distributing our film through film festivals, DVD, Hulu, iTunes, and Amazon. Additionally, we've had forty individuals or groups from six nations sign up to stage screenings in their own communities. We think we can get that number to 300 in the first year. Folks from Vancouver to Sydney are ready not just to see the movie, but also to really *use* the movie to create change. We often say this isn't just a movie; it's a movement.

Founding a new Non-Profit[252]

It can be a highly targeted movement to the people who need to hear its message most. That's why we decided to incorporate the Blue Ribbon Foundation as a 501(c)(3) non-profit organization to lead a three-pronged mission in awareness (the documentary), education (the Blue Ribbon Fellowship), and fundraising for research (Step Up for ME).

---

251 www.youtube.com/watch?v=Tp7Z4eZseHI (accessed June 28, 2016).

252 www.youtube.com/watch?v=uxCRP_axGw0 (accessed June 28, 2016).

We want this film to have an immediate impact for families, nurses, doctors, local organizations, and large-scale advocacy initiatives.

Nicole will serve as the first Director of the Foundation. I currently serve as president of the Board. Other members of our Board of Directors include:

- Linda Tannenbaum (Executive Director, Open Medicine Foundation)

- Joey Tuan (Co-Founder, HealClick.com)

- Hannah Tsui (Silicon Valley Entrepreneur)

- Giridhar Subramanian (Analyst, CSX Transportation)

With our 501(c)(3) arm now formed (pending IRS determination), we can outline several exciting ways to make this documentary's message stick.

How *do* we do that?

First, numerous healthcare filmmakers have partnered with Continuing Medical Education (CME) providers so that doctors and nurses who watch their films can receive CME credit. We're embracing that. It's the perfect incentive to engage the medical community. Much of the educational material physicians would absorb from The Blue Ribbon documentary, *Forgotten Plague: M.E. and the Future of Medicine* would pertain to the definition (with an emphasis of the Canadian Consensus Criteria), prevalence, symptom severity, bio-markers (low NK cell function, immune dysfunction, low V02 max, mitochondrial dysfunction, etc.), cost to society, latest therapies (such as antivirals) and coping mechanisms.

Second, we would like to create a system and an information package by which patients can systematically distribute the film via local support groups so that patients can partner with their physicians in seeking adequate care. Such a package might give patients a set of talking points in how to direct the conversation. It would provide doctors with brief, yet detailed information that could prepare them to watch the documentary, receive CME credit, and better help the patient.

Third, we have been laying the groundwork for a medical fellowship by which current medical students can spend their summers studying and researching at the top ME/CFS institutes in the world. The Blue Ribbon Fellowship will enable them to experience the thrilling sights and sounds we get to experience on the film set every single day. They'll get a glimpse into the future of medicine, observing and participating in innovative collaboration spanning Big Data, gene expression, molecular biology, and translational medicine.

Reaching practicing and future doctors[253]

Both the Blue Ribbon documentary (*Forgotten Plague: M.E. and the Future of Medicine*) and the Blue Ribbon Foundation strive to reach doctors at each stage of their careers. Practicing doctors can receive CME credit. Future doctors can apply for our fellowship program, a program that could inspire and equip them to build a career and a practice fighting neuro-immune diseases.

The Blue Ribbon Fellowship proposal calls for $50,000 to fund ten fellows for eight-week summer internships funded at the rate of $5,000 per student. At a time when many of the first generation of the ME/CFS pioneers is nearing retirement, we believe the Blue Ribbon Fellowship program delivers the best bang for the buck to light fires in the minds of the next generation of neuro-immune visionaries. In a future article for Phoenix Rising, we'll outline our new initiative, Step Up for M.E,[254] which will empower patients, families, and communities to build awareness and help raise money for research, each in their own unique way. Together we can team up to make CME credits, physician education, and the Blue Ribbon Fellowship a reality.

This is our vision not just for making a film, but also for implementing an innovative, scalable, and sustainable approach to 21st century physician education.

Update | November 2014 | Ryan Prior

The production team has raised $100,000 to support production and post-production of *Forgotten Plague*. Productions of this size and ambition can often cost three to five times as much, but we assembled a great team passionate about the film and the cause, and willing to work for less. The production took about sixteen months and required travel to nine U.S. states. It also included four trips to San Francisco, CA and two trips to Boston, MA.

On October 26th, we held a private preview screening of the working cut at the Chinese Theater in Hollywood (the same theater where films like *The Wizard of Oz* and *Star Wars* held their premieres). Upon final completion in January 2015, we expect a world premiere at a major film festival in spring 2015. We have garnered support for over 100 screenings of the film all over the world.

During or after our festival run, we hope to make the film available on streaming platforms like Netflix, iTunes, and Amazon, as well as DVD/Blu-Ray. We plan to make it available in multiple languages as well.

253 www.youtube.com/watch?v=PofBJow2Vfc (accessed June 28, 2016).

254 For more information on the initiative, go to stepupforme.causevox.com (accessed July 19, 2016).

Update | October 2015 | Note from Valerie

Public screenings of *Forgotten Plague* have been held in a number of locations in the U.S. and internationally. It has been well received. If you would like to host a screening, contact www.forgottenplague.com for more information. The film has also been released on DVD and other media as of December 2015.

∼୨

Update | July 2016 | Note from Valerie

Things have been busy with the *Forgotten Plague* team as they work to get the film the broadest possible exposure. The well-deserved accolade from Huffington Post, calling it a "Must-See Documentary," was much appreciated and the feedback from viewers has been enthusiastic. Public screenings of *Forgotten Plague* have been held to coincide with the #MillionsMissing protest on May 25, 2016, and DVD copies of the film have been sent to many in Congress to continue raising awareness about ME/CFS and its impacts.

The film has been released on DVD, iTunes, Google Play and Amazon. As of June 23, 2016, it was officially available at iTunes in 80 countries (including many European countries). The translations are downloadable via iTunes in Norwegian, Spanish, Dutch and Italian.

The Blue Ribbon Fellowship is also off to an encouraging start.

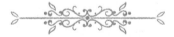

CHAPTER 8

Recovery, Improvement, and Hope

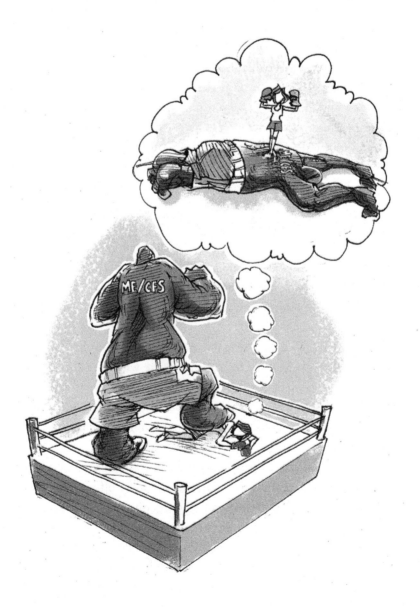

Thriving after ME/CFS

Chris Carruthers | March 2013 | Alberta, Canada

My name is Dr. Chris Carruthers, and I am a consultant with a large Canadian provincial healthcare system. I am a kinesiologist with an MSc in Coaching and Cardiac Exercise Physiology and a PhD in Integrative Healthcare.

Today, I am a woman of abundant energy and mental clarity, and every day is a gift. I say that with deep gratitude, because for seven and a half years, I suffered with extreme pain and overwhelming fatigue every moment of every day, along with acute environmental sensitivities whereby I was overwhelmed by loud noise, bright lights, new fabrics, and common smells. Having previously been perfectly healthy, I was stunned with the extent of my sudden illness and the rude realization that my illness was a mystery to my extensive healthcare team. This was followed by what seemed like endless years of non-recovery, hope, hopelessness, fear, and a full spectrum of emotional ups and downs.

My illness started suddenly in 1993 with a severe flu, which didn't go away. I was thirty-eight years old at the time. Gradually, I lost fifteen pounds and developed dull headaches, severe inflammation along my thoracic spine, and severe food sensitivities. My pain was a constant eight out of ten, and my fatigue oscillated between five and ten. At times, I would collapse to the floor with a sudden muscle failure and be unable to get up. I couldn't tolerate medications and fell into a sleep dysfunction, living in a state where my muscles themselves felt nauseous and where I could eat nothing but steamed vegetables. I was never really awake and never really asleep. I felt lost in a vague universe where no one could reach me.

Thankfully, I had a very compassionate doctor who recognized the change in my normally pleasant and energetic demeanor and believed me when I told her that I was not depressed and that I was trying desperately to regain my work, family, and sports life.

Coming to a diagnosis took over eight months. Eventually, an internal medicine specialist diagnosed me with chronic fatigue syndrome and fibromyalgia, and I was forced to accept that I was very ill.

Over the following seven years, I tried every therapy, eating plan, and complementary, alternative and conventional treatment that medicine had to offer. Some things worked a little, but nothing worked a lot. There was no clear path and no clear answers. My life as I knew it was on hold, and I was heartbroken. Over this period of time, my disability insurance ended, my unemployment insurance ended, and my savings were depleted.

The challenge and many frustrations that came with repeating my story over and over again made me realize how important the little things were in terms of patient care: a gentle smile, a kind word, compassion, and empathy. One of the kindest things one of my physicians said was, "Together, we will get you better." It didn't happen for so many years, but it was the kind of interaction that helped me heal. People with ME/CFS need to be respected, heard, and supported just as any other individual dealing with illness.

In the depths of despair one night, I had an out-of-body experience, where I felt pain-free for the first time in four years. It was then that I realized that I was so much more than my body; that even though by body was failing me, my spirit was still strong. Experiences like this one helped me cope better with symptoms and detach myself from them.

My slow recovery was a mystery and a surprise. As I reached a gradual acceptance that perhaps I was not going to recover, I learned to accept myself and began to explore spirituality, which to me was acceptance and self-love. I learned to meditate and developed breathing techniques to manage pain. I practiced relaxation techniques such as a body scan to help me fall asleep. As I addressed the sleep disorder, I began to get better, almost imperceptibly. It took well over one year.

Now I can look back and appreciate that my experience of illness has made me a wiser person and a more compassionate health professional. The lesson I learned was that my physical, mental, emotional, and spiritual needs were to be respected and honoured, not submerged – something I still struggle with when stress in the workplace makes me mentally foggy, unfocused, and fatigued. I do not override these signs now, but honour them and quickly move into self-care practices and skills that I know will restore me to a balanced state.

My daily practices to maintain health are expressive writing (journaling), laughter in whatever form I can find it, lots of solitary time in nature, prioritizing sleep, removing myself from stress, and deep breathing and meditation. I promote my own health by recognizing early on when my energy begins to fail, by saying "no" when necessary, and by asking for help. I listen to the messages that my soul sends me and honour them.

I am now happy to announce that I have completely recovered, have been healthy for over ten years, and have returned to competitive tennis and ballroom dance. I am privileged to be able to give back professionally. I work full time as a health consultant, educator, and professional speaker in cancer care, spirituality, self-management of chronic illness, and sleep health. I have a deeper level of compassion for ill people and work from the perspective of patient and family-centered care. I use the integrative health approaches, which combine the best practices, practitioners, and systems of medicine into a personalized healing plan that honours the individuality of the patient. I wrote a book, *Sleep Well Tonight,* and I deliver webinars and conference programs for educational institutions, healthcare, and the corporate sector on a regular basis.[255]

Many people do improve and recover completely from many serious illnesses. I lived this experience and have seen this many times professionally. I encourage people to focus on health promotion, and not on illness. It helps to disregard the labels given by the

---

255 www.chriscarruthers.com (accessed June 29, 2016).

healthcare system and simply continue to focus on what helps you feel better. Allocation of funding and resources to research the characteristics, treatments, and other circumstances of those who recover, is much needed.

I wish for everyone an outcome such as mine. It is possible.

From Being Sick to Being of Service

Johannes Starke Interview, the Creator of
"CFS Recovery Project"
Introduction and Interview by Valerie Free | March 2014

Johannes Starke was born in Kiel, Germany and spent his childhood playing soccer and wind-surfing – and doing as little schoolwork as possible.

Like many other young people, he took a gap year between high school and college to travel, in his case to New Zealand, along with his best friend. He met his future wife, Erin, an American, at a backpacker hostel there.

Back in Germany in 2007, Johannes enrolled in chemical engineering. He was always interested in making people's lives better and felt that, through chemical engineering, he could ultimately take on some of the world's environmental challenges. Unfortunately, soon after, he came down with mononucleosis and then began to develop monthly "colds" and other recurring symptoms that eventually turned into full-blown ME/CFS. This was the beginning of a very difficult and dark time.

Convinced he would never be able to work again, and with barely enough mental capacity to manage his basic needs, Johannes did contemplate suicide, but made the decision to give it two years. He was willing to try many different things, had the financial and family support to do so, and fortunately began to improve.

He married Erin in June 2009, and with Johannes well enough to travel, they moved to her home state, California, U.S. where Erin works as an engineer. In addition to the warm climate, more suited to Erin, they felt that the U.S. had better doctors and more treatments available for ME/CFS than Germany.

Johannes feels he has reclaimed his life. He is able to work twenty hours a week and has a fulfilling relationship with his wife, a wonderful family, and the support of his best friend. Aside from the blessings of emotional and familial support he is fortunate to have, he attributes a great deal of his recovery to the mind-body techniques he has learned, and he created the CFS Recovery Project in 2012 to share his knowledge with others.

The following is extracted from our written interview in 2014.

What does the word "Recovery" in the CFS Recovery Project mean?

I mean recovering one's ability to be content, to function, and to feel well. I call it the Recovery Project, because with chronic fatigue syndrome, no one is sure how far someone will get on the healing journey. Unfortunately, many people with CFS don't ever regain their full health. However, even some of these people, through mind-body techniques and lifestyle changes, can recover a sense of well-being and better functioning.

What was the onset of your illness like?

I came down with mononucleosis soon after I started university. I was very weak for six weeks, and my liver was also affected. However, I was eventually able to resume my studies and social activities. A couple of things weren't right, though. I remember coming down with a cold for a few days about once a month. Six months after I recovered from mono, I did some strenuous exercise and got what I assumed was another one of my "monthly" colds. This time, the brain fog stayed, and I became very sensitive to light and sound and got many food sensitivities. I had trouble sleeping at night and woke up with muscle aches and tension headaches.

During the third semester, the classes got a little more difficult, and my situation worsened. The brain-fog bothered me the most, because my plan was to read books to make the time pass until I felt better, but now I could really do nothing. I failed most of my classes, noticed that studying worsened my condition, and decided to give the studying a break. My life felt very difficult, and stopping university was the only way for me to reduce my symptoms to a level that was bearable.

Leaving the university was only one of so many stages of loss that I experienced during the first year of my illness. I could no longer do my hobbies, my studies, exercising, really anything that I used to enjoy in life.

What illness label do they use in Germany (ME, CFS, or both), and what was the attitude toward CFS or ME at the time you were there?

They refer to the illness as CFS. Coincidentally, it turned out that my primary care doctor, Dr. Bueckendorf, is the foremost CFS specialist in northern Germany. After I had the symptoms for more than six months, I asked him if I would ever get better. He said, "We don't know, but we'll work on it." That's when I realized that I had a chronic illness.

Dr. Bueckendorf gave me some homeopathic medicine, herbs, and probiotics. When none of this helped, he didn't know what else to do. He was better at diagnosing than at treating it.

When, eighteen months into my illness, I saw Dr. De Meirleir, Europe's foremost ME/CFS expert based in Brussels, Dr. Bueckendorf was willing to help me implement the suggested treatment by writing the necessary prescriptions for me when I was back at home. Also, he was really good about writing to my health insurance company and to my university explaining why I had to drop out after one year.

I would say that few doctors know how to diagnose CFS in Germany, but many doctors were willing to co-operate on my treatment once I told them that I was diagnosed with it. I had some very kind doctors, though they were pretty clueless about the treatment options I found.

How did your family cope, seeing you in this new way?

My family was very supportive, and they always believed me. The substantial financial security and support they provided was very important for me to be able to rise above the challenges of the illness. Of course they were sad and worried about me. I felt especially well supported emotionally by my mother and my sister. My dad had faith that I would get better and was there to support me financially in any way, including paying for a treatment when I wanted to do it. My brother also played a very important role in my life at the time because he could lead the life I no longer had, so it felt like he was living it for both of us.

What I wished for, but didn't have, was my dad or my brother sitting down with me and helping manage my treatment regime. I felt alone in managing it – a task not really suited for my foggy brain.

I only realized how much my mom was affected when I had improved somewhat, two years into my illness. I noticed how sad and worried she looked. I told her, "I am no longer suffering so much, Mom. You look like I am still going through hell and like you have to watch me without being able to do anything." It took her a couple of months after that conversation to really get that I was no longer [as sick] and for her face to light up again.

In your blog, you mention that you felt as though you were living through hell in the first stages of the illness, but in January 2008 you decided to give yourself two years to regain your health or at least learn how to enjoy life again. Why?

The reason I made that decision to press on was for my family and my girlfriend. I thought it would break their hearts if I took my own life. I don't think I was that optimistic and didn't think I would actually be able to enjoy life again. However, there were lots of things to try, and I just tried one after the other.

I luckily found something that helped, [and] I slowly improved. By January 2009, I was quite happy again. I remember because as soon as I loved my life again, I started thinking about a shared future with my girlfriend.

Eventually, I know that, even though you were skeptical that mind-body techniques would help a physical condition, you decided to explore their power. What modalities did you utilize, and how did they help you?

When I started, I was very new to the mind-body approach to chronic fatigue syndrome, which was probably an advantage because I didn't have any prejudice against it. I was skeptical, but not prejudiced.[256]

What started me out and gave me a great foundation was the Gupta program.[257] Ashok Gupta, the creator, asks you to give the program 100 percent for six months. Luckily, I had some very quick results. Around the same time, a friend gave me a book by Buddhist teacher, Thich Nhat Hanh, on mindfulness.[258] The concept of mindfulness has grown bigger and more beautiful over time. I've learned to tweak these techniques for my special needs, as someone who is easily distracted and easily fatigued.

Another big influence has been my coach's training, which works a lot with visualization and changing one's state of mind. I still visualize and get into a healing hypnotic state almost every day and have developed a technique that my clients and I can do with each other. I love it because it puts me in a perfectly healthy and happy state at least once a day.

I've written in detail about many of the techniques and influences on my blog, so I invite you to have a look there to learn more.[259]

How did you decide to become a coach in these modalities? What strategies and coping skills have you developed to keep up your motivation and attitude?

I noticed before I decided to become a coach that, while engineering still tired me out in a heartbeat, speaking with my friends energized me, and I could do it for an hour or two at a time. I didn't really have to learn that much for coaching other than finding ways to get well myself (although I did take several coaching seminars). Most of what I teach, I initially learned trying to get better.

Now that I'm running a business, writing articles, and designing classes, I spend several (up to twenty) hours a week on tasks that don't energize me as much as speaking with

---

256 As Johannes noted in his blog of October 23, 2013, "I never thought that psychological techniques would help me to improve my well-being and sense of happiness, let alone my health: ME/CFS and fibromyalgia are physical conditions! How's that psycho stuff supposed to help? At the time, I was studying engineering in school and didn't believe in anything that couldn't be seen or measured in some way by a scientist." www.CFSrecoveryproject.com (accessed June 4, 2016).

257 The Gupta program is based on the belief that "ME/CFS is a neurological condition, and may be caused by abnormalities in brain structures called the 'amygdala' and the 'insula'." www.guptaprogramme.com/causes-of-me (accessed June 4, 2016).

258 Thich Nhat Hanh is thought by many to be the father of mindfulness in the West. He has authored many books on the subject. He teaches how to meditate and to live with peace and joy, right here, right now.

259 CFSrecoveryproject.com (accessed June 4, 2016).

people. However, I have learned over the last couple of years to bring the same flowing energy I get from speaking to these activities. That being said, I am still careful not to write for more than two to three hours a day, which is my current limit for this activity. My whole day is filled with healing activities, some of which I co-created with my coaching clients! My favorites right now are:

- Creating beliefs that make my life seem easy and happy. I am still very sensitive to stress, so when I notice something stressing me out, I change my mind's story and beliefs about it with Byron Katie's technique called "The Work." [260] I don't think I'd be able to run a business without practicing this technique.

- Meditating a few times a day.

- Taking mini-steps. It took some practice but I'm now very good at cutting any big task down into simple mini-steps.

- Check-in times with a buddy every ten to thirty minutes.

My latest, and definitely one of the most powerful discoveries, has been the power of communities for healing.

It can be difficult for someone with chronic fatigue syndrome to be part of a community because of our limited energy and mobility. Once I recognized the need for community in myself, I could just start one and see if my coaching clients wanted to join me.

The healing community I created has been a big success. The first six months, it was only a few people, but still a very tightly knit community. I got as much out of it as everyone else and almost pinched myself because I couldn't believe how lucky I was that, all of a sudden, I had people to practice my self-care techniques with.

In the online self-care hour I created, we also meet in community, either in a chat room or on the phone, and practice all of the healing self-care techniques we've discovered.

How has ME/CFS affected your relationship with your wife? How, when she is healthy and you are limited in some ways, do you stay connected and caring of one another?

Soon into my illness, I realized that the biggest strength I had was to be a healing presence for the people around me. While Erin has to focus a lot on her work to provide the vast majority of our income, I make sure we are happy and relate to each other in a calm, loving, and supporting way. CFS made me a more sensitive person, and I really learned to get in touch with my inner love and positivity in order to heal. Today, I think that "being

---

260 The Work of Byron Katie is a "process of inquiry that teaches you to identify and question thoughts that cause all the suffering in the world." www.thework.com/thework.php (accessed June 4, 2016).

different" actually makes me a better husband. I don't think many of my friends can relate to their partners with as much positivity and love as I can.

I can work from home and cook Erin healthy, yummy meals when she comes home from work.

Of course, I'm sharing right now from a place of having overcome my illness to a comfortable degree. It wasn't always that easy.

Can you tell us what a day in the life of Johannes looks like now?

I get up around 6:30 a.m. and do a little phone check-in with a "healing buddy" to get my motivation and brain going. Then I wash, brush my teeth, and dress.

From 7:00 a.m. until 8:00 a.m., I work a bit or do stuff around the house or go on a walk. I make a yummy, healthy, but simple breakfast (oatmeal with apples and bananas and flaxseed oil).

Then I meet with a healing buddy for thirty minutes of mindfulness sharing or "Perfect Health Experience."

From 9:00 until 10:00 a.m., I prepare for the first client. After the session, at 11:00 a.m., I take notes and usually do twenty or thirty minutes of mindfulness with my healing buddy.

Then I prepare for the next client at noon. After that client, I usually work on some client notes for thirty minutes and some other work for another thirty minutes. From 1:00 p.m. until 2:00 p.m., I eat lunch and go on a twenty to thirty-minute walk.

At 2:00 p.m., a friend and I meet on the phone and we meditate or practice what I call the "Perfect Health Experience," traveling in my mind into a completely healing space and forgetting about my work and my body. This time in the middle of the day is important because I feel it completely recharges my energy and resets my nervous system, which would get too stimulated without this break.

In the afternoon, I also focus on things around the house and make dinner for Erin.

I take another ten to twenty-minute break around 4:30 p.m., and then another thirty to forty-five minute break after dinner.

Johannes, do your practices and attitudes help with your symptoms? Are you back to your pre-illness level of health?

They make a difference of night and day. If I do them, I feel little to no fatigue or irritability. I feel very well. I also believe they have been essential in allowing me to exercise again.

While these practices have not returned my body to 100 percent pre-illness health (only sixty-five percent I think), my practices allow me to be nearly symptom-free for as long as I stay within my limits.

Overall, I feel good in my body and very happy. I occasionally have light headaches and some fatigue and am easily distracted and sensitive to noise at times. But through the healing techniques, I am able to embrace all of that and feel very good in my skin.

What is your mission with the Recovery Project?

One big part is to bring authenticity and love into the way mind-body techniques are presented for people with CFS and fibromyalgia. I think that a lot more people can have access to these techniques and get some relief.

Also, I want to bring the way that people with CFS can be supported or helped to the next level. Just in these two years, I've discovered so many ways to make mind-body techniques work better for me and other people with ME/CFS or fibromyalgia. For example, practicing "mindfulness sharing" together with a friend on the phone is a little tweak to mindfulness meditation that makes it become more fun and no longer feels lonely.

Do you enjoy working with individuals or do you prefer the broader picture of advocacy in politics and medicine for positive change?

I very much prefer the work with individuals and groups on their healing. That's what energizes me. I think advocacy is extremely important too, but since it drains my energy, I choose not to go there. However, I have a huge place in my heart for people who engage in advocacy, and I support them where I can. For example, I was able to support ME/CFS awareness when I jumped out of an airplane (yes, with a parachute) at a fundraiser in 2012 for ME/CFS Awareness Day. You can see a video of it on my website.

Update | May 2015 | Note from Valerie

Johannes experienced a serious relapse in the fall of 2014, which required him to take a break from his work. He's now back to his pre-crash levels, but realized during his time out that he needed to further change his lifestyle. He told me that his mistake was to pour all of his new energy into his work. He had to minimize the time he spent hanging out with friends, taking care of his marriage and his body, and the pursuit of fulfilling hobbies. Although his self-care practices worked well during the first two exciting years of building a successful website and coaching practice for people with CFS, it became a problem when his work became more like work.

As Johannes emerges from his sabbatical, he hopes to always make enough time to date his wife, hang out with his friends, enjoy his music (sing in a choir and play the piano), walk his dog, and give his body a stretch in a gentle yoga class. When he can, he will continue to devote time to his work and his website, cfsrecoveryproject.com.

Update | July 2016 | Note from Valerie

I asked Johannes for a brief update because it had been a while since I checked in on how he is doing. He tells me he is feeling much better than when he was in his last "dip" and he has made further diet and lifestyle changes – the biggest of which is that of fatherhood! Johannes is now the proud father of a baby girl. With support fom his wife, neighbour and in-laws, he is able to focus on parenthood and says, "I find it very, very healing to be around my cute, curious, happy, and sometimes very funny Eva."

Hope: Double-Edged Sword or a Light in the Darkness? [261]

Jody Smith | December 2013 | Ontario, Canada

Hope is essential – especially when things look darkest. And yet, when you're living with ME/CFS, stirring up hope can be the hardest thing to do.

Having hope is no guarantee of success, and fanning that wee flame takes the courage of a warrior. It takes a certain recklessness that can be in short supply when you feel surrounded by the darkness that is ME/CFS. Indeed, daring to hope can feel like you are setting yourself up for more pain. And let's face it, you are.

As I'm hunkered down bracing myself for more disaster, raising my head can seem like the ultimate in foolishness. What if the good things I am setting my sights on never happen? I was broken before. Will I now find myself shattered into pieces, ending up in an irreparable state?

When you can't get up from your bed, the idea of rising up can seem ridiculous. Maybe you've forgotten how. Maybe every time you've done it before, you've been slammed back into a worse situation than you were before.

But without hope, what really do you have? And without hope, how will you ever have a chance of moving forward?

That is the dilemma. There is no guarantee that hope will be fulfilled. But without it, I was almost assured of staying where I was.

For a long time, I had no hope of things ever changing. One day dragged after another, each one dreary and heartbreaking. My waking hours of effort were spent on things like breathing and trying to stop the vibrating, the nausea, and the whirling vertigo. Will I chance a shower? Is there a point to wearing myself out by getting dressed? Eat something. Sit in a chair, if I was lucky. Drag back to the bed when the interminable day is over. To sleep…Or not.

To live like this for weeks, months or years, bound by the chains of ME/CFS, changes a person. The lauded plasticity of the brain seems only to work in reverse as your mental powers and thought patterns seem only to shrink and atrophy.

When a bad ME/CFS crash gradually subsides, you can't remember who you were before it hit. Or maybe you are able to remember that good things used to happen, that

261 Originally posted on Phoenix Rising on December 9, 2013. phoenixrising.me/archives/21168 (accessed June 4, 2016).

you were at one time capable and productive. But it can seem as if these memories are not really your own; it can feel like you are thinking about someone else's life.

Were you ever strong, active, happy? Can you ever be so again? How do you get there from where you are?

The road seems unclear, the means out of reach.

∿

I spent months in bed, rousing only to drag myself out to see my family for short periods, and only on "good" days. I progressed to sitting in a chair, staring out a window, at a world that had forgotten me and was now irrelevant to me, in my new life as a vegetable and cripple. [Although] too sick to read a book or watch TV, I was well enough to be suffocated by the endless sameness of empty days.

Eventually, I was well enough to rail against the void. For several years, I would spend my evenings in my bedroom, after managing to eat dinner with the family, talking to myself.

My conversations were repetitive and full of rancor and anger. I complained about the unfairness of my fate. I felt shame and guilt about the possibility that I somehow had done this to myself, at my inadequacy in being able to pull myself together and take care of my family.

After a long time, all this venting brought me to a kind of crossroads. I had no idea how to get out of this mess. I had no energy to follow a plan if I'd had one. But somewhere, my direction changed. And I decided to expect things to get better.

It sounded foolish, even to myself. How could expecting improvement lead to anything but frustration and disappointment?

I didn't have an answer that brought any comfort or reassurance. I just knew I couldn't go on like this in the unrelenting dark. So, metaphorically speaking, I lit a candle, which got extinguished more times than I care to remember.

My hope, in retrospect, became a lifeline. I didn't get any quick rescues and didn't find myself suddenly being pulled up into the light. But things did eventually improve.

What did it?

I changed my diet and worked with a compassionate naturopath who wanted to help me above and beyond the norm; I learned to rest and met people online (some of them on Phoenix Rising[262]). And I'd like to believe that each of these pieces to my puzzle fell into place in part because I hoped for them – because I was open to, and looking for, new possibilities, even though I knew there were no guarantees.

---

262 phoenixrising.me (accessed June 29, 2016).

If anything, hope made my days lighter: Telling myself that things would not always be like this made it easier to survive. And that, in and of itself, was better than where I'd been for so long.

CHAPTER 9

The Tightrope of Multiple Illnesses

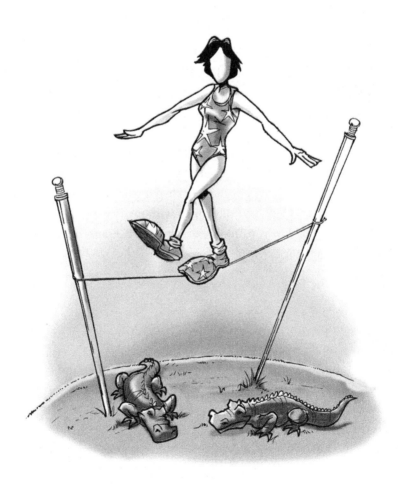

Trapped: Living with ME/FM/MCS

Jeanne Samonas | March 2014 | Ontario, Canada

As I enter the store, I am hit by the scent of perfume. I inquire about the shampoo that's on sale and try to educate the employee about ME/FM/MCS and why unscented products are needed for quality of life and health. I also suggest that carrying these products would be beneficial for the store. I'm told that unscented products are not selling well, and that's why they're priced on sale.

I feel a little dizzy, and the perfume has triggered a headache, so I check out. On my way out of the store, I am affected again as some person is spraying himself with the sample bottle!

I get to my car and sit for several minutes. In addition to the headache, I have the shakes, and I am not feeling well enough to drive just yet. I give up on the grocery store and bank – the other things I was going to do while out.

After waiting for my head to clear, I drive towards home. I pull into my driveway and know I have to leave the shopping bag in the car and get into the house. I head for the bathroom. I just make it to the toilet, my bowels let go, and I am in terrible pain. I know I am going to vomit, so I reach for the garbage can. I still have the shakes, my heart is racing, and I have hot and cold flashes and terrible gut pain. My jaw hurts. I am very close to crying, but I know that I will have more pain with my jaw if I do.

I clean myself up and slowly, painfully walk to my bed and collapse. I still have my coat and shoes on. I pray for relief.

I live with Multiple Chemical Sensitivity (MCS), ME/CFS, fibromyalgia, and tem-poromandibular joint disorder (TMJD).

My name is Jeanne Samonas. I was born in 1957 in the province of Nova Scotia in Canada. The valley where I grew up is the most beautiful place on earth, wonderful for growing fruit and vegetables, for the sea air, and for changing of the tides. It is where part of my heart will always be.

I live in Ontario now with my husband, three almost-grown sons, and our dogs.

Let's go back a few years. I was self-employed in a great profession: team coordinator and crisis management in the field of children's mental health conditions. We were living in a great neighborhood, volunteering at several organizations, and involved in activities for the children and our church. Life was great, money was good, and everyone was fairly healthy.

I started developing some issues with unusual things – for example, scents like gasoline or those that come out when opening packages of pantyhose. Usually in the cold weather, I also experienced pain in my hips, lower back, and elbow; and I was not sleeping well. My family GP sent me to a rheumatologist, who diagnosed me with fibromyalgia syndrome (FMS), gave me a cortisone shot for my elbow pain and told me to use over-the-counter medications if I had pain. "Just live your life," he said.

Several years later, a car accident completely changed my life; my list of issues grew longer, and my career and my fairly good health ended. Whiplash, soft tissue damage, and TMJD were new problems. This was the start of severe multiple chemical sensitivity syndrome (MCS) and severe fibromyalgia, as well as the need for oxygen from a tank so I could breathe easier and be more functional for my boys.

Along the way, I also got diagnosed with myalgic encephalomyelitis/chronic fatigue syndrome (ME/CFS).

∽

A very lengthy court case due to my accident took over six years to settle. What a terrible situation; I could barely manage to get up and walk to the bathroom due to dizziness, excruciating pain, and immobilizing fatigue. I can describe fibromyalgia pain as equivalent to taking a sledgehammer to varying parts of my body repeatedly and consistently. Narcotics for pain have become my best option despite the long-term repercussions.

Even with the help of a woman who was looking after the children and me full time, it was a very difficult time for our family. Our children were ages three, five, and seven, and we needed to live on one income.

We survived! We stayed married, the children grew, and we learned a lot. We did spend time and money "chasing the cure" ($80,000 – $90,000) only to find out that the lotions and potions not only didn't help, but in some cases, added new problems. I even went outside the country to see what was possible, only to learn that we are guinea pigs for the most part.

Many people who didn't understand that I was disabled dropped out of our lives. They wanted the "other woman" who used to live in my body, the one who was the "go-to" girl, always on top of the game, always active and involved. So did I! I cried for the loss of my former self and for what my family was facing.

I feared for us. How would we manage? Could we keep the house? Did we have enough money to buy groceries? I remember having to choose not to buy hamburger meat because I needed to buy second-hand boots for my son.

∽

Through the darkness came some light: ME/FM/MCS support groups and provincial and national organizations. I found a doctor specializing in these illnesses who gave me the tools I needed to cope. The kind, wonderful people living with these illnesses shared their knowledge about everything from disability tax credits to therapeutic pool programs and coupons. They even gave me winter coats for my children that their children had outgrown. I deeply appreciated the second-hand stores and the people who gave us food and help when we really needed it.

Often, the battle consists of facing doctors who don't believe that you are really ill, along with employers, insurance companies, lawyers and the Canadian Pension Plan. The list goes on and on. Most of us lose these battles because we lack the support of the medical community or family and friends. I can count on my hands the number of people who respect me and understand some of what it takes to attempt to live a life with any quality.

❧

The most misunderstood of all these illnesses is MCS (Multiple Chemical Sensitivity). MCS falls under the umbrella of Environmental Sensitivities or Environmental Illnesses (ES or EI). "What do you mean, you have chemical sensitivities? Why can't you just 'not' have that problem?"

I never know when, or if, I will become sick from something that I come in contact with. NOWHERE is totally safe.

I remember watching an old black and white movie about London during the war, and everyone walked around with gas masks, knew of the obvious danger, and were doing what they could to protect themselves. But today, even so-called "safe" substances can create or trigger an environmental illness, and cause violent physical reactions for those with MCS. These include vomiting, dizziness, shaking, disorientation, fainting, falling down, and severe headaches.

Maybe those of us with MCS and similar illnesses are like the canaries that the miners would take into the mines to warn of the invisible dangers of mining. When the canary stopped singing or died, they knew to get out.

There is no such thing as a simple trip to the grocery store. Meet my friends for coffee? As I have severe reactions to the scent of coffee, my poor husband has to drink his coffee at work and then brush his teeth with unscented toothpaste. Even my three teen sons must use only scent-free products: shampoo, deodorant, soap, and toothpaste.

Then there are the laundry products and cleaning items – for example, dryer sheets, with their perfumed scents blowing through the vents of your next-door neighbor's homes into your open windows which exacerbates asthma, allergy, eczema, and MCS conditions.

Even on sale, most scent-free products tend to be much more expensive than the "poison" kind (as I call them). To make matters worse, they must generally be purchased from health food or specialty shops, some of which burn incense and sell other scented products. I try to avoid those things I already know cause a reaction. However, every new item creates a potential problem with my health, and I can't predict them all. I certainly don't want to live my life in a bubble, but the amount of energy it takes to try to live safely in my own home with my own family is tremendous!

Doctors' waiting rooms – not for me. Parent/teacher meetings, church or dinner out with the family at a restaurant hardly ever happen. I have had to leave restaurants so many times when someone dove into their perfume, body sprays, or hair products just before going on their outing. My husband then must ask for the food to be wrapped up, and I go wait in the car.

He also has to put the gas in the vehicle, because I cannot deal with the scent of the fumes. I am so grateful to him and my sons for understanding that MCS makes me very ill, and for helping and supporting me.

❧

Many people cannot find an environmentally safe home. Many suffer from severe reactions to molds, chemical "off-gassing" from furniture, flooring, and paint, and from agricultural chemicals including pesticides and fertilizers. Dry cleaning solutions and items manufactured using glues and solvents are also problems. Electromagnetic (EMF) sensitivity is another trigger for reaction to some individuals and can be caused by cell phones, computers and even home electrical systems.

Prevalence of MCS is surprisingly high – even more people report being diagnosed with it than with chronic fatigue syndrome or fibromyalgia, according to the latest Canadian Community Health Survey (CCHS).[263] And there is a surprisingly high overlap between the conditions. The numbers of people with one or more of these disorders, as reflected in the survey of 2010, was over one million Canadians.

❧

A small group of people, suffering with these illnesses, has been working hard to bring awareness in our province of Ontario through the annual International Day of Awareness for the illnesses on May 12th. I am one of them. I have chaired the Awareness Day group, and I have been president of the provincial organization.

The group has been meeting with government agencies, trying to get them to address the issues of ME/FM/MCS. This is a slow and difficult process because everyone involved with the group either has the illness or lives with someone who does. Most support groups are at the grass roots level with limited resources. Provincial and national organizations are also doing what they can; but there are too few people attempting to meet very big needs.

---

263 The survey is available in Appendices B and C.

I have witnessed three generations of acquaintances with environmental and overlapping conditions like mine, and these affect everyone.

When will they be acknowledged and addressed?

From a Blue Ribbon to a Pink One

Doris Fleck[264] | June 2013 | Alberta, Canada

It was a wonderfully warm Valentine's Day in Vancouver. It was 1986, and I recently celebrated my twenty-fifth birthday. Though I usually enjoyed these rare sky-blue days amongst the drizzle of February rains, the past few weeks had dragged me down with unusual flu-like symptoms. Dizziness, nausea, blurred vision, and a strange type of fatigue were weighing me down. I decided to take a break from my university classes and drove to my parents' house in Abbotsford for some of my mom's tender loving care.

Illness was not the norm for me. In my youth, I had been an athlete and an academic. My roommates called me Superwoman, since I juggled a full-time class schedule with two part-time jobs and extra work in the thriving Vancouver film industry. I was active in my church, continued to hone my photography skills, and found time to spend with family and friends. I was firing on all cylinders and loving every minute of it.

But after twenty minutes of negotiating Vancouver's busy streets, I knew I was in grave danger. An intense burning sensation started at the base of my neck, like someone putting a steaming hot cloth there. My eyes felt like boulders and kept closing. My head was so heavy it nodded back and forth uncontrollably.

The burning turned into a tingling sensation that felt like tiny needle pricks all over the top of my head. I became dizzy and felt faint. I panicked. My heart was racing, and I began to gasp for air. The tingling rapidly changed into a progressive numbness that cascaded over my neck and down my arms. I could see my hands gripping the steering wheel, but they felt like cotton balls.

This must be a stroke, I thought. I began praying out loud, begging God to spare my life. I stopped the car, called an ambulance and was rushed to the nearest hospital.

This was the beginning of six years of confusion, questions, emergency room visits, and medical testing. My symptoms confounded over forty doctors and specialists until I was finally diagnosed with CFS as it was known then. I couldn't continue my studies, gave up my two jobs, and needed my family to feed me, drive me to doctors' appointments, and help me take baths. I spent most of the time in my bedroom, totally isolated.

I had dozens of bizarre symptoms that neurologists, endocrinologists, and internists couldn't explain: from hypersensitivity to sound and light, to nausea, to numbness, and

---

264 Doris is a Canadian journalist who lives in Red Deer County, Alberta. She also blogs about her experiences at doris-fleckimages.blogspot.com (accessed June 6, 2016).

recurrent fatigue. Over the six years, I was tested for multiple sclerosis, brain tumors, lupus, rheumatoid arthritis, diabetes, thyroid disease, cardiac problems, and a host of other ailments. Each time, I was pronounced "healthy."

Many physicians thought I was clinically depressed or concluded my symptoms were emotionally induced and advised me to see a psychiatrist. I already thought I was going crazy, so I readily agreed. But after just three visits, the psychiatrist told me my mind was sound and advised me to seek medical help.

I began to see naturopaths and allergists. By sticking to a strict diet that eliminated sugar, white flour, yeast, cheese, and fungal foods, I saw some improvement. Within two years, I had moved to Calgary to live with a friend and found a part-time job with flexible hours. I managed to work two hours a day, but needed to rest or sleep through much of the other twenty-two hours just to make it to work again. During the next three years, my energy slowly increased until I was able to work five hours each day and socialize on weekends.

I noticed that my symptoms got worse when I encountered strong smells or airborne fungus. When I researched this disease I found studies that implicated environmental factors, like fungi and pesticides, as potential risk factors for acquiring CFS. Not surprisingly, during the first eighteen years of my life, I lived in a mold-ridden home. On top of that, I was exposed to many different experimental pesticides when I worked for Agriculture Canada, during the three summers leading up to my illness. I am convinced this made my risk of getting CFS even greater.

❧

Unlike many people with CFS, I have the unconditional support of family and friends.

In 1990, at the age of twenty-nine, I married an exceptional man with boundless energy. Peter has been compassionate and understanding with my many limitations and relapses, but it has not been without huge concessions and tough decisions.

I had a relapse a few weeks before our wedding. I mistakenly assumed once the honeymoon started, I would be well on my way to recovery. But I progressively became more debilitated until I was bedridden again a few months into our marriage – this time with the most debilitating symptoms I had ever had.

Peter had been working long hours on the fledgling newspaper he founded, as well as doing all the cooking, cleaning, and grocery shopping. He coordinated the requests of friends and family that wanted to see me and help out. I required assistance to get to the washroom and could no longer give myself a bath. Peter knew I needed twenty-four-hour care – more than he was able to provide.

Some friends who were naturopaths agreed to take me in. On New Year's Eve, 1990, Peter dropped me off at their house and left for an event he was covering for his newspaper. The next six months, while I was living there, were the hardest of my life. I was totally bedridden, and Peter could not be with me for much of the time. I was eating six healthy meals each day, yet watched the pounds melt off my normally robust frame. Even with all the care I was receiving, I was seeing no improvement.

I began to sink into a deep depression. On my thirtieth birthday, I was imagining the rest of my life in an extended care facility. I came to the conclusion that I couldn't put Peter or myself through this kind of torture and, for the first time, began to think of ways to kill myself. But I didn't want to die, even if that meant decades of debilitating illness. It was then that I began to enjoy simple pleasures again.

Courage filled me and slowly dragged fear from my body. Finding a deep well of thankfulness for the love and support I had helped me fight my way out of that two-year long relapse, as well as each and every relapse that followed.

Although my CFS was diagnosed as severe, a friend who has been disabled by CFS and fibromyalgia for a decade says I have lived a "charmed" life. She is so right! Even though I have had numerous relapses lasting a year or more, I have always been able to claw and crawl my way back to living a fairly normal life. But even though I can get my energy levels back to 70 percent of a healthy person, I have had to give up many things, including travel, my sport activities, and driving.

༄

In 2012, just after I turned fifty-one, I was physically attacked by another disease: After feeling a hardening of my right breast and the growth of a lump, I went for an ultrasound and mammogram and found out that I had breast cancer!

Earlier, the doctor who diagnosed me as having CFS also warned me I was at greater risk for thyroid disease and cancer. As I began to understand the science of CFS, I realized my immune system was severely compromised, and the killer cells in my body were disabled. Since my cells were not able to metabolize oxygen properly, getting cancer was a definite risk. I have a family history of leukemia and always thought if I were to get a cancer, it would be leukemia. Being diagnosed with breast cancer was a total shock.

I quickly got chest and spine x-rays, a bone scan, and an abdominal ultrasound. My team of doctors wanted to see how aggressive the cancer was and how far it had spread. The bad news was, the only type of cancer that matched my symptoms was inflammatory breast cancer, a lethal form of the disease. Most women with this diagnosis have, at most, a year or two to live.

My oncologist hadn't even done a biopsy before she indicated this was probably a highly aggressive form of cancer and the first course of treatment would be chemotherapy – hard, fast, and long. After explaining that I had CFS and a compromised immune system, I asked if they did low-dose chemo or provided beneficial therapy for people with immune disabilities.

"You are no different from any other woman," she said. "Some people can handle the chemo and some just can't." This news totally demoralized me. I knew that I would never survive such a treatment plan.

But all eight biopsies indicated that I had a type of non-invasive breast cancer (ductal carcinoma in situ-DCIS). I was so relieved, I was in tears. Surgery was scheduled immediately. I made it through the radical mastectomy and recovered without having a CFS relapse. Amazingly, there was no need for radiation or chemotherapy.

❧

Breast cancer is a visible, provable disease – ME/CFS, for the most part, is not. Women who battle breast cancer are hailed as heroes and survivors. Those who fight ME/CFS daily, often for decades, may be misdiagnosed, medically alienated, or even abandoned by family and friends. It is much harder for friends of ME/CFS sufferers to know how to support them. How do you encourage someone to get up and fight a disease when there is no fight in them?

As a cancer patient, I was contacted by a group of nurses who provided me with information, met me at every doctor's appointment, called to see how I was doing, visited me in the hospital, and provided discounts on medical apparel I now needed. I could phone anytime, and they would be there. The pretty pink ribbon that represents breast cancer awareness is everywhere: on T-shirts, calendars, pens, notepads, dinner napkins, balloons, banners, yoga mats, license plate frames, and even dog apparel.

ME/CFS is represented with a royal blue ribbon, something I was completely unaware of until I was researching for this article. It was good to see that ME/CFS, one of the most invisible of diseases, has some symbol. But unfortunately, it does not have a very high profile: That royal blue ribbon had been elusive to me for decades.

❧

As I write this story in June 2013, I am in the middle of another lengthy relapse, struggling to climb my way back up to the life I am used to – my 70 percent. But this time, I am resting much more, not pushing myself as hard on the way back. I've had this unpredictable disease for twenty-seven years now, and I realize most people with severe ME/CFS remain much more debilitated than me.

Even though my local medical doctor knows nothing about this disease, when I bring in papers or books on the subject, she readily reads them and is interested in providing the best care possible for me.

Peter and I have recently moved to forty acres of wooded land in Red Deer County, and we take time to watch the sunsets and marvel at the deer, beaver, moose, foxes, and porcupines that call this land their home. We canoe the creek that runs through our property and spend time in our huge garden. My life is a gift, and I now choose to enjoy the simple moments that happen each day, even the days filled with illness.

Diseases That Get No Respect
White Coat, Black Art Radio Show

Dr. Brian Goldman[265] | May 2011 | Canada

When it comes to patients, people like me are trained to respect them all. As for the diseases patients carry, that's a very different story. This week on *White Coat, Black Art* [266] [WCBA], "Diseases that get little respect inside the hospital's sliding doors," I speak with a Vancouver woman whose medical condition has generated everything from skepticism to outright disbelief from many of the doctors who've treated her. And, a medical historian explains why some diseases get a lot of respect while others don't, and whether marketing can change that.

In medical circles, there are diseases that command respect among physicians. Multiple sclerosis, rheumatoid arthritis, and strokes are three such examples. These and many others have two things in common. First, they are serious conditions in that they are either life threatening or cause serious disability. Second, they can be confirmed objectively through blood work, CT scans, MRIs, and other forms of testing.

Cancer may well top the list. Even so, some forms of cancer get more respect than others. As reported by *CBC News*, in terms of fundraising and research dollars, we tend to respect breast, prostate, childhood cancers, and leukemia far more than lung, colorectal, and stomach cancers. That's surprising since it's the latter three types of cancer that are among the most common and most deadly.

Then again, there's a category of medical conditions you'd swear people like me are trained or acculturated to disrespect if not view with outright contempt – no matter how much that makes you suffer.

Comedian Rodney Dangerfield made a successful stand-up career out of getting no respect. It's fair to say the Rodney Dangerfield of diseases is one called fibromyalgia (FM). It's a condition that causes pain, stiffness, fatigue, and poor sleep, plus trouble thinking and concentrating. According to a recent review article, roughly five percent of the population has FM, with the highest prevalence occurring in middle-aged women.

---

265 Dr. Brian Goldman is the host of the CBC radio show "White Coat, Black Art" (WCBA). This is his blog about the 2011 WCBA radio show episode called "Diseases That Get No Respect."

266 Dr. Goldman's blog was originally posted online on www.cbc.ca on May 27, 2011. His blogs, at the time this was posted, were called "Dr. Brian's Side of the Gurney." The full WCBA, "Diseases That Get No Respect" show, can still be heard at www.cbc.ca/player/Radio/White+Coat+Black+Art/Full+Episodes/2011/ID/2170992213 (accessed May 12, 2016).

Researchers are zeroing in on the cause of FM. It is now seen as a biological neurosensory disorder characterized in part by abnormal processing of pain signals in the central nervous system. Along with a new understanding of the biological basis of FM, have come new drug treatments to relieve the symptoms. Not only that, in 1990, the American College of Rheumatology published guidelines on how to make the diagnosis.

Still, it's hard to find a disease with less respect among people like me. None of this is news to Susan MacLean, a patient with FM and president of Myalgic Encephalomyelitis and Fibromyalgia Society of BC (MEFM) who began by battling the disease and ended up battling many of the doctors who treated her.

"I've had a number of very negative reactions from doctors," MacLean told WCBA. "I'd like to describe my experience when I actually received the diagnosis of FM. I was seeing a doctor for a number of months before a referral to a specialist was actually made. The reaction of the rheumatologist was that this was an illness of high-strung, uptight, middle-aged women, [and] that I should buy new shoes to alleviate the excruciating pain in my feet and legs.

"They did a very cursory physical examination, handed me a brochure, told me not to seek out any support for the illness from any of the local support groups in town, because that was simply a bunch of people sitting around, holding hands feeling sorry for themselves. I was patted on the back, escorted out of the office, and was told that they hoped they never saw me again," recalls MacLean.

If Susan MacLean's current physician is helpful, that's the exception and not the rule. More often than not, I hear patients say their doctors fail to even recognize they have a disease.

Dr. Jacalyn Duffin, a hematologist and medical historian at Queen's University in Kingston, says FM is only the latest in a long line of diseases that are greeted with contempt by members of the medical profession.

"You can go back a long, long way to the nineteenth century," Dr. Duffin told WCBA. "There were people who experienced accidents when railways came along. The trains were going faster than other vehicles had ever gone before. If there was a sudden stop or a jarring, then people would develop some kind of musculoskeletal injury, and there was actually a condition called 'railway spine.'"

Other modern-day illnesses that have been disrespected by physicians include chronic fatigue syndrome and – at least until recently – concussion.

Diseases that are dissed by physicians have several factors in common. The first is that they can't be confirmed with objective testing. When it comes to cancer, you can do a biopsy. You can diagnose a stroke with a CT or MRI scan of the brain. A heart attack can be detected with a blood test that measures troponin. By contrast, FM is diagnosed by asking about symptoms and by examining the patient for tender points on the body.

The most charitable explanation given [by] my colleagues is that the symptoms of FM are non-specific and could apply to many other conditions. In addition, tender points can be elicited in people who haven't been diagnosed with FM.

But some MDs have a more sinister way of explaining away their reluctance to endorse a diagnosis of FM. Recently, I heard a colleague refer to a patient with FM as having "Faker-myalgia." What's worse, my colleague made this flippant comment to a resident who my colleague was mentoring.

"That's pretty depressing and, I would think, a poor modeling example for the student," says Dr. Duffin. "It's become interesting from a medical philosophical perspective. In the eighteenth century, to be sick, you had to feel sick. Nowadays, because of various technologies, to be sick, the doctor has to find something."

In other words, back then, all we physicians had to go on were your symptoms. Had FM been discovered in the eighteenth century, it would have fit the definition of a disease to a 'T.' But not today. Today, if a condition has a lot of symptoms but not a lot of objective proof, we doubt the condition is genuine.

"Not a real disease, or, it's all in your head, and therefore, it's a psychological disease," says medical historian Dr. Duffin. "And if a disease is caused by mental distress, then it's to be respected less."

Another reason why doctors disrespect FM is that they fear it. More specifically, they fear they'll have to stick their necks out endorsing a claim for long-term disability that many sufferers of FM request. There are two reasons for this. First, they worry that a colleague will write a report that flat-out contradicts the physician's endorsement of the claim of disability. Second, right or wrong, many of my colleagues nurse a suspicion that patients are constantly trying to bamboozle them into writing sick notes when they aren't particularly ill or disabled.

Hate to say it, but the third reason why FM and other similar diseases get little respect is the perception among many physicians that the people who suffer from such conditions tend to be difficult patients.

It's a charge that makes FM patient and MEFM President Susan MacLean bristle with anger. "I think that doctors are perceiving difficult patients when in fact they should be perceiving a difficult, complex illness," MacLean told WCBA. "Patients face a multitude of problems. It's not just a chronic pain syndrome. There are other problems with the illness that cause great difficulty in the patient's life. Doctors have a tendency to see chaos when in fact they should be seeing complexity."

I'm struck by something medical historian Dr. Duffin said to me during our interview. With our boundless fascination for technological progress in medicine, the way doctors treat people with FM shows just how out of touch emotionally we are with our patients. In my opinion, it's time MDs get back to the idea that our job is not just to treat diseases, but also to help people who are suffering because of them. Expressions of disbelief – much less scorn – have no place in the consulting room. Objective proof is essential in measuring response to therapy. But it should never be used as a stick to beat patients whose only misfortune is to contract a disease that's difficult to verify.

Comment on "Diseases That Get No Respect"

Dr. Ellie Stein [267] | Alberta, Canada

Thank you for this show on disrespected conditions. As one of a handful of physicians in Canada caring for over 338,000 patients with myalgic encephalomyelitis/chronic fatigue syndrome and a similar number with fibromyalgia, I have reached the conclusion that the medical profession is being willfully blind. These conditions are not taught in most medical schools. Therefore doctors do not learn the criteria (which have been around for over twenty years as mentioned) and do not know what tests to order to prove that there is an objective problem.

For example in ME/CFS, research for over twenty years has shown immune dysfunction, specifically a defect in an ancient defense called natural killer cell function. However, the necessary test [for] "natural killer cell function" is not available in any province in Canada. As a result, patients pay out of pocket for this and other tests in U.S. labs to help them gather evidence of the severity of their condition and to track progress when they try various treatment approaches.

Similarly in both ME/CFS and FM, cognitive testing offers objective evidence of the problems. In Alberta, patients with ME/CFS and FM are specifically (by name) denied access to neuropsychological testing through Alberta Health Services – presumably because it would overwhelm the system and because they are not considered "as important" as people with dementia or traumatic brain injury. I hope this program helps generate "respect" and that access to timely diagnosis, objective testing, and compassionate management will follow.

---

267   E. Stein, MD, FRCP (C), Alberta, Canada: Expertise in ME/CFS, FM, and MCS.

My Lyme Disease Story

Mary Logan | January 2013 | CO, U.S.
Introduction by Valerie Free

Lyme disease remains a largely hidden illness much like ME/CFS. Because Lyme is often difficult to diagnose due to the lack of knowledgeable medical practitioners and inadequate testing, it often ends up undiagnosed or misdiagnosed. In fact, sometimes people who have been diagnosed with ME/CFS find out much later that they, in fact, have Lyme disease. After the acute stage of Lyme infection, if antibiotic treatment has been given but does not help, patients may end up with both a chronic Lyme and ME/CFS diagnosis. Mary very clearly demonstrates in this story how undiagnosed, late stage Lyme disease can lead to life-long health struggles and disability. (See Part III, Stanza 27 Notes for more details on Lyme disease.)

Winter, 1982: it is a beautiful, blue-sky day in the mountains of Colorado — a wonderful day to be working outside as a professional ski patroller. My husband, Nick, and I are enjoying our work, which includes avalanche mitigation with explosives, as well as evacuation of injured skiers and snowboarders down the mountain with patrol sleds. Feeling strong and healthy, we are happily unaware of what the near future holds for us.

During my pregnancy with our second child, I was able to continue professional ski patrolling. At that time, I was 29 years old. As the due date approached, I anticipated taking a week off before the birth. To my surprise, I worked my last day, went into labor that evening, and delivered a healthy, beautiful daughter early the next morning!

Six weeks after her birth, I developed an unexplained fever. I also presented with heart issues, including episodes of extremely high heart rate (160 – 200 beats per minute), and missed heart beats. Extreme joint pain soon followed. Thus began 10 years of declining health. Visits to many doctors and specialists gave no concrete answers to our questions about my decline. Pain, fevers, and severe fatigue became my everyday existence. Eventually I was unable to ski patrol any longer.

Pain and joint destruction led me to apply for disability compensation, which was approved. I appreciated it because I could no longer perform my duties as a professional ski patroller of 17 years.

An eventual diagnosis of "mild rheumatoid arthritis" was made by a rheumatologist. This diagnosis led me to the standard immune suppressing treatments offered for rheumatoid arthritis. The treatments, even at very low doses, caused the arthritis and pain to spread to joints never previously affected. During the time I was on these medications,

I went from being a fairly mobile person to someone having difficulty walking due to increased pain. My local general practitioner encouraged me to stop the medications, and I followed his advice.

From the research I did, I realized that I could fit into any diagnosis including lupus, multiple sclerosis, and chronic fatigue syndrome. Nothing would have surprised me at that time.

My mother, a registered nurse, watched my decline with much worry. By this time, I was bedridden for days. At one point, pain levels sent me to the emergency room at the local hospital. The morphine given to me did not touch the pain. Luckily for me, when she and my dad came to Colorado on vacation, she brought a nursing magazine with her. In it was an article about Lyme disease and its symptoms.

My mom saw similarities between the symptoms listed in the article and my own. She asked if I had ever been bitten by a tick, and that question changed my life. My answer was "Yes"! Years before, I had travelled to Minnesota to visit my parents. That is where I remember being bitten by a tick. It was a very small but very engorged tick by the time I found it. I remembered pulling it off of my scalp and hoping that I would not get sick. I had heard of other tick-borne illnesses, such as Rocky Mountain spotted fever, but not Lyme disease.

The article my mom brought for me contained a checklist of signs and symptoms for Lyme disease, and I suffered from 90 percent of them. Included were pain and joint inflammation, impaired neurological and cardiac function, fever and fatigue. My mom arranged for me to visit a neurologist in northern Minnesota where they lived and where I grew up. The doctor did a clinical evaluation of me. Her diagnosis was late stage, untreated Lyme disease of 10 years duration. I started intravenous antibiotic therapy that day.

One thing that began to make sense from this diagnosis of Lyme was that the immune-suppressing properties of the drugs for rheumatoid arthritis, which I had received in the beginning years, caused the flaring of the Lyme disease infection. Thus, it is very important to get an early and accurate diagnosis.

This was the beginning of a "recovery" that still continues 30 years later. During this time, antibiotic therapy has been the basis for my treatment, but never a cure. My condition improved and some of my strength returned, but I was far from my previous level of good health.

Over the years, I have sought out alternative and traditional treatments from doctors in eight different states and Mexico, at my own expense. Through my travels, however, I met my friend, Valerie Free, the author of this book. We have continued our phone friendship to this day. When Valerie was diagnosed with celiac disease along with chronic fatigue syndrome, I explored it as well. I found out that I carried two genes for it and also have celiac disease. The gluten free diet I maintain has alleviated some symptoms and the need for some medication.

I am luckier than many because I have an amazing support system. My late mother, our daughters, and my husband have all been through this with me. Their support and love have carried me through the times I did not think I could make it. We have struggled together, and we are surviving this horrific disease. I am now 60 years old. It has been 31 years since the birth of our second daughter and the onset of this illness.

I am one of many people who have been struck down by a misunderstood and debilitating illness. We are everywhere, but remain mostly in the shadows and fringes of life. Our hope is to have others recognize our need for their help and understanding, as well as their advocacy for more research efforts into the many facets of Lyme disease.

My personal story is evidence for how critical it is to get a proper diagnosis early on in the course of this complex illness. Being undiagnosed, then misdiagnosed, for 10 years has left me disabled and still struggling for a stable and fulfilling quality of life. As an example, my husband kindly typed this out for me because one of the consequences of chronic Lyme is joint destruction. I have had multiple surgeries, including hand and wrist surgery. I am left with hands and fingers that are deformed and painful. It is difficult to write and type.

Winter, 2013: I continue to need consistent antibiotic, and some alternative, treatment. I have good and bad days as well as good and bad seasons. I continue my research for any and all ideas to improve my situation.

My gratitude remains strong for the life I am able to live and my ability to enjoy my growing family, which now includes two lovely granddaughters. I have the occasional treat of skiing the Colorado slopes with my husband. During those times, we try to forget about the disease, even if just for that glorious moment.

Update | August 7, 2016 | Mary Logan

I continue to struggle with the day to day pain and disability caused by long term, late stage Lyme disease. I am seeking out the help of a doctor who specializes in treating late stage Lyme disease with unconventional methods. His approach is quite different than most practitioners, as he addresses the immune dysfunction (autoimmunity) as well as the infections. His treatments include genetic testing, appropriate supplementation, homeopathy and use of a Rife machine. I am hopeful, that with his guidance, I can slowly gain a better quality of life. I am blessed to have the love and support of a very compassionate husband. My gratitude for each day and the joy I find is what is most important to me.

CHAPTER 10

So Many Hats and Dead-ends

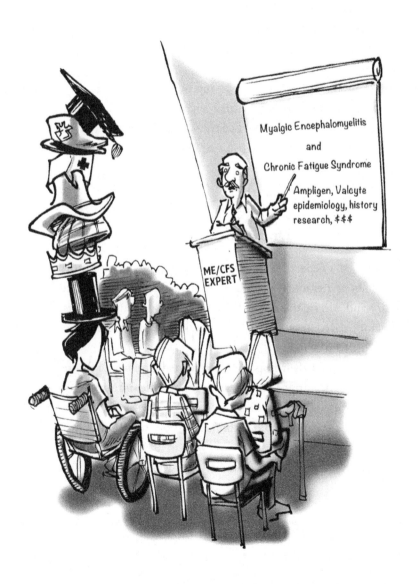

So Many Hats and Dead-Ends

Valerie Free | November 2011 | Alberta, Canada

In May of 2011, I attended a public lecture: "New Advances in the Diagnosis and Treatment of Myalgic Encephalomyelitis/Chronic Fatigue Syndrome," by Drs. Daniel Peterson, MD and Logan Chamberlain, PhD. As Dr. Peterson is a world-renowned ME/CFS clinician and researcher from the U.S., and he was coming to speak in my home city in Canada, I was eager to hear what he had to say.

In the weeks following the event, I thought about what I had heard. As my thoughts unraveled, I realized that my reactions were on many levels: mental, emotional, physical, and spiritual.

My feelings came from two broad areas: my hopes for effective treatment, which too often end up dashed; and the realization that I had taken on many roles as a patient with ME/CFS (in my case, for more than twenty years). From there, I came up with two illustration ideas depicted in this book: "Dead-ends," Section 1, Part III; and "So Many Hats," the cover for this chapter.

Dr. Peterson's Lecture

Dr. Peterson provided a general overview of the illness, including history and prevalence, before he spoke about treatment and research. Dr. Chamberlain shared his expertise in Complementary and Alternative Medicine (CAM) such as supplements, herbs, and acupuncture. He emphasized that patients need to keep experimenting to see what makes them feel even a little bit better.

Both speakers expressed their hopes for better medicine in the future for all ME/CFS patients, while noting the current limited state of available options.

Dr. Stein, our local expert/doctor who arranged the event,[268] was inundated with patients who, after the lecture, had new hope for more testing and treatment options. I was one of them. Unfortunately, just because we had all learned about these options did not mean we had access to them in our country – at least not at that time.

---

268 The public lecture was only one piece of a weekend-long event on ME/CFS, called "ME/CFS Diagnosing and Managing: The basics and beyond." Aside from the lecture, it included a number of events for clinicians to learn from international experts. This, I thought, would have been a great opportunity for traditional and alternative medical providers to meet and learn from ME/CFS experts and patients. Unfortunately, I heard that none of the professionals who attended the program felt compelled to enter the field of ME/CFS – a hard realization, considering how many patients were so desperately awaiting their help and support in our province.

Dead-Ends

I was inspired by the medical progress and the knowledge that the lives of some patients improve through the methods Dr. Peterson shared; but then I realized that this information, no matter how I looked at it, was leading to more of a dead-end, at least for me personally.

I know that I cannot access most of the research lab testing or treatment options that are currently available outside my country due to the strain of repeated travel and the exorbitant cost of the treatments. However, hearing about the latest laboratory testing and experimental treatments now available in the United States and elsewhere in the world is comforting. For the tests and treatments that are available in my country, there are very few doctors in mainstream medicine who have the experience to interpret the tests or to manage the interventions. Some examples which are not available here are the drugs Ampligen, Rituximab, or high-dosage antivirals.

Some of the medications mentioned by Dr. Peterson are administered intravenously on a weekly basis or more, and for long periods of time. For those treatments to have a chance to work, I would have to consider the option of a long-term move to the United States. Treatment obtained in another country often does not have follow-up care available in Canada since medical professionals are not experienced in the illness or the treatments.

And there are no guarantees. If I knew that these therapies would make me well in a year or two, I would consider them. But they, for now, come with no assurance of improvement, and some come with substantial risks.

This was not the first dead-end I had experienced in my search for recovery. I, in common with most patients, have faced impasses at every stage of the illness. These can include every aspect of care such as:

- Finding a doctor interested or experienced in ME/CFS.

- Getting a proper diagnosis and follow-up.

- Ordering appropriate lab tests, inside and outside of our home countries.

- Having the financial means for the tests or treatments long-term.

- Receiving informed and up-to-date interpretation from the recurrent lab testing.

- Finding a safe and effective treatment/combination of treatments.

- Sustaining follow-up monitoring and care.

So Many Hats

The lecture also confirmed how multifaceted dealing with this condition is: Patients need energy to sort it out, process it, understand what is happening, and take appropriate action. In other words, the fact that we are still in the early stages of understanding this illness forces patients to be responsible for their own care and for developing their own knowledge base – to be their own advocates.

Here are some of the hats I need to wear which are depicted in this section's illustration (aside from those of mother, wife, daughter, and friend):

- The top hat – Understanding history and politics.

- The crown – Acting as a decision-maker on difficult health issues.

- The military helmet – Being a warrior both in battle with illness and to regain health.

- The cowboy hat – Being an advocate and an activist.

- The nurse cap – Understanding medicine and treatment options (both traditional and alternative).

- The police officer's hat – Keeping the peace between the ill and the healthy.

- The graduate's cap – Learning about science and research.

We're so busy "making it real" so we can heal, which means supporting at least some of these roles at times. Sometimes I feel that we are alone taking on these responsibilities, and that unless healthy people put on these hats too, there will be no improvement, no supportive infrastructure, and no solution.

While my poor health tempts me to give up all hats (except for a nightcap – the drink, not the hat), what I really wish for is to put my healthy hat back on. I hope I can sport it soon.

My Job and ME/CFS: Fading Away [269]

Carol Lefelt | November 16, 2013 | New Jersey, U.S.

We humans define ourselves in terms of what we can DO. With CFS you have an existential crisis, because you think, "If I can't DO, who or what AM I?" ~ Chris B

I walk to the wooden cubbies in my school's front office to pick up my mail. Usually my box is stuffed with notices, pamphlets, messages from the guidance department, invoices, catalogues, book samples – so much stuff that there's an overflow box for the Humanities Department on the floor. But I can't find my name. It goes from Lassiter to Meyers. There's no Lefelt.

What's going on? I've been working in this high school for twenty-five years, checking my mailbox every single day. "Good morning," I say to the other teachers crowding the office.

They smile vaguely, surprised to see me there. I approach Edie, the secretary I've known forever. "I can't find my name," I tell her. I've looked and re-looked. She flashes her warm smile but doesn't answer. Then I remember that I haven't been receiving my salary checks for a long time. She explains that she's called the business manager and superintendent many times, but no one seems to know anything.

I try to see the principal, but his office is empty. I stand bewildered. Lost.

And then, I wake up.

I'd been part of this school community for my whole professional life. I'd taught every course in the English Department: all levels of ninth and tenth grade English; electives like Lively Arts, Poetry, Modern Novel and Satire back in the 'seventies and 'eighties; most recently Creative Writing and Advanced Placement English. I'd become the writing guru.

One year, when Highland Park decided to move the seventh grade from the middle school building into the high school building, parents rebelled and insisted they'd only agree to the switch if I were the seventh grade English teacher. I was flattered but furious; I wanted to teach upperclassmen, not the little middle school pishers with their raging

---

269 Excerpted and adapted from the story "My Job: A Chronic Fatigue Syndrome Chronicle #15" on Health Rising, posted on November 16, 2013. www.cortjohnson.org/blog/2013/11/16/job-chronic-fatigue-syndrome-chronicle-15 (accessed June 29, 2016).

hormones and concrete thinking, and I cried when the principal, who had the right of assignment, gave me the news.

Then I actually came to adore this group of kids, many of whom I taught in grades seven, nine, eleven, and twelve. I still communicate with some of them. Thank you, Facebook.

I had a reputation in the community for being hard but effective. Some students loved me; some hated me. A sophomore, Kerrianne, tormented me daily with her refusal to do anything in class but curse at me. But Nancy bragged to her mother about how she loved *Romeo and Juliet* and knew all the dirty jokes because she had Mrs. Lefelt for English. Many wrote me letters from college thanking me for teaching them to write and to love reading.

I advised *Dead Center,* the literary magazine, which won all kinds of awards, including the much-coveted "Superior" rating from the National Council of Teachers of English (NCTE). We met evenings in my basement, and I baked chocolate chip banana muffins with wheat germ, which the staff ate and teased me about the next day in school. (She made us healthy muffins!) I started a student-run writing center named a "Center of Excellence" by NCTE. I trained these students during the day in a course I originated and developed called "Writing and Responding."

I saw parents all over town. In the supermarket and the beauty parlor and the B-B-Big convenience store, people stopped me and asked, "Aren't you Mrs. Lefelt? My daughter talks about your class all the time!" Steve, the Superior Court Judge, became better known as "Mrs. Lefelt's husband" in the homes of Highland Park. I'd taught some of his law clerks. "Are you related to Mrs. Lefelt?" they'd ask him.

Many times, I entered the front office where some stranger sat waiting for something: maybe a job interview or a meeting with an administrator to demonstrate a new software package to enhance scheduling or record keeping. I'd known everyone else in that room for years. Unlike this outsider, I was a part of things, an important part.

The Flu Shot

Then came the cold January morning, the school's broken heating system and the resulting day off. So I took the opportunity to go to the doctor's office for my yearly flu shot. I had never had any sort of reaction from the shot in prior years. However, this time was different – life changing. Three days after the shot, I developed a severe sore throat and chest, body aches stronger than anything I'd ever experienced, pounding temples, a head-spinning sensation, and sinus congestion. These symptoms did not recede and sent me wandering from doctor to doctor in search of a diagnosis and treatment. For the next year-and-a-half, I tried to keep working. I'd feel well enough one day, but then the exertion would accelerate my symptoms, and I'd find myself back in bed the next.

When I finally couldn't struggle to continue working anymore, I rolled around in my sickbed in fear and panic: fear and panic from this unnamed illness, but also from suddenly being no one, nothing, severed from all my routines, from the people I'd related to every day for twenty-five years – from all the connections I'd made.

Who was I now? Like Macbeth's rival Macduff, "from his mother's womb untimely ripped," I'd been untimely ripped from my life.

My colleagues celebrated their retirements with special evening dinner parties and lots of hoopla. I was too sick for that.

I forced myself to attend an after-school farewell party. The superintendent had assured me I wouldn't have to stay long, and so I searched my closet for something to wear, since I had lost enough weight that everything looked baggy. Feeling scrawny and wobbly, I walked into the high school cafeteria to enthusiastic greetings from many colleagues, but didn't have the strength to get around to everyone.

After the preliminary chatting and cake eating, came the speeches…The superintendent made a sweet and flattering speech, as did Steve Heisler, my colleague, friend and around-the-block neighbor. They presented me with a few retirement gifts, and then waited for me to say something. Speech? I had to talk?

I have no memory of what I babbled, but I know that I failed to thank people for their kindnesses, especially the ones who had taught my classes for the semesters I had been missing. After a twenty-five-year career, I blew the final minutes with some impromptu drivel that glossed over my very real and complicated feelings.

For all the years since that afternoon, I've regretted that I hadn't thought to prepare something. There's a lot I should have said, but at the time, I was so uncomfortable and ill, I just wanted to go home. I was in lockdown.

At fifty-five years old, I just faded away.

Today

I miss dreadfully the sea of eager and intelligent faces I stood before each day. I miss the hilarity, the warmth, the excitement, the probing of a good class; the creativity and honesty of good student writing; the crafting of engaging and challenging lessons; the more personal and private discussions during individual conferences.

I drive by the school building now and feel little connection. There's my parking spot; here are the windows of the classrooms in which I taught; that's the door to the hallway of what used to be the English wing where kids would hide to smoke a joint in the 'seventies. I've gone inside a few times to see drama productions. But that was in a former life that I can barely conjure on these pages, a sequence of days and weeks and years that added up to something meaningful but now is distant and indistinct.

For years, the opening of school in September brought an especially powerful depression. But I've mellowed with time, and I'm grateful to no longer feel such deep September sorrow and estrangement.

I am also grateful that I actually had a fulfilling career for so many years, unlike many whose disease started when they were too young to have established themselves. I've watched videos of youngsters like Jessica (The World of One Room[270]), Sazra[271] Claire,[272] and Ben.[273] CFS/ME so tragically trapped, restricted and isolated them when they were teenagers. Imagine the profundity of their loss.

Because I worked for twenty-five years, I also have great health insurance from the state of New Jersey in addition to Medicare, along with a pension. Again, so many sufferers younger than me do not have these benefits.

I try to remind myself of this "luck" in my darkest moments of self-pity. Sometimes it helps.

---

270 www.youtube.com/watch?feature=player_embedded&v=VH-puNCQxh4 (accessed June 4, 2016).

271 www.youtube.com/watch?v=j5tE0BHiyWc (accessed June 4, 2015).

272 www.youtube.com/watch?v=cPH3kKkEYAI (accessed June 4, 2016).

273 www.youtube.com/watch?v=NRrGVL_TVVk (accessed June 4, 2016).

Adapting [274]

Jennie Spotila | August 2012 | Pennsylvania, U.S.

I have been an ME/CFS patient for more than eighteen years, but it was not until I had two cardiopulmonary exercise stress tests (CPET), spaced twenty-four hours apart (referred to as the Stevens Protocol), in 2012 that I truly began to grasp my limitations. I have attacked ME/CFS the way I attacked everything in my healthy life – college, law school, or a career as a litigation attorney. I pushed myself to the limit, working to exhaustion until bed was the only choice. Then I would get up and do it again the next day. I believed that pushing myself was the only way to make the most of my ME/CFS limitations, even though that meant increased pain and misery. But the exercise testing I went through showed that I was much more disabled than I knew. I was operating over my anaerobic threshold (AT) [275] just by sitting still on the second test day. By pushing myself so hard for years, I had become habituated to being over my AT, and this led to severe overexertion and crashes. The exercise testing gave me the actual parameters of my functionality, and I began wearing a heart rate monitor to signal when I was over my limit. [276]

I was shocked at how frequently the alarm sounded and how little activity could set it off. I despaired that the things I had thought I was capable of pushing myself through would now be off limits. Take, for example, making and canning jam, one of my hobbies. Working in a hot kitchen for several hours clearly seemed out of bounds.

But could I bring the art of jam making within my limitations? There is a way to adapt some of our activities to make them feasible and it usually requires the sacrifice of other things. For me, making peach jam was worth the effort and the changes.

I remember my mother and grandmother canning every year. My grandmother would put up jars of peach halves and applesauce, and my mother made strawberry jam. It always seemed like a silly waste of time to me, since you can buy all those things in a store. But canning is a "thing" now, and on a whim, I decided to try it a couple years ago.

---

274 Excerpted and adapted from the blog Occupy CFS, "Adapting." www.occupycfs.com/2012/08/31/adapting (accessed June 6, 2016).

275 The level of exercise at which the rate of oxygen uptake into muscle becomes limiting and there is an increasing proportion of anaerobic metabolism to yield lactate.

276 By measuring respiratory gases and monitoring the heart rate, one can determine the maximum heart rate to stay under in order to avoid acid buildup, which is part of post-exertional malaise (PEM).

I made one batch of strawberry jam, and I was hooked. I can't explain it, but there is something extraordinarily satisfying about hearing the ping of jars sealing: Because then, you know you've done it right.

But canning is a high-energy activity. There are several places in the process where you can't stop for a break. The boiling water in the canner heats up the kitchen. Many recipes require constant stirring. I always dissolved into a puddle on the floor after a canning session. The day I turned fifty pounds of tomatoes into thirteen quarts of tomato sauce comes to mind as an example of the insanity.

When I started using the heart rate monitor, canning was one of many hobbies that seemed completely incompatible with this new way of pacing. Certainly my old way of canning was now impossible. But could I adapt the process to be more heart rate friendly? My husband bought a peck of peaches at our local farmer's market, so I decided to give it a shot.

Here's what happened:

1. Gather equipment (canner, funnel, tongs) and wash jam jars. Move very slowly so you don't set off the heart rate monitor.

2. Sit down for 10 minutes.

3. Blanch peaches.

4. Sit down for 5 minutes.

5. Peel peaches and chop. Mix peaches with lemon juice and hope they won't turn brown while you rest.

6. Lie down for 15 minutes.

7. Drink a large glass of water.

8. Drag chair over to stove so you can sit while you stir the jam. Make jam.

9. Wonder how sick women managed to survive on the frontier. Decide that they didn't.

10. Remove jars from boiling water. Wonder why no one has invented a better jar lifter that makes you less likely to scald yourself.

11. Fill jars with jam. Quietly exult that there is one half-jar of jam that will have to be consumed immediately.

12. Add lids and move jars back to the canner.

13. Drink a large glass of water. Resist the burning urge to do all the dishes. Lie down for 10 minutes instead.

14. After jars have boiled for 10 minutes, remove lid and turn off heat. Start the dishes.

15. After 5 minutes, remove jars from the canner and wait for that lovely PING! As the lids seal, finish the dishes.

16. Collapse on the couch.

17. Test jam on a piece of toast.

18. Wonder how you got a splatter of jam on the *back* of your T-shirt.

19. Admire your lovely jars of jam.

Did taking rest breaks make it easier? Yes. My heart rate monitor went off a couple times, but never for very long, and the highest it went was 100 beats per minute. I was still exhausted at the end of the process, but I don't think it was quite as bad as previous canning sessions. That may just be wishful thinking since I don't have hard data from past years for comparison. My pre-heart rate monitor canning would have taken 1.5 hours. Adding in the rest breaks extended it to 2.25 hours.

I think I'll pat myself on the back for giving this a try. Rather than assume that this hobby is off limits because of the way I used to do it, I tried to adapt it to my limitations. It's bittersweet because I was happy to be doing it, but also frustrated that I couldn't work as fast as I did before. It would be easier if I could recruit help. (Anyone want to wash my dishes?) And I doubt I'll be tackling monster projects like thirteen quarts of tomato sauce any time soon. But I'm really proud of my peach jam, and it will taste even better for the effort that I put into it.

Having a Regular Day

Kelvin Lord [277] | February 2013 | U.S.
Introduction by Cort Johnson

In 2010, Kelvin Lord dragged himself into Dr. Lapp's office in a last-ditch effort to recover his failing health. A year of Ampligen infusions and thirty-plus often hilarious and poignant blogs later, he signed off with a blog in January 2011, "Learning to Fly Again," charting his gains. He wasn't fully recovered, but they were still impressive: brain fog and orthostatic intolerance gone or almost gone, working six hours a day, able to do forty-five minutes of resistance training. In short, Kelvin had a life again, and a pretty productive one at that. Next on his agenda was to take up past passions, such as parasailing and gliding.

He then disappeared from the Internet for two years. Now he's back.

The timing of the blindness couldn't have been worse. It was 5:30 a.m. I was driving in a new town, on a frozen highway, in the cold pre-dawn morning darkness, when it crept up on me.

I had just left the all-night pharmacy, having picked up a few items my wife said we really needed, when I struggled to get the defroster on. For some reason, the windshield wouldn't clear completely. But I motored on anyway.

I had been finished with Ampligen for almost a month and had moved to this city in the Rockies to live my post-Ampligen life in health and clean air. Amazingly, my very first day here, by divine providence, I found one of the best doctors in the region who was more than familiar with ME and more than ready to start me on a detox program and Methylation Protocol. So I had been on both treatment plans for a couple weeks, with no noticeable side effects. That is, until that moment.

As I passed a big intersection lit up by Las Vegas-style signage, it became obvious: The defroster wasn't the problem; my right eye was! Just like a bathroom mirror fogs over with steam, the vision in my right eye was completely whited out. But surprisingly, I didn't panic. After having dealt with this disease for over two decades, nothing surprised me anymore. Besides, it wasn't my first experience with temporary blindness.

The last time one or both of my eyes stopped working was back in Charlotte, during the Ampligen trial. I was initially freaked out about it, but Dr. Lapp reassured me that when the drugs and the immune system start defeating the bugs or viruses, their decaying

---

277 Originally published on Health Rising, Feb 27, 2013. www.cortjohnson.org/blog/2013/02/28/kelvin-lord-returns (accessed June 7, 2016).

corpses are often so toxic to our systems that side effects, like temporary blindness, are not uncommon.

So although driving with one eye is tricky, that morning, I was neither worried nor concerned. After all, I'd been there before. The blindness would pass, I told myself. Besides, this was evidence that the detox and Methylation were working! So I continued down the road, Foo Fighters music blaring through my car speakers, oblivious to the trooper behind me – until the red and blue lights in my rear-view mirror lit up my car and every car in front of me.

With 100,000 lumens radiating from that officer's light bars, the remaining vision I had in my left eye was now also [temporarily] ruined. Knowing that the police don't normally let guys like Stevie Wonder or Ray Charles get behind the wheel, I forced my eyelids open in an effort to look "normal" to the officer.

The sheriff's deputy who approached my window was very nice. He kindly explained the speed limit situation and offered that, as I was new in town, he'd let me go with a warning – but he first needed to see my proof of insurance.

Now I don't know about you, but even on a good day and with clear vision, finding registration paperwork in my glove compartment is a challenge. That morning, I just used the sense of touch and felt for what I *thought* was my insurance paper. I cheerily handed it to him with an overly enthusiastic, "There you go, officer!"

Minutes later, he was walking back to my car with my warning in hand. But wait! Did I sense him chuckling as he approached my drivers' side window again? Sure seemed like it. When he spoke with a giggle in his voice, I knew something was up.

"Sir," the sheriff said, "here's your paperwork back, and the warning for the speed. If you'll just sign here we'll get you safely back on your way."

As I grabbed the paperwork back and signed the ticket, the sheriff added, "By the way sir, you may want to get that proof of insurance card in order. The next officer who stops you may not want what you're offering."

Looking down at the document in my hand revealed why the sheriff was chuckling. On top of the paper I thought was my proof of insurance, in big, bold 14-point Arial type was the Walgreen's Pharmacy coupon headline staring back at me: "Save $5 When You Buy Four Fleet Enemas!"

With the deputy still grinning and stopping traffic for me, I slowly merged into traffic going about one mph, still incredulous that I had given the officer a coupon for an enema. Yet, the moment was not lost on this amazing officer. As I pulled away with my window still open, I heard him yell to me, "Have a super regular day, sir!"

I got the joke, and chuckled out loud, even though I thought to myself, *No one with this disease EVER has a regular day, sir.*

CHAPTER 11

Looking for Clarity in the Confusion

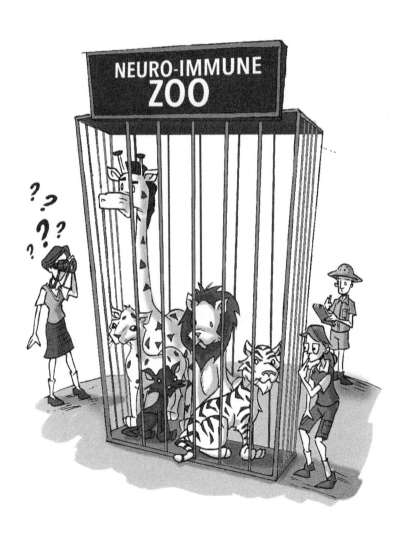

The National ME/FM Action Network and the Canadian Consensus Criteria

Lydia Neilson Interview by Maureen MacQuarrie
March 2015 | Ontario, Canada
Introduction by M. MacQuarrie

Lydia Neilson is the founder and chief executive officer of the National ME/FM Action Network, an all-volunteer, registered Canadian charity founded in 1993 to provide support, advocacy, education, and research for myalgic encephalomyelitis/chronic fatigue syndrome (ME/CFS) and fibromyalgia (FM). In the following interview, which has been edited and condensed, Lydia answers a few questions regarding how she ended up being part of the creation of the Canadian Consensus Criteria and what her thoughts are about the future.

I know you founded the National ME/FM Action Network, but I don't know anything about your personal history. What can you tell us?

There are dates in your life you never forget. For me, it's October 17, 1986, and the last day I worked for a living. It all started when everyone in the law office where I worked was exposed to a co-worker who thought she had the flu and only decided to see her doctor when she wasn't getting better. She was diagnosed with high titres of the *Epstein-Barr virus* (EBV). By that time, everyone in the office was ill. Though they took weeks to recover, all bounced back to normal – everyone, that is, except me.

My doctor sent me for tests that came back positive for high titres of EBV, along with the comment that it was not of significance. She told me I needed to rest, and I would be well in three months or so. Fat chance, I found out later.

What followed were three years of doctors' appointments, visits to the hospital, specialist appointments, and tests. Nothing showed up on any of the diagnostic tests, except for the EBV, so for all intents and purposes, I was extremely healthy. Really?

As my health and spirit deteriorated, my doctor told me that she knew I was ill, but she'd run out of options as to what it might be. However, she had received a letter from Dr. Byron Hyde who had written a letter to doctors in Ottawa advising them to watch out for something called myalgic encephalomyelitis (ME). Dr. Hyde had recently been on a trip to England and had familiarized himself with this condition, and he had patients in Ottawa who were in the same shape as me.

Since I had nothing to lose, I asked to see him. Dr. Hyde sent me for tests; what came back indicated an active Coxsackievirus. ME was then confirmed as the diagnosis. My spirits were lifted as I felt I would be taken seriously and I would be on my way to recovery. This turned out to be a good news/bad news situation. Sure, I had a diagnosis, but the bad news was there was no treatment available.

In the three years following my diagnosis, my life mainly consisted of sleeping in my bed or on the couch, dressing, and struggling to make it from one room to the other, followed by more rest. Watching television and reading became things of the past, as did seeing friends or any kind of entertainment. My husband Al (who I am sad to say passed away in 2008) and my two sons somehow managed to hold our household together.[278]

Many people have a similar illness story, but what prompted you to start an organization?

With trial and error came small discoveries that helped me function better. They did not cure me, but gave me a quality of life and I wanted to share what I had learned with others. So I decided to try and set up a support group, and I put a notice up on a grocery store bulletin board. I was amazed when fifty people showed up for a meeting of what would become the Ottawa MESH (Myalgic Encephalomyelitis Self Help) group. I also became the Communications Director at The Nightingale Research Foundation,[279] the charitable organization founded by Dr. Hyde to research ME and similar illnesses. This got me in touch with not only people from Canada and the United States but from around the world.

It became very clear that what had happened to me had happened to many people. What we all had in common was that we needed help and support with our daily lives. I felt less alone, but MESH was not enough to help others. We needed to unite. I knew that the issues facing people with ME and fibromyalgia (FM) are very similar and that we had to look at it from the national and international perspective. Thus, in 1993 the National ME/FM Action Network came to be.

Can you tell us more about the National ME/FM Action Network?

The Network now has a national and international following. It collaborates with support groups, organizations, and the medical and legal communities. *QUEST,* our quarterly newsletter, contains research, legal, and support information. In September 2011, we

---

278 Lydia Neilson's full story can be found at unheardvoices.mefmaction.com/?cat=1 (accessed June 7, 2016).

279 The Nightingale Research Foundation can be reached at www.nightingale.ca (accessed May 22, 2016).

hosted the tenth International IACFS/ME Research and Clinical conference in Ottawa for ME/CFS, FM, and related illnesses. In 2008 Margaret Parlor took on additional responsibilities as the president of the organization as well as newsletter editor and I continued as the chief executive officer.

Our logo is the Canada geese flying in V formation. I chose the Canada geese because they flew over our house on their way going to the south for the winter or returning from there. The geese pick up speed by flying in V formation and this also makes it easier on the other flyers. Our motto has become *DO NOT REACT TO UNFAIRNESS BUT ACT FOR CHANGE.* Like our logo demonstrates, by uniting our efforts and taking turns to lead, we also make it easier for each other.

I started the Network because I saw a need, so it was a great honor that I was presented with the Governor General's Meritorious Service Medal.[280]

The Canadian Consensus Criteria (CCC) are so important in the history of our illness. We are interested in how they came to be.

These criteria are perhaps the Network's most important project to date. They began in the late 1990s, when we sent a questionnaire to doctors in Canada asking them what they thought was the most important aspect in diagnosing and treating people suspected of having ME and FM. Their response was, "standardized clinical definitions."

Armed with that information, Drs. Anil Jain and Bruce Carruthers, two physicians experienced in the diagnosis and treatment of ME and FM patients, were recruited to draft the definition. The project was coordinated by one of the National ME/FM Action Network's then directors, Ms. Marj van de Sande. Health Canada supplied the terms of reference and selected the Expert Consensus Panel, which would make the final determinations. Between them, the experts had seen more than 20,000 patients with ME and/or FM.

The Consensus Workshop was held March 30th to April 1, 2001. With the expert panel's unanimous consent, the documents for ME and for FM were established: "Clinical Working Case Definition, Diagnostic and Treatment Protocols." They were published in medical journals in 2003.[281]

In these documents, the conjoined name "myalgic encephalomyelitis/chronic fatigue syndrome" was used to define a very specific illness; an illness focused, not on fatigue, but on post-exertional malaise. In response to requests for shorter, easier to read versions, Dr. Bruce Carruthers and Ms. Marj van de Sande produced the Overviews of the ME/CFS and of the FM definitions and protocols in 2005.

---

280 Lydia was presented with the Governor General's Meritorious Service Medal (MSM) in 2005, and in 2011 the Special Service Award by the IACFS/ME.

281 The ME/CFS definition and protocols were originally published in Haworth's Journal of Chronic Fatigue Syndrome and the one for fibromyalgia was in Haworth's Journal of Musculoskeletal Pain.

The CCC are well-respected around the world. You must be very proud of that achievement.

Although an international expert panel created it, the ME/CFS clinical case definition has become known worldwide as the Canadian Consensus Criteria (CCC). It has gained the respect and support of clinicians and researchers, and it has been tested both clinically and in research.

The clearest example of this support came in the fall of 2013 when over fifty ME/CFS clinicians and biomedical researchers sent a letter[282] to the Honorable Kathleen Sebelius, U.S. Secretary of Health and Human Services. This letter was to advise the Secretary of Health that these experts had reached a consensus that the CCC should be used as the case definition for this disease. This advice was not put into action.

What are your thoughts about the future?

We need research and a unified [set of] criteria worldwide for diagnosing and treating ME/CFS and for treating FM. I feel that the future is bright as we are all on the same page regarding the things that matter. Let's not quibble about the things that will not assist in finding the answers.

---

282 The letter and signatories can be found at dl.dropboxusercontent.com/u/89158245/Case%20Definition%20Letter%20Sept%2023%202013.pdf (accessed July 25, 2016).

Reality Check: CFS and the Ugly Side of Our Public Health System

Mary Dimmock | May 2014 | U.S.
Introduction by Valerie Free

In 2015, Mary Dimmock and her son, Matthew Lazell-Fairman, prepared a well-referenced background paper, "Thirty Years of Disdain."[283] It examines the policies created, and the actions taken, by HHS as well as health agencies from other countries over the last thirty years. It exposes the impact they have had on how ME is understood, studied and treated.[284] Here Mary gives us some personal background and a look into their important paper.

In 2010, my son Matthew developed myalgic encephalomyelitis (ME) – a disease that causes profound neurological, immunological, and energy production dysfunction – after contracting giardia[285] while backpacking in Asia. Since then, I have watched, helpless, as this disease has ripped his life to shreds, turning the promise of a vibrant and spirited future into a soul-crushing existence that has been so unrelentingly harsh and circumscribed, so brutal, so cornered and with so little hope that I have wondered how he manages to keep going.

But worse than the heartbreak, it has been profoundly disturbing and surreal to watch as the world around my son, especially the medical community, not only dismisses his disease, but also ridicules and even brutalizes him for believing that it is real and serious.

When my son first became sick, I struggled to understand what was happening to him physically. Then I struggled to understand why there was such a disparity between what he was experiencing and the response of doctors, the public, and especially the U.S. Health and Human Services (HHS) — the government agency responsible for our nation's public health. I naively thought that perhaps patients and advocates just needed to do a better job of helping CDC, NIH, and FDA understand the disease.

But after four years of talking to ME patients and researchers, reading about ME science, history and politics, and trying to engage with Health and Human Services (HHS) on more occasions than I can count, I am left with the simple fact that HHS has

---

283   For more information on background, history, and politics, refer to the entire paper at http://bit.ly/The_Burial_of_ ME_Background (accessed July 25, 2016).

284   To get an idea of the main criteria used over the years, you can refer to Appendix E of this book.

285   Giardia is a parasite that infects the intestines of humans and animals. The infection from this parasite is called giardiasis, or "beaver fever."

known about ME for over thirty years – since before my son was even born – and has utterly failed to take ME seriously or provide even a small fraction of the funding needed to address this crisis. HHS has provided erroneous medical education that has trivialized ME, confused doctors on the nature of ME and harmed patients, including my son, with inappropriate treatment recommendations.

Worst of all, HHS' actions have buried ME inside of chronic fatigue syndrome, a man-made waste-bin of medically unexplained fatiguing conditions inextricably linked to psychiatric illness.

The impact on ME research, medical care and patient lives has been devastating – and entirely predictable. I spent my career in the pharmaceutical industry, and everything I know about science says that the failure to carefully define what you are studying – in this case, to correctly and precisely define the disease – is bad science that will drown your work in conflicting, un-interpretable results. Yet for the past thirty years, such bad science has held ME hostage and destroyed the lives of ME patients – one million Americans and 17 million worldwide!

The story of this disease is about the ugly side of public health policy in this country – the politics, the personal agendas, the bad science, the neglect and arrogance, the lack of transparency, and the utter refusal to listen to ME patients and their doctors. It is the story of how thirty years of failed U.S. public health policy toward ME has sentenced ME patients to an inescapable living hell devoid of hope and support.

What has happened to ME patients is morally and scientifically wrong. For this to continue into the future would be outrageous, especially given what is known – what has been known – about the biology of this disease. For the sake of ME patients everywhere, HHS' public health policy for ME must change. But that will not happen until we find allies in the media, Congress, and the public. To do that, we will need to counter the misinformation and misunderstanding that has held ME hostage. I hope "Thirty Years of Disdain" can help with a small part of that by documenting how ME has been buried inside of the waste-bin called "chronic fatigue syndrome."

This Illness Cannot Be Ignored Any Longer

Matthew Fairman | CFSAC Testimony [286]| June 14, 2012 | U.S.
Introduction by Valerie Free

~∾

At age twenty-four, Matthew Fairman – the son of Mary Dimmock, who authored the last piece – provided a moving statement on the impact of ME/CFS in his testimony[287] at the Chronic Fatigue Syndrome Advisory Committee meeting on June 14, 2012.

∾

I never imagined, before becoming sick, that an illness could so completely redefine my life. Instilled with the inspirational ideal of the disabled who rise above their limitations to achieve great heights, I imagined that disabilities were obstacles that could be overcome, at least to some degree. One only had to pull oneself together and rise above the obstacle. It was to my horror, then, to become sick with ME/CFS, an illness that I could not rise above, an illness that wrecks both body and mind, rendering victims living shells of their former physical and intellectual selves and leaving them forever to languish on the margins of an unaware and uncaring society.

No description can do justice to the experience of this illness.

To those with only healthy points of reference, ME/CFS can only be described as feeling at <u>all</u> times like you have just finished running a marathon, while extremely hung over and severely sick with the flu, after having not slept in at least three days. And even the slightest exertion – brushing teeth, showering, reading the newspaper, washing dishes – amplifies that feeling to even more unbearable levels, to the point where you can only lie on your back, face-up in a dark room not to feel worse.

And the longer you are sick, the more ragged and worn out you feel. To state that ME/CFS is comparable to late-stage AIDS, congestive heart failure, and multiple sclerosis does not begin to convey the severity of this illness. The harsh, soul-crushing reality of an incurable illness that straitjackets the bodies and minds of its victims is lost in translation.

For me, the change from vibrant life to pallid sickness was frighteningly abrupt. I graduated from Connecticut College Phi Beta Kappa and summa cum laude, after

---

286 Excerpted from the full testimony, which can be found at www.hhs.gov/advcomcfs/meetings/presentations/fairman_061412.pdf (accessed June 7, 2016).

287 As Matthew noted at the beginning of his written testimony: "It took me more than a week and a half, and assistance from my wife and mother, to write this testimony. Reading or writing more than a couple sentences wears me out, making it difficult for me to understand sentences and unable to piece together words. It makes my eyes burn, makes me feel more zoned out, brings on headaches and unrelenting exhaustion. This was a painful labor of love."

winning awards in my final years for outstanding achievement and writing a 275-page honors thesis on the evolution of wartime repression in America.

After college, I backpacked across Asia for five months, traveling alone for two and a half months through an unstable part of western China, India, and Southeast Asia...I also met the wonderful woman who has become my wife. A life of joy and promise lay in front of me.

Today, the sense of boundless opportunity is gone, replaced by never-ending sickness that totally dictates the boundaries of my life. Only two years later, I am unable to work, am largely housebound and cannot read or write for more than a few minutes without developing headaches and becoming confused. I cannot sustain any significant physical or mental exertion without suffering a severe crash.

On days when I crash, I am often so sick that I cannot even leave on the TV, as the light and noise aggravate my symptoms. On those days, being too sick to do *anything at all*, I just lie in bed, lightheaded and zoned out, with my head aching, my eyes burning like fire, my muscles sore and weak, and exhausted to a degree the healthy have never known, yet unable to sleep. My every experience of reality is mediated by pain and incomprehensible fatigue, from the moment of waking till the moment of sleep...

Had I only lost an arm or a leg, I could still enjoy my old Sunday ritual of drinking coffee, reading the newspaper, and listening through my stacks of vinyl records, which now gather dust. Had I only lost my hearing or my sight, I could spend my time advocating, or at least find the right words to express my travails. I might even still pursue a career in academia. But, with this illness, those possibilities are off limits for me. My *only* hope is that they will not always be so.

You must know that ME/CFS is one of the most severe illnesses in America today. This illness is not the "Yuppie Flu," as popularly imagined. Nor is it "all in my head," as our uneducated medical community too often believes. Rather, it is a serious, life-robbing illness that is so torturous and difficult to bear that some choose suicide to escape it.

It is beyond travesty, then, that ME/CFS receives such an outrageously small sum of taxpayer funds for research while other illnesses of similar severity (and often smaller patient populations) receive hundreds of millions and even billions of dollars for research. When this illness is one day solved, it will no doubt be obvious to all, as it is to the doctors, patients, and advocates here today, that those we trusted as stewards of the public health system were too busy, too inattentive, too locked into erroneous, outmoded preconceptions to realize how vastly they were failing to meet the trust we put in them...

It is time for our government to...embrace this illness with a seriousness and vigor that characterized the fight against HIV/AIDS. For that to happen, public officials responsible for ME/CFS must take seriously the trust implicit in their position, for it is their *moral responsibility* to break down the doors that we sick patients cannot reach, to give form to the outrage we patients, doctors, and advocates feel by savagely working the message to Secretary Sebelius that this illness cannot be ignored any longer.

All in the Mind? Why Critics are Wrong to Deny the Existence of Chronic Fatigue

Sonia Poulton[288] [289] | May 2012 | U.K.
Introduction by Valerie Free

Sonia Poulton is a journalist, writer and broadcaster, based in Britain. She began her career as a music journalist but, in 1997, expanded her horizons well beyond the music industry. As she states: "I run the journalistic gamut from the socio-political to popular culture." Her work has appeared in Britain as well as internationally.

This week is Myalgic Encephalomyelitis (ME) Awareness Week. That may not mean a great deal to you. Certainly, it didn't to me.

Oh wait, yes it did.

Based on no personal knowledge whatsoever – fortunately neither I or my loved ones have ME – my judgment was gleaned from how the world has portrayed the illness. Like millions of others, I have seen ME through the eyes of the medical establishment, the government, and the media. The picture has not been good.

Here is what I have previously understood about ME and those who have it.

ME sufferers are work-shy malingerers. They whine, constantly, about feeling tired. They are annoying sympathy seekers.

Damn it. We're all tired. Especially those fools like me who work all hours God sends (and even some he doesn't) to support the type of people who say they are too tired to work.

Oh, and most importantly, ME is "all in the head" and can be overcome with a bit more determination and a little less of the "poor me" attitude.

That, generally, is what I thought about ME.

Until, that is, a reader sent me a DVD of a British-made film about the illness titled *Voices From The Shadows*.

I receive dozens of clips and films each month, and I try and see as many as I humanly can, but there was something about *Voices*...that stopped me in my tracks.

---

288 More can be found at Sonia's website, soniapoulton.co.uk (accessed August 9, 2016).

289 Originally published in the Daily Mail, United Kingdom, May 8, 2012. www.dailymail.co.uk/debate/article-2141230/All-mind-Why-critics-wrong-deny-existence-chronic-fatigue.html (accessed June 7, 2016). Another article on ME was posted on her blog on September 19, 2012 entitled, "ME is no more in the mind than Multiple Sclerosis. When is the world going to get that?"

One of the reasons the film had such an impact is because it challenged my deep-seated preconceptions about ME. Through *Voices...* and the subsequent research I have conducted – I have come to realise that what I thought I knew about the illness was a fallacy, but, more importantly, it was actually detrimental to those affected.

So, as a naturally curious individual (I'm not a journalist by mistake), I began to question why I had been furnished with one version of events – and inaccurate ones at that. The more I began to delve into the subject, the more curious it all became.

Like for example, why are records pertaining to ME locked away in our national archives in Kew for seventy-five years? The normal period would be thirty years. Seventy-five years, the period generally used for documents of extreme public sensitivity and national security, is excessive.

The reason given, that of data protection, is nonsense as it is perfectly acceptable, and easy, to omit names on official documents. The excuse, supplied in Parliamentary questions by the Department of Work and Pensions, didn't wash with me.[290]

Why, I thought, were they making such an exception?

It got me thinking about what information the files actually do contain. And, seeing as the topic of ME is still beset with misunderstanding, we could all benefit from some enlightenment on the subject.

So, to this end – and seeing as it [is] ME Awareness Week – here is my personal guide to shattering the myths and blatantly peddled untruths about ME.

Myth No. 1: ME is a mental illness

Not so. It is a neurological one. It is not a case of "mind over matter" despite many GPs [General Practitioners] and health professionals still thinking it is. Psychiatrists have bagged it as "their thing" and the General Medical Council has been somewhat remiss in supporting it as a physical condition.

I spoke with one ME sufferer, who asked to remain anonymous for fear of upsetting the medical professionals who are currently treating her. She said a new GP at her practice had suggested she take up meditation to help her combat her decades-old condition.

Thankfully there are some doctors, few and far between admittedly, who really understand the physical nature of ME.

Dr. Speight, a medical advisor for a number of ME charities, does. Commenting on the wide-ranging debilitation of the illness, he has said:

---

290 You can find the files at www.meactionuk.org.uk/The-MRC-secret-files-on-ME.htm (accessed August 6, 2016). The Medical Research Council's secret files on ME/CFS, Margaret Williams, December 10, 2009. valerieeliotsmith. com/2015/01/20/the-secret-files-unwrapped-part-i-the-importance-of-fair-and-accurate-records (accessed March 13, 2016). valerieeliotsmith.com/2015/03/02/the-secret-files-unwrapped-part-2-control-not-collaboration (accessed March 13, 2016).

"The condition itself covers a wide spectrum of severity, but even the mildest cases deserve diagnosis and recognition because if they are given the wrong advice or don't handle themselves correctly, they can become worse.

"At the more severe end of the spectrum, there's a minority of patients who are truly in a pitiable state...some of them in hospitals, some of them at home. And this end of the spectrum is really one of the most powerful proofs to me of what a real condition this is and how it cannot be explained away by psychiatric reasons."

Sadly, there are still many health professionals who buy into the notion that ME is a psychological disorder and should be treated as a form of insanity.

In Denmark, only last week, the Danish Board of Health sought to remove a twenty-three-year old woman, Karina, from her family home on the grounds of mental illness despite the fact that what she really has is ME. Karina, bedbound, light and sound sensitive, and too weak to walk is considered to be insane, rather than physically sick, and her family has been repeatedly told by Danish doctors that the diagnosis of ME is not recognised.

Myth 2: ME is just extreme tiredness, right?

Wrong. Despite falling under the chronic fatigue syndrome category – as does fibromyalgia, which has its own Awareness Day next week – it is entirely wrong to assume that ME is merely about lack of energy.

This confusion arose over the past twenty-odd years and is due to the condition being re-classified as a fatigue syndrome. The result of this has been to trivialise the illness which has served as fodder for ill-informed public commentators who have used ME and fibromyalgia to talk about "scroungers" in the benefits system who are "too lazy" to get out of bed. For those who know about the illness, this type of commentary is viewed as dangerous rhetoric that deserves to be classified as a form of hate crime.

Myth No. 3: ME is just like a bad flu

Oh, if only. ME is a complex, chronic, multi-system illness that affects the body in similar ways to multiple sclerosis. In addition, inflammation of the neurological system can lead to heart disease, extreme muscle pain, and other debilitating and life-threatening conditions.

As one doctor put it, comparing ME to an illness like flu is like comparing emphysema to a chest infection. It seriously undermines the extent of ME.

Myth No. 4: ME sufferers should just "pull themselves together"

Many sufferers have found themselves abandoned by health professionals, struck off of registers and even rejected by their own families when they have failed to respond to "tough love." Too many people assume that ME can be overcome with the right mental attitude. This consequently leaves ME sufferers even more vulnerable to issues like depression as they are further isolated. ME is not a case of the mind being able to heal itself with determination. ME breaks the body down, and that also includes the brain.

Myth No. 5: Only adults have ME

Children have ME and their childhoods are destroyed as a consequence. Margaret Rumney of Allendale, Northumberland watched as her eleven-year-old daughter, Emma, was reduced to a shell of her former self when she was struck down with ME nine years ago:

"Since then it has been a continual rollercoaster of emotions and has been one fight after the other," says Margaret. "It is very hard for my daughter being ill. She is virtually housebound, often reliant on a wheelchair, and to have to cope with disbelief and ridicule on top of this makes this illness even harder to bear.

"Our experience of my daughter's school was an awful one. When my daughter was receiving home tuition organised officially by the Education Welfare Officer we were threatened by one professional that if my daughter didn't return to school that it would be classed as a psychological issue and social services would get involved."

Threats and intimidation of this nature at the hands of the authorities are a constant feature of those in the ME community, and particularly those caring for children with the illness. Naturally, this pressure merely adds to the overall anxiety that sufferers are already experiencing. Education is key. Bullying is not.

Myth No. 6: You can "catch" ME

A hotly contested issue: Data suggests it's possible, but the true cause is still subject to much debate among the more knowing professionals. What appears clear, however, is that ME seems to follow on from various viral infections, including meningitis. More research is needed.

Myth No. 7: Real ME sufferers are few and far between

There are currently 250,000 recognised cases of ME in the U.K.. That's 1 in 250, so that's hardly an insignificant number, is it?

Myth No. 8: Only severe cases of ME are worth acknowledging

Terrible misconception. ME ruins people's lives even if the patient is not entirely bed-bound. The media tend to concentrate on the worst-case scenarios, but this does not help the full situation, as it leaves others who are still able to move at times with the stigmatisation of not being "ill enough."

Claire Taylor-Jones, a mother of one from Rhyl in North Wales, has been unable to pursue her ambition of becoming a solicitor after she was diagnosed with ME. In common with other sufferers, Claire has good days and bad days, but she is not consistently well enough to pursue her goals and she is left in a type of Limbo land. Her plans are on hold.

Myth No. 9: Children with ME have neglectful parents

There's the notion that children with ME are actually victims of mothers who have Munchausen's by proxy – the illness where parents act as if the child is sick, to further their own need for attention. This is a particularly dangerous belief system as it leaves the true ME sufferer without sufficient support and diagnosis, and the carer is treated as the problem.

Myth No. 10: Physical exercise will benefit ME sufferers

Absolutely not true. Worse still, enforced "graded exercise" can escalate the condition to dangerous and irreparable levels for the patient. During the research of this subject, I have watched footage of hospital physiotherapists literally bullying ME patients to stand and walk. It is pitiful to witness. The physios say things like, "Come on, you can do it. You just have to put your mind to it" and, at worst, "You're not trying hard enough."

Julie-Anne Pickles, who has had ME for the past seven years, has experienced a serious deterioration in her condition as a consequence of wrong diagnosis and ineffective medical response. She is now ninety percent bedbound and has been diagnosed with depression, diabetes, and angina.

She told me: "Cardiology phoned me with an appointment the other day, and they told me to wear trainers because they want me running on a treadmill while on an ECG!

I said, "You do know I have ME?" They said they did, but not to worry as I won't be running for more than five minutes! Running? I crawled on my hands and knees to the loo this morning!"

This idea among some of the medical professionals, that enforced exercise will help the condition of ME, belongs to a darker time in our history – a period when we thought that autistic children were a result of being born to cold and detached women, or "refrigerator mums" as they were heinously and immorally labelled.

Myth No. 11: ME is not life-threatening

It is, although the true mortality rate of ME is mired in great confusion.

Recently, Labour MP [Member of Parliament] George Howarth asked Paul Burstow, Minister of State for Care Services to supply details of deaths to arise from ME. Mr. Burstow replied, that "this information is not available and is not collected centrally." As with so many issues regarding our sick and disabled, the Coalition had this wrong, too. According to figures obtained from the Office of National Statistics, there have been five deaths listed [with] the cause of ME in recent years.

For campaigners this is nothing less than a fudge of the true scale.

Figures are easy to massage with ME because it triggers so many other illnesses, such as heart disease. Given that many health professionals still deny that ME is a physical condition, they are unable to list it as a cause of death even if it is.

Myth No. 12: ME is an excuse not to work

Despite recognition from the World Health Organisation in 1969 that ME is a neurological disorder, many governments – including our present Coalition – have chosen to ignore this. Consequently, ME sufferers are subject to a battery of controversial fit-to-work assessments. The anxiety and physical exertion this requires generally worsens the condition.

When the ME sufferer is unable to work, because of their illness, they are removed from disability benefits and are plunged into poverty.

So, for ME Awareness Week, let us be clear. ME is comparable to AIDS and cancer and all the other vicious and uncompromising diseases that savage the body and, in some extreme cases, kill it completely. The fact that it is still so widely misunderstood is a modern day travesty that must be addressed without further delay. Or is it convenient that we still view ME as being "all in the mind"? I believe that we, as a nation, deserve to know the truth. Not only for those still battling the disease, but for those poor souls who have already been lost to it.

CHAPTER 12

Science, Research, and Progress

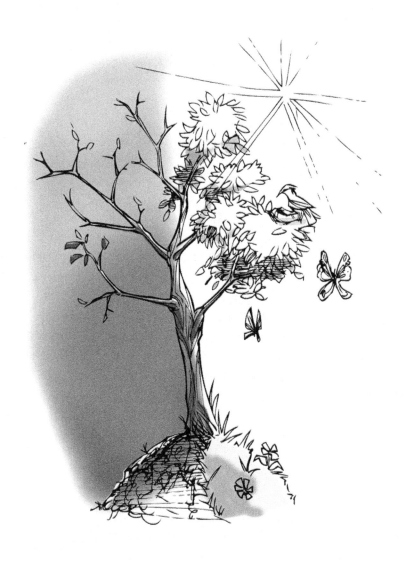

From Darkness to Progress

ME/CFS: Global Perspective and Overview

Transcript of remarks by Daniel Peterson, MD [291]
at a seminar held by the Swedish National Society for ME Patients
at the Swedish Parliament | October 15, 2013 | Stockholm, Sweden
Introduction by Valerie Free

Daniel L. Peterson, MD is an internist in Incline Village, Nevada, and a recognized medical expert on ME/CFS. Dr. Peterson has devoted more than twenty-five years of his clinical career to diagnosing and caring for patients with ME/CFS and related neuro-immune disorders, as well as collaborating with researchers to better understand the illness. His repository of more than 1,000 patient biological samples and records is a rich resource for research studies. Dr. Peterson is a Scientific Advisory Board Committee member of Simmaron Research. He has been described as a pioneer in the treatment of myalgic encephalomyelitis/chronic fatigue syndrome since the 1984 cluster outbreak at Lake Tahoe, Nevada.

Dr. Daniel Peterson: Well, thank you very much for the introduction. And it's such a pleasure to be here again. I've seen the progress in Scandinavia over the past ten years in terms of recognizing chronic fatigue syndrome, or ME, and the importance that you're now assigning to this very disabling and serious disease that I have spent my career [on]; both in basic research and in care of patients…

Just as a brief introduction…The federal diagnostic criteria[292] were established twenty-five years ago, so this is not a new thing to the scene. They have been revised several times, and they continue to be debated, and that's a problem in the field. There really is a need for one set of diagnostic criteria accepted worldwide. We have proposed[293] – and I hope that the people in decision-making positions in Sweden decide to join the bandwagon – to accept the Canadian Consensus Criteria as how the disease should be diagnosed. But, really, we should forget the nomenclature, and we should get on with diagnosing and treating patients.

---

291 The original remarks with the slide presentation can be found at www.youtube.com/watch?v=AAnR2nIrkF4 (accessed June 16, 2016). The footnotes and square brackets with text have been added by V. Free and M. MacQuarrie. For more information about the research being done by Dr. D. Peterson and others at Simmaron Research, see www.simmaronresearch.com.

292 As Dr. Peterson mentions later, the first federal diagnostic criteria were the CDC's 1988 Holmes criteria.

293 The open letter (October 25, 2013) from 50 ME/CFS experts can be found at dl.dropboxusercontent.com/u/89158245/Case%20Definition%20Letter%20final%2010-25-13.pdf (accessed July 20, 2016).

So the prevalence is a question that always comes up because it has been viewed as an orphan disease around the world and actually doesn't meet [the] criteria for orphan diseases. The prevalence in the United States, by conservative counting, is 400 patients per 100,000[294] or over a million patients, making it much more common than multiple sclerosis, for example. And the prevalence in Sweden has been estimated at 40,000,[295] but that's probably underestimated because many patients go undiagnosed…And the prevalence worldwide is 19 million;[296] and I stress that this disease has been found in every country where it has been looked for.

It's costly to treat. And I always like to talk to the politicians about this, because the direct cost in medical care in the United States is $9 billion a year.[297] The indirect costs (when you add missed work, disability payments, and things like that) are $51 billion.[298] So it's actually one of the most costly diseases to deal with. One of the reasons for that is, most of the patients are disabled, in contrast to other chronic diseases (HIV, diabetes, etc…), which are devastating diseases, but people continue to work. It also has quite a young onset, so you're looking at disability for many, many years. So that adds to the cost as well.

There [are] problems with it though, as we have a problem with the diversity of presentation [and] the pathogenesis. Clinicians and researchers have really been confounded with this problem over the years. What we know about this – and I think it's important to emphasize – and what we've found worldwide is that the symptoms are the same, the presentation is the same, the physical exam is the same, and the immunological abnormalities are basically the same around the world.

There's a high degree of limitation of activity.[299] These patients are very, very disabled, even by U.S. Federal Government standards. They have difficulties with things like showering, bathing, cooking, getting out of bed. What other disease can you mention where people have trouble getting out of bed? People who don't have personal experience have trouble grasping that.

---

294 Jason L, Richman J, Rademaker A, Jordan K, Plioplys A, Taylor R, McCready W, Huang C and Plioplys S. 1999. "A community-based study of chronic fatigue syndrome." Archives of Internal Medicine 159(18):2129-2137.

295 iacfsme.org/PDFS/0412-Attachment-7-report-from-Sweden.aspx (accessed August 6, 2016). Report dated March 20, 2012.

296 Prevalence figures vary widely by country and by study. Worldwide prevalence figures are based on estimates. A more commonly reported figure worldwide is 17 million, which appeared in the now retracted XMRV paper – Lombardi, Vincent C., et al. "Detection of an infectious retrovirus, XMRV, in blood cells of patients with chronic fatigue syndrome." Science 326.5952. 2009. 585-589.

297 Reynolds K, Vernon S, Bouchery E, Reeves W. 2004. "The economic impact of chronic fatigue syndrome. Cost Effectiveness and Resource Allocation," 2(4).

298 Lin J, Resch S, Brimmer D, Johnson A, Kennedy S, Burstein N and Simon C. 2011. "The economic impact of chronic fatigue syndrome in Georgia: Direct and indirect costs. Cost Effectiveness and Resource Allocation" 9(1).

299 The limitation of activity and socioeconomic impact has also been demonstrated in the data coming out of the Canadian Community Health Survey (CCHS) in 2005 and 2010 as analyzed by the National ME/FM Action Network Quest 80 and 88. www.mefmaction.com (accessed August 6, 2016).

There's a great socioeconomic impact. Most of the patients are permanently unable to work. The average income in the United States is $15,000, and that's from disability payments; so you can't really survive on that. There's insecurity about food, they have no sense of what community they belong to, and there's difficulty with socialization...It's very common for these patients to end up living in the basement of their parents' home, which is a very sad outcome. There are many unmet medical needs and unmet home care needs in all the systems.

A brief history: In the pre 'eighties, as some of you may know, when the disease was first named by Ramsay in the U.K., he termed this "ME." And I will use them [CFS and ME] simultaneously because about five years ago,[300] it was decided that we'd combine ME with CFS and then ultimately decide on a better name. But unfortunately, the "ultimately" has never arrived, so we're still stuck with these names...

Then in the 1980s and early 1990s, the focus was on fatigue, and the definition surrounded fatigue because that was the outstanding symptom...The Holmes criteria, which was established by the CDC in 1988, was a very restricted diagnosis. It was revised in 1994 [to the Fukuda criteria], and [the focus] became signs and symptoms – malaise – and it is a definition that we still live with for research purposes. So if physicians are publishing papers or something, we use the 1994 Fukuda criteria.[301]

In the 'nineties, the definition broadened because the emphasis became on the neurological complaints, immunological, the recurrent infections, the endocrine abnormalities, and particularly post-exertional malaise, because it's one of the few diseases that is characterized by fatigue worsening with physical or mental exertion. Many chronic diseases actually improve with physical exertion...

There was a consensus diagnosis criteria established in 2003 called the "Canadian Consensus Criteria," which is what we mostly use. [The oldest] criteria [in North America] have been in place for twenty-five years. For the physicians in the room, we've got to stop arguing about this [whether the disease exists] and move forward...

This [the Institute of Medicine (IOM) contract[302]] is a recent development in the United States. We have the patients and researchers who are in advocacy groups, and they give their input to the Chronic Fatigue Syndrome Advisory Committee, which directly advises the HHS [Department of Health and Human Services], which is our central agency that controls health in the United States. They [HHS] recently gave an independent contract

---

300 ME/CFS was combined in the 2003 Canadian Consensus Criteria. In October 2010, the Chronic Fatigue Syndrome Advisory Committee recommended that the term myalgic encephalomyelitis/chronic fatigue syndrome (ME/CFS) be adopted across HHS (the U.S. Department of Health and Human Services).
     wayback.archive-it.org/3919/20140324192813/www.hhs.gov/advcomcfs/recommendations/1012-142010.html (accessed July 7, 2016).

301 For the full Fukuda criteria definition, go to www.cdc.gov/cfs/case-definition/1994.html (accessed July 25, 2016).

302 The IOM report, the product of the process Dr. Peterson is describing, was released in February 2015. It suggested new diagnostic criteria as well as suggesting that the name of the disease be changed to Systemic Exertion Intolerance Disease. www.nationalacademies.org/hmd/Reports/2015/ME-CFS.aspx (accessed June 16, 2016).

to the Institute of Medicine, in order to redefine the disease and to use standards of care, evidence-based medicine, and then they're going to proselytize this to the whole world.

This is their [HHS's] ambitious plan, that over the next eighteen months…this change [redefining the disease] will be made, based on evidence-based medicine, and there will be new recommendations. We'll have to wait and see if that takes place.[303]

So the model of ME/CFS now is that patients have a genetic predisposition[304] – that has been demonstrated many, many times – that an infection, trauma, stress, or toxins can then set off the chain of reactions that's mediated by changes in the endocrine system and in the immunological system that results in the symptoms that we call "ME/CFS".[305]

So in medicine, we try to make the most accurate diagnosis, we determine how severe it is, and we try to do therapeutic interventions. There [are] challenges to this in chronic fatigue though, in that the population is very heterogeneous. There's not a good bio-marker. That means there's not a simple test for this where you can order one test and make the diagnosis. There [are] different clinical definitions; there [are] different view points, [depending on] whether you're practicing in the U.K., the United States, or Japan. There's no licensed drug, and if you think about it, a lot of diseases are kind of defined by the therapy for the disease. And there [are] no really good surrogate markers.

However, what we've realized over years and years of research is that we really need to concentrate on subsets of patients[306] that match each other – that are homogeneous – and we can establish an ideology and a treatment. That's pretty much accepted.

The FDA, you know, is our agency that approves drugs; and drug development takes eight to fifteen years and $100 million. So there is no licensed drug for chronic fatigue/ME right now. This is going to be a long process, unfortunately. They require well-doc-umented and validated endpoints, and we don't have very good endpoints at this point in time.

So how do we approach these challenges? Well, one of the ways … to do this is through computational analysis and bioinformatics. What that basically means is you take a whole bunch of information from thousands and thousands of patients, and then you look sta-tistically for correlations and potential interventions. And that has been done. We have

---

303 The IOM report has been released, as noted in the previous footnote, and still to this day, August 2016, is awaiting official government response.

304 See IACFS/ME Primer for some studies: IACFS/ME (International Association for Chronic Fatigue Syndrome/Myalgic Encephalomyelitis). 2014. ME/CFS: Primer for Clinical Practitioners. Chicago, IL: IACFS/ME.

305 Some of the articles supporting this hypothesis are cited in Brenu E, Driel M, Staines D, Ashton K, Ramos S, Keane J, Klimas N, Marshall-Gradisnik S. 2011. Journal of Translational Medicine. "Immunological abnormalities as poten-tial biomarkers in Chronic Fatigue Syndrome/Myalgic Encephalomyelitis." 9:81.

306 See IOM report p. 57 Box 3-1 "ME/CFS Research Subgroups" and Chapters 4, 5 and 6 for evidence relative to certain subgroups.

now a worldwide database.[307] It started in the United States, and it has now spread to most countries. And I'm trying to encourage the Swedish doctors and the institutions to join so that you can participate in this. We're looking for novel pathogen discovery, for new agents; we're looking for immunological biomarkers, endpoint evaluation so that drugs can be approved. And in spite of the slow progress, drug development and clinical trials are going on.

There are biological markers that most physicians in the world agree with. Chronic Fatigue/ME is called "low natural killer-cell disease"[308] in Japan, and the most common abnormality worldwide is impairment of NK cell functioning. And, interestingly, natural killer cells were actually first described here in Sweden many, many years ago. So you have the scientific expertise here to drive this research forward.

We have associated with Griffith University, Australia: Sonya Marshall[309] who is doing some really innovative work in terms of biomarkers and micro RNAs. Physicians in the room know that that's a really hot field right now, and its utility remains to be determined.

---

307 Such as OpenMedNet and the OMI-MERIT Initiative. See www.healthrising.org/blog/2013/06/18/medicine-for-the-21st-century-the-open-medicine-institute-takes-on-chronic-fatigue-syndrome-me-cfs (accessed August 6, 2016); and www.openmedicinefoundation.org/2015/01/27/andreas-kogelnik-md-phd-comments-on-a-busy-and-progressive-year-of-research (accessed August 6, 2016). For more information, go to the OpenMedNet website, www.openmednet.org (accessed August 20, 2015).

308 This name, or the alternate, "low natural killer-cell syndrome" (LNKS), was for some time widely attributed as the name used in Japan (including in a Newsweek article in 1990) as a result of work done by Japanese researchers in the 1980s. LNKS is a condition very similar to – but not the same as – CFS. Aoki T, Usada Y, Miyakoshi. 1985. "A novel immunodeficiency: Low NK syndrome (LNKS)". Jap J Med 3212:14-17, Also see Aoki T, Miyakoshi H, Usuda Y, & Herberman R. 1993. "Low NK Syndrome and its Relationship to Chronic Fatigue Syndrome." Clinical Immunology and Immunopathology, 253-265. Indeed Japanese researchers have been involved in research into ME/CFS. Nakatomi Y, Mizuno K, Ishii A, Wada Y, Tanaka M, Tazawa S... Watanabe Y. 2014. "Neuroinflammation in Patients with Chronic Fatigue Syndrome/Myalgic Encephalomyelitis: An 11C – (R) –PK11195 PET Study." Journal of Nuclear Medicine, 945-950.

A Japanese CFS prevalence study was published in 2011. Hamaguchi M, Kawahito Y, Takeda N, Kato T, Kojima T. 2011. "Characteristics of chronic fatigue syndrome in a Japanese community population: Chronic fatigue syndrome in Japan." Clinical Rheumatology PMID: 21302125.

309 Dr. Sonya Marshall-Gradisnik's research expertise is focused on ME/CFS, natural killer cell function, and signaling pathways, T regulatory and B cell phenotypes and cytokine production, and transcriptional profiling and gene expression. She teaches immunology at Griffith University, Australia. Dr. Peterson collaborated on papers coming out of Dr. Marshall-Gradisnik's laboratory including: Brenu E, Ashton K, Driel M, Staines D, Peterson D, Atkinson G, Marshall-Gradisnik S. 2012. "Cytotoxic lymphocyte microRNAs as prospective biomarkers for Chronic Fatigue Syndrome/Myalgic Encephalomyelitis" Journal of Affective Disorders 141 (2):261-269, doi: 10.1016/j.jad.2012.03.037; and more recently, Brenu E, Ashton K, Batovska J, Staines D, Marshall-Gradisnik S, 2014, "High-throughput Sequencing of Plasma MicroRNA in Chronic Fatigue Syndrome/Myalgic Encephalomyelitis". PLoS One. 9(9) doi:10.1371/journal.pone.0102783.

Right here, Dr. Yenan Bryceson[310] is focusing his research on NK cell function. There are many other people in your local community here – I'm impressed – the virologists, and the chemists, and proteomics…and there's a lot of the basic science here that could contribute to the research worldwide. We're looking for global collaboration, as I mentioned.

There are more than 5,000 peer-reviewed articles. So this is not a new field. This is not speculative. And I just listed [in the slide Dr. Peterson is showing] some of the recent publications with respect to NK cell function and dysfunction.[311]

Well, the FDA, in January, declined the provisional approval of Ampligen. That's a drug that has been used in chronic fatigue since 1988. And the reason they did that is they said it was a safe drug, but there weren't objective endpoints. So, we physicians really have to work hard at designing better clinical trials – multi-centered [trials], meaning international; this can't be some little study that was done in the United States and then expect the rest of the world to accept that. And we're working on some endpoint markers for that in the future.

Now, you've all probably heard about the Norwegian Research Council that has allowed a Phase III trial of Rituximab just across the border here, and the initial results are kind of positive.[312] We're looking for more studies. Some have been proposed: one in California at the Open Medicine Institute; and the Invest in ME charity in London, U.K.[313]… The Open Medicine Institute in Mountain View, California …has very ambitious research and treatment planned for the future,[314] with some grants, outside funding and a mix of governmental funding, to achieve some of these goals that I mentioned.

---

310 Dr. Bryceson is an assistant professor at Karolinska Institute, and his laboratory is located within the Center for Infectious Medicine at Karolinska University Hospital Huddinge. He leads a research group that aims at understanding the complex regulation of cytotoxic lymphocyte function in health, infection and disease in the setting of human genetic variability and environmental factors. The group also hopes to develop new conceptualization of immunological disorders like CFS and new ways to treat them.

311 An example is a paper (on which Dr. D. Peterson collaborated) Brenu E, Driel M, Staines D, Ashton K, Hardcastle S, Keane J,… Marshall-Gradisnik S. 2012. "Longitudinal investigation of natural killer cells and cytokines in chronic fatigue syndrome/myalgic encephalomyelitis." Journal of Translational Medicine 10:88.

312 Phase 3 clinical trial started in 2014 available at clinicaltrials.gov/ct2/show/NCT02229942 (accessed August 6, 2016). In July 2015 the positive results of Fluge and Mella's open label trial were reported and commented on in an article on Phoenix Rising phoenixrising.me/archives/26930 (accessed August 6, 2016). The article can be found at Fluge Ø, Risa K, Lunde S, Alme K, Rekeland I, Sapkota D,… Mella O. 2015. "B-Lymphocyte Depletion in Myalgic Encephalopathy/ Chronic Fatigue Syndrome. An Open-Label Phase II Study with Rituximab Maintenance Treatment." PLoS One, doi: 10.1371/journal.pone.0129898.

313 The 2012 work being done by the Open Medicine Institute on an off-label trial of Rituximab was reported in various sources including phoenixrising.me/treating-cfs-chronic-fatigue-syndrome-me/immune/antivirals-and-immunemodulators/rituximab-rituxian (accessed August 6, 2016). See www.ukrituximabtrial.org/home.htm for a description of what's happening with the proposed U.K. trial (accessed August 6, 2016).

314 See www.openmedicineinstitute.org. Also phoenixrising.me/archives/17128 (accessed August 6, 2016). "Open Medicine Institute: Big Plans and a Sense of Urgency," article by Sasha. July 1, 2013. Along with many other respected physicians & scientists, Drs. Marshall-Gradisnik and Bryceson are signators to the OMI-MERIT initiative.

The Centers for Disease Control set up a study[315] to see how physicians define the disease and if we can find a better phenotype or a better way of describing patients. They proposed a five-year study. We're now in year two of that study…What they did is they took the physicians who see a lot of patients, and we were consulted with respect to entrants into this.

Their conclusion is that there's a great deal of difference between sites, and that a clinical definition is probably not going to be sufficient to diagnose and treat these patients. But they are developing instruments that will be helpful for all of us to measure various things about these patients.[316] And I would encourage all the Swedish patients and physicians to join in this network rather than try to reinvent the wheel and do things that have cost millions and millions of dollars to set up when now, simply with the Internet, you can just join with the databases that are there…

So the novel pathogen study[317]…Dr. Ian Lipkin of Columbia [University, Mailman School of Public Health] – who is called the virus hunter and has discovered over 500 new viruses – is looking in depth at these patients, their blood, their saliva, their urine, [and] tears to see if there are any novel pathogens.

He has some preliminary results that were very exciting to people, and he's completing those studies. He's doing high throughput sequencing,[318] and that's an exciting project. He looks at the communication system; how your immune system communicates with your brain and the rest of your body, and he has found some very interesting abnormalities there.[319]

---

315 Multi-site Clinical Assessment of CFS: to characterize patients with CFS or myalgic encephalomyelitis (ME) in clinical practices of clinicians with expertise in CFS/ME. There are seven participating clinical sites. The project started in 2012 and aims to enroll 450 patients. www.cdc.gov/cfs/programs/clinical-assessment (accessed June 16, 2016). An interview with the CDC's Dr. Beth Unger on the Multi-site study was posted on Phoenix Rising on January 31, 2014. http://phoenixrising.me/archives/22889 (accessed August 6, 2016).

316 Preliminary results were reported at the April 26, 2013, FDA meeting on ME/CFS. www.fda.gov/downloads/Drugs/NewsEvents/UCM353570.pdf (accessed August 6, 2016) with preparation of formal papers for publication underway. See "A Breakthrough for ME/CFS? Dr. Unger on the CDC's Multisite Studies" by Cort Johnson. www.healthrising.org/blog/2014/11/09/breakthrough-mecfs-dr-unger-cdcs-multisite-studies (accessed June 16, 2016). Some of the results have now been published including Klimas N, Ironson G, Carter A, Balbin E, Bateman L, Felsenstein D… Komaroff A. 2015, "Findings from a clinical and laboratory database developed for discovery of pathogenic mechanisms in myalgic encephalomyelitis/chronic fatigue syndrome." Fatigue: Biomedicine, Health & Behavior, 75-96. More information was given by Dr. Unger in a CDC Patient - Centered Outreach and Communication Activity (PCOCA) telephone call on February 23, 2015 and reported on by Cort Johnson on Health Rising, "Big Studies – Big Possibilities: Montoya and Unger on their big Chronic Fatigue Syndrome Projects." April 1, 2015. www.healthrising.org/blog/2015/04/01/big-studies-big-possibilities-montoya-and-unger-on-their-chronic-fatigue-syndrome-programs (accessed August 10, 2016).

317 Simon McGrath: "Lipkin and Hornig go hunting for ME/CFS pathogens," February 27, 2013. phoenixrising.me/archives/16081 (accessed August 6, 2016).

318 A DNA sequencing method that analyzes full sets of protein interactions.

319 Hornig M, Montoya J, Klimas N, Levine S, Felsenstein D, Bateman L, Peterson D, Gottschalk G… Lipkin I. 2015. "Distinct plasma immune signatures in ME/CFS are present early in the course of illness." Science Advances.

We began a new study of the cerebral spinal fluid.[320] Many of these patients have what they call "brain fog" and they have difficulty concentrating and difficulty performing tasks, and the theory is that they have a problem probably with cytokines or other inflammatory markers within their brains. So we went to the source and are looking at the spinal fluid. That has been done in other places in the world as well.[321]

He [Dr. Lipkin] has found some interesting markers indeed, suggesting that there's inflammation in the brain of these patients. There's a lot of work to be done. This is underfunded as well. Dr. Lipkin made an appeal for increased funding. We'll see if that happens so we can complete that study.

So, in summary, very briefly, worldwide collaboration is really necessary. We need to define the patients better. It needs to be universal. Everybody needs to define this the same way. We need to determine a specific diagnosis.

The prognosis, we know. I'm treating the prognosis as bad. People do not recover. They can be treated, and they can have an improved quality of life, particularly if they have experts. And I would encourage the healthcare system here to consider Centers of Excellence[322] where the patients could be treated by experts and returned to their primary care physicians for ongoing care.

We need to find the pathogenesis and the mechanism of disease. I showed you the research that's going on with that. The research is ahead of the clinical care in the United States. We're actually doing more research than we are taking care of patients. We need to design appropriate interventional studies that meet regulatory agencies' requirements, because even if there was a successful drug right now, it probably wouldn't be licensed. We

---

320 The study was published in March 2015. Hornig M, Gottschalk G, Peterson D, Knox K, Schultz A, Eddy M… Lipkin W. 2015. "Cytokine network analysis of cerebrospinal fluid in myalgic encephalomyelitis/chronic fatigue syndrome." Molecular Psychiatry. doi:10.1038/mp.2015.29.

321 Peterson D, Brenu E, Gottschalk G, Ramos S, Nguyen T, Staines D, and Marshall-Gradisnik S. 2015. "Cytokines in the Cerebrospinal Fluids of Patients with Chronic Fatigue Syndrome/Myalgic Encephalomyeltitis. Mediators of Inflammation," 1-4. doi 10.1155/2015/929720. Also Marshall-Gradisnik S, Gottschalk G, Ramos S, Brenu E, Staines D, and Peterson D. 2014. "The role of cytokines in the cerebrospinal fluids of patients with Chronic Fatigue Syndrome/ Myalgic Encephalomyelitis." Cytokine, Vol. 70 (1):31, doi: 10.1016/j.cyto.2014.07.22.

322 Centers of Excellence are medical facilities that would combine research and treatment to care for CFS patients. As Cort Johnson said in his article: CFS patients "don't fit well into our medical system and special measures need to be taken if they're going to get treated properly. A network of Centers of Excellence would be the perfect place to produce a good definition, to methodically assess treatments, and to train young physicians and medical students." www.cortjohnson.org/blog/2015/02/01/case-centers-excellence-chronic-fatigue-syndrome (accessed June 16, 2016).

need to create Centers of Excellence.[323] This is going on in the United States. And we have an open invitation to collaborate with the clinics here that are in existence in Sweden, and if there [are] proposals for new ones, we're happy and open for collaboration.

---

323 Here is what Dr. Peterson said about Centers of Excellence in an interview by Deborah Waroff in October 2013 on Episode 50 of ME/CFS Alert. When asked what he would do if he had all the money in the world, he responded: "I would invest the money in Centers for Excellence. The reason for that is I don't think that primary care physicians can really manage this disease. I think it's too complex, too time-consuming, and they have too many other things to do. If we could get primary care physicians to recognize the disease, to qualify the patient, then they have to have some place to refer them to. I see a great need all around the world for people to seek specialty care, which is appropriate until it [the disease] becomes cookbook...simpler." Dr. Peterson concluded that it will be a long while before ME/CFS becomes as manageable as AIDS.

"End ME/CFS" Mega Chronic Fatigue Syndrome Project Begins [324]

Cort Johnson | October 2014 | U.S.

Now *this* is exciting.

The Open Medicine Foundation (OMF) announced on October 7, 2014, it has created a project called "End ME/CFS" [325] and is raising funds for it. They're looking for five million dollars a year to fund it…That's a really ambitious project. Could they actually pull it off?

I think they could, and the reason why starts with Ron Davis, PhD, the originator and leader of the project (Director, OMF Scientific Advisory Board). His son, Whitney, introduced us. Whitney was quite ill then, but since then has gotten much worse. He now has one of the worst cases of ME/CFS I've heard of [326]…

Ron Davis, PhD, has directed the Stanford Genome Technology Center for twenty years. He has a long list of firsts by his name including one – using restriction fragment polymorphisms to construct genetic linkage maps – that helped launch the field of genomics in 1980 and ultimately made the Human Genome Project possible.

He's won numerous awards and prizes (Eli Lilly, Distinguished CIT Alumni, and NAS Awards and Dickson, Gruber, and Warren Alpert Foundation Prizes). He won the Lifetime Achievement Award from the Genetics Society of America ten years ago. PubMed lists over 500 publications for Dr. Davis – the most I've seen for a researcher.

At the presentation of the Warren Alpert Prize last year, Harvard Medical School geneticist Clifford Tabin concluded that Davis's contributions were so seminal in the world of genetics and disease that it was "impossible to quantify the impact" he and his colleagues had had. In 2013, Davis was pegged in an *Atlantic Monthly* article as one of eight

---

324 This article is excerpted and adapted from Cort Johnson's article originally published on Health Rising. You can find the entire story at www.cortjohnson.org/blog/2014/10/11/end-mecfs-mega-chronic-fatigue-syndrome-project-begins (accessed June 28, 2016).

325 The END ME/CFS Project was founded on the idea that a comprehensive, interdisciplinary effort is needed to produce breakthroughs in our understanding of ME/CFS and neuro-immune diseases.

326 Ron Davis is not the only one on the OMF team with a personal stake in finding answers as quickly as possible. Linda Tannenbaum, Executive Director of the OMF, has a daughter who lives with ME/CFS. As the OMF press release announcing this project notes, "Personal dedication can be a powerful force for making breakthroughs in difficult to understand diseases."

inventors tomorrow's historians will consider the greatest inventors today. "He's not just a one-hit wonder," said Church. "He's a frequent provider of disruptive core technologies."

Frequent is the word. Three years ago, Dr. Davis talked about the urgent need to assess the role the HLA region of our genome plays in ME/CFS. No one, however, had been able to figure out how to analyze this very complex region of our genome. In the interview below, he reports his lab has developed a low cost means of doing that.

It's safe to say that nobody with this kind of background and reputation has worked in the ME/CFS field before.

❧

Now Davis is engaged in the biggest challenge of his career: solving chronic fatigue syndrome. He's best known for his ability to devise creative solutions that clear up technological impasses. He likes nothing better than to attack complex problems…

Davis believes both the field and medicine itself are ripe for breakthroughs. He's been making the rounds telling everybody that ME/CFS is the field to be in now. This is the place to make big breakthroughs that resonate throughout the medical field. He is convinced that cracking ME/CFS will [also] provide key insights to the other puzzling neuro-immune disorders that dot the medical field.

❧

The idea is to get experts from inside the field and from outside the field. The ME/CFS experts will lend their deep knowledge from inside this field. The experts from outside the field will bring a rigor and creative approach to problem solving that has made them experts in much larger fields than ME/CFS.

Thus far, Davis has been able to gather a group of partners the likes of which we haven't seen before in ME/CFS. How many boards boast two Nobel Laureates? The Scientific Advisory Board includes (and the list will grow over time to include ME/CFS experts and more outside researchers):

- **Mark M. Davis, PhD**, who runs his own immune lab at Stanford. One of the things he's doing is characterizing what a normal immune system actually looks like.

- **Mario Capecchio, PhD**, a molecular geneticist, Nobel Laureate and Lasker Award winner.

- **Craig Heller, PhD**, a Stanford exercise physiologist and inventor of "the glove," (which reduces body temperature to increase muscle performance).

- **Baldomero M. Olivera, PhD**, a University of Utah neuroscientist focusing on how the ion channels and receptors affect nervous system signaling.

- **Ron Tompkins, MD, ScD**, who has produced ground-breaking work on the process of inflammation.

- **Andreas Kogelnik, MD, PhD**, an ME/CFS expert and founder of the Open Medicine Institute.

- **James Watson, PhD**, the Nobel Prize laureate, who with Francis Crick, uncovered the structure of DNA.

…Ron Davis is a stickler on scientific rigor. Time and again in our discussions over the years, he's emphasized the need not to be beholden to any preconceived notion – to be open to where the science leads you…

Don't be surprised if their efforts overturn some ideas regarding ME/CFS. In fact, be surprised if this effort doesn't yield completely novel ideas about ME/CFS…By the time this consortium has completed its mission, you can expect a new field to emerge. Expect ME/CFS to be completely redefined. Expect several subsets or perhaps disorders inside of it to pop out. Expect them to illuminate numerous pathways that lead to the production of "ME/CFS."

This is research on a different level than we're used to. It's a $5 million a year project. For ME/CFS, it is a lot of money but it's not a lot of money for the NIH. It's not a lot of money for medical research, and it's definitely not a lot of money for an often-disabling disorder that affects a million people or more in the United States and many millions more across the world…

This is a long-term effort. Don't expect answers overnight. New technologies will need to be developed. But give this Consortium the funding and time it needs, and it's hard to imagine it won't succeed.

❧

Cort Johnson Interviews Dr. Ron Davis: About six months ago, I asked Dr. Ron Davis to answer a few questions:

You've been engaged in high-level research at Stanford for many years. Now you're working on ME/CFS. What is different about working in the ME/CFS field as opposed to other fields? Another way to ask this is, What is missing in ME/CFS which is present in other fields that is keeping the ME/CFS field from progressing the way other fields do?

What is missing in ME/CFS research is long-term stable funding. Short-term funding is okay for specific small projects, but what is needed is a total attack on the problem. This includes developing new technology, which may take time.

For example: a number of laboratories have measured gene expression from cells in the blood. However, blood is a complex mixture of many types of cells. It is obvious that gene expression from every cell type in the blood measured independently would be much better. It could give us more information and may yield a molecular diagnostic test.

Unfortunately, there is no technology available to reliably accomplish this for every cell type. This technology needs to be developed. It is important to note that this does not have to be solely funded by ME/CFS research dollars because the technology is generic and is useful for many diseases.

For example, we are currently sequencing the HLA region in the human genome. This region controls many aspects of the immune system. It's a very complex locus and is not revealed by "whole" genome sequencing. We have developed a very accurate technology that can sequence this region at very low cost. This technology was developed using funds from the navy and NIAID. Now it can be used in ME/CFS research at very low cost.

Another serious problem is there is no molecular diagnostic test for ME/CFS. This can result in grouping similar diseases into one group. Such a heterogeneous grouping will make it difficult to get unique quantitative molecular information and understanding of what is wrong. This problem is confounded by each set of investigators collecting a new set of patients for every study. It would be far better to have one large set of patients that is used for every study. Validation would then be done on a second or third large set of patients.

The problem is further complicated by having a loose and non-specific definition of the disease. Including patients that have some of the symptoms but not the disease can result in considerable confusion about treatment. If treatment helps those patients with some of the symptoms but not the disease and does not help those with the disease, this could result in a mistaken mandate that all patients be treated in this manner, which could actually harm those with the disease.

You've worked in consortiums before and would like to put one together for ME/CFS. What can consortiums accomplish that individual researchers or even research groups cannot, and what kind of consortium do you envision for ME/CFS?

For ten years I worked on a large consortium (Inflammation and the Host (human) Response to Injury) funded by the NIH (NIGMS) and involved sixteen laboratories (most of the laboratories that worked on trauma) in the U.S. It was chaired by Ron Tompkins, MD, at MGH. He did a marvelous job and I think this should be the model for other consortiums. I was the head of genomics for the project. We all met at the O'Hare Airport (Hilton) every three months to go over new data and plan the next experiments.

There were several principles that we used:

- We wanted the right answer no matter whose theories we destroyed. Some of our results have upset a number of researchers. But we have a massive amount of data supporting our conclusions.

- We wanted the best experimentalists to do the experiments. When we did not have the best we recruited the best. Not everyone in the consortium had to do experiments. In fact very few of the members did experiments. Everyone had to come to the meetings and share their knowledge and expertise and give suggestions.

- All these contributors were on all the publications. This last point is very important. At the beginning many researchers wanted to collect their own patients and collect their data in their own laboratory. This would have been a disaster. The experimental variance by this method would have been so great that it would have obscured most of our results. In the end only a few researchers collected data (ten percent of the group). It is one of the largest and best molecular data sets ever collected on humans. Aside from the hundreds of thousands of facts about individual genes, we discovered that the main theory of trauma taught in medical schools was totally wrong. We also found that the mouse model for trauma used in research laboratories throughout the world showed no relationship to human trauma and should not be used to model human trauma.

I think something like this consortium should be used for ME/CFS. It should include physicians that treat ME/CFS patients. It should also include the best experimentalists and thinkers from several scientific disciplines regardless of any experience with ME/CFS.

This group should work together to design a total attack on ME/CFS and focus on understanding the disease, finding diagnostic markers, and devising treatments.

Medicine and science have neglected and misunderstood ME/CFS for so long that they really need to make up for their mistake by inspiring and supporting the most high-powered scientists available and funding a large group of experts in different fields to generate the best data and analysis possible.

The millions of suffering ME/CFS patients are owed an apology and a concerted urgent effort to find effective treatment.

Update | June 2016 | Note by Valerie

Already, there are encouraging findings emerging from the ME/CFS Severely Ill Big Data Study:

"Professor Ron Davis presented new findings from his Big Data study at Friday's Invest in ME 2016 conference. Davis's preliminary data shows serious problems with the biochemical processes needed to convert sugars and fats from food into energy the body can use. If these findings are replicated, this could prove a major step forward in understanding ME/CFS." Posted June 4, 2016 at www.meaction.net/2016/06/04/ron-davis-errors-metabolism.

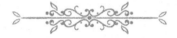

2015 Onward

Massachusetts CFIDS/ME & FM Association[327] | December 2015

More than ever before, 2015 has been a year that has brought fresh hope to Myalgic Encephalomyelitis (ME) patients. The Institute of Medicine (IOM) and NIH Pathways to Prevention (P2P) reports confirmed the neglect and disbelief that have held the disease hostage for decades and strongly recommended action to improve patient care. Publications from Stanford, Columbia and Haukeland (Norway) Universities brought new insights into the biology. World-renowned scientists have joined the fight. Stories about severely ill patients like Dr. Ron Davis's son have created more public awareness. And the Tuller series brought greater exposure to the concerns with the PACE trial and psychogenic theories. For the first time, there is a sense that we have huge opportunities to change the future for ME patients. And just as importantly, there is a sense that if we want to turn those opportunities into reality, then we need to find new ways to work together to increase the impact of our voices. To that end, the U.S. Action Working Group (USAWG) has formed as a way for a number of organizations, bloggers and independent advocates to identify and discuss those areas where they can agree on goals and work together to achieve what is needed for patients.

Thus far, we have identified common goals to focus on, including the need to dramatically increase funding, to advance the research agenda, to resolve the definitional challenges, and to improve clinical care through quality medical education. We expect that this will lead to actions directed toward Congressional leaders, HHS and its agencies, and public awareness through the media.

To achieve these goals, we are going to need broad participation inside and outside the community. Collaborative efforts taken by members of the USAWG will be posted on various individual advocacy sites including www.meaction.net.

---

327 Excerpted and adapted from the Advocacy Announcement published by members of the U.S. Action Working Group, December 2015 – permission by Massachusetts CFIDS/ME & FM Association. www.masscfids.org.

CONCLUSION

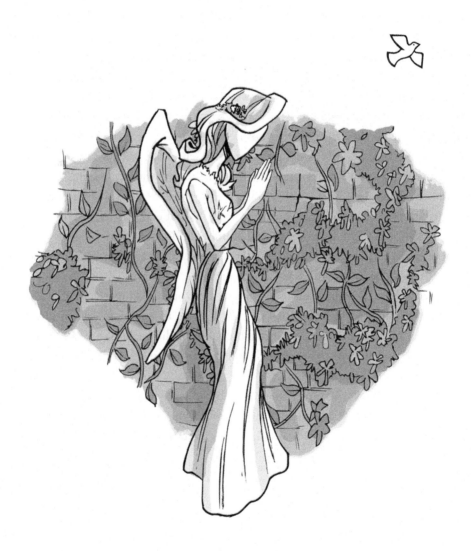

The Time to Heal

Valerie Free

So progress is being made, and many people are working toward a better outcome for ME/CFS and other neuro-immune illnesses. Chapter 12 and Section 3 primarily outline a very busy scientific community in need of funding, new researchers and doctors in the field, as well as public support. We are moving forward!

It is time to learn from, and to let go of, the past in order to make way for something new. As I say in "The Chronic-Call," the outcome will be what we do.

Telling the historical ME/CFS story has been both a longer and more interesting project than I ever imagined. Moving from a personal focus to one of community pulled more strings than I knew existed. I hope exploring it with me has been helpful to you in some way. It has certainly been helpful for me – although not always an easy ride.

Although my health has not been restored… yet, I do feel that there has been some form and level of healing after sharing my experiences and those of others. When I finish this book, I hope to focus more on my personal health and my loved ones.

Thank you for reading and helping by simply opening your mind and your heart, and by becoming better informed. I hope I have provided some of the tools that are needed to accelerate care, cure, and prevention for myalgic encephalomyelitis/chronic fatigue syndrome, along with other poorly understood complex illnesses, across the globe.

> "…Truth in all its glory, harsh and uncompromising, beautiful and nourishing, a lightning bolt that shakes us awake or a soft light that gently draws us from our sleep."
>
> — *Sarah Varcas*

SECTION 3
How To Help

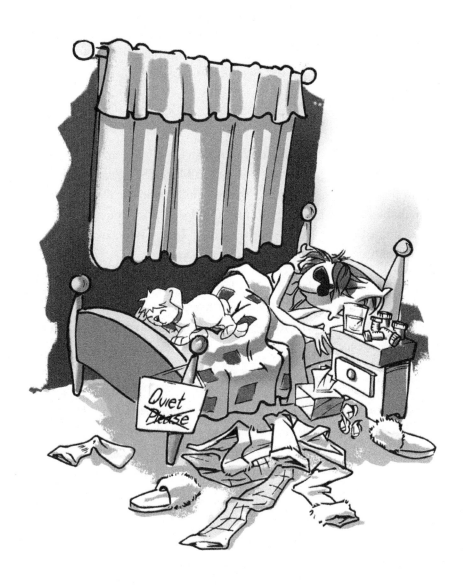

How to Support Yourself or Others with ME/CFS

Ten Frequently Asked Questions
Doris Fleck | August 2015 | Red Deer, Alberta, Canada

After the story about my sudden onset of ME/CFS was published on the Internet, I received hundreds of emails from people asking for help. Here are the top ten questions I have put together arising from these requests as well as from my own experience. The answers contain some practical ways you can help yourself, friends, or loved ones who are suffering from this disease. These suggestions are primarily aimed at people with mild or moderate ME/CFS: They will need to be modified for those who are in the severe category.[328]

1   Do you know a good doctor in my area who understands ME/CFS?

This is a widely asked question. Unfortunately, training for doctors in medical schools is lagging when it comes to ME/CFS, so you may have a hard time finding a practitioner that is familiar with the illness. Don't give up, however. A good way to find the closest practitioner to you is to reach out to an ME/CFS support group. They may be aware of the doctors who are ME/CFS competent in your area.

Your own doctor may be willing to learn, and could benefit from, the 2014 *IACFS/ME Primer for Clinical Practitioners*.[329] It is an excellent resource written by experts for experts, although no doubt you will find it helpful as well.

2   What can I do to improve my health?

An important objective is to get educated and informed about ME/CFS or to have a loved one do so. There are many good resources out there, but unfortunately there are also some that are not. Exercise caution and check the source of the material. Two respected resources that I would recommend are: *Hope and Help for Chronic Fatigue Syndrome and*

---

328 "The Severely Ill/Lowest Functioning Patient: Special Considerations" (section 6.1) pp. 27, 28 of IACFS/ME (International Association for Chronic Fatigue Syndrome/Myalgic Encephalomyelitis). 2014. "ME/CFS: Primer for Clinical Practitioners." Chicago, IL: IACFS/ME.

329 IACFS/ME (International Association for Chronic Fatigue Syndrome/Myalgic Encephalomyelitis). 2014. "ME/CFS: Primer for Clinical Practitioners." Chicago, IL: IACFS/ME.

Fibromyalgia by Dr. Alison C. Bested,[330] and *Let Your Light Shine Through* by Dr. Ellie Stein.[331] Dr. Stein's work is a manual with helpful strategies including diet considerations, medication and supplement options, as well as self-management skills such as pacing.

3   Are there any practical things I can do to help my friend/loved one who has this illness?

No matter where on the severity spectrum people are, there are opportunities to help with the things they are unable to do. Ask how they are managing and about the degree of disability they are experiencing. You can use this information to assess what they can and cannot do. Don't be surprised if they have difficulty figuring out what they can do for themselves because this may fluctuate within a day or over weeks, months and seasons.

Unfortunately, sudden serious illness can leave people in a financial bind, and they may require outside financial support short or long-term.

Some practical ways you can help people with this disease are to: pick up groceries (you may need to make the list); make a meal they can eat (many people with ME/CFS develop allergies or may be gluten intolerant); help with laundry; shop for vitamins, supplements or pick up their prescriptions; drive them to a doctor's appointment; call for a short encouraging chat; do their dishes; take care of their kids for an afternoon; or, if they will let you, clean their house. It is important to keep in mind that they may need quiet and rest while you are with them. Having a conversation while you are helping may be taking away the good that you are trying to do because it can drain the patient's energy.

4   How can I support a person with ME/CFS mentally and emotionally?

Validation that the disease is "real" [332] is critical, as is encouraging the feelings of being needed, worthy, and important. Remember, people with this disease were productive, active, and intelligent in good health. Their feelings of loss in these areas need to be acknowledged. What they are

330 Bested AC, Logan AC and Howe R, "Hope and Help for Chronic Fatigue Syndrome and Fibromyalgia" (2nd ed.), Nashville, Tenn. Cumberland House Publishers. 2008.

331 Stein E, MD, FRCP(C), "Let Your Light Shine Through – Strategies for Living with Myalgic Encephalomyelitis/ Chronic Fatigue Syndrome, Fibromyalgia and Multiple Chemical Sensitivity." 2012. Calgary, AB. It is available as a hard copy or e-manual at www.eleanorsteinmd.ca/manual-2 (accessed March 2016).

332 See, for example, Komaroff A. 2015. "Myalgic Encephalomyelitis/Chronic Fatigue Syndrome: A Real Illness." Annals of Internal Medicine Ann Intern Med, 871-871. annals.org/article.aspx?articleid=2322808 (accessed July 20, 2016).

experiencing is frightening and incomprehensible to them (let alone to a well person). Listening to their concerns is important. Remember these people want to be well and thriving. Support those ideals by understanding the disease and how it affects your friend/loved one and those around him or her.

5   What is the best way to encourage self-reliance and independence?

First, it's important to avoid comparing their/your current state with pre-illness health. Levels of self-reliance and independence can be very different for a person with ME/CFS than that of a healthy person. Small tasks like showering and cooking or driving short distances may seem trivial to the average healthy person, but they can be big accomplishments to ME/CFS patients. Make sure to recognize them as such! As well, remind them that improvement is possible over time.

6   How can I advocate for my friend/loved one and for better recognition of the illness?

You can go to a doctor's appointment with ME/CFS patients to listen or even explain their symptoms if they are too sick to do so themselves. You can help them deal with the paperwork needed to apply for disability income or to make financial decisions. Sometimes people have to deal with the legal system, which can be very intense and confusing. Helping to sort things out and communicate with lawyers can be so helpful in a stressful time. Gain knowledge about this condition and share it with other friends or relatives. Join others who advocate for people with this illness and share ideas.

7   What type of environment is best for someone with ME/CFS and related illnesses?

Stressful and difficult environments are two factors that can exacerbate illness. A healthy environment could be one free of scents, loud sound, and bright light. A person with this disease can easily do too much in a day and push him or herself into a relapse, and these factors can add to that. Relationships with family or friends who question or undermine the disease can cause arguments and emotional repercussions, which can turn into a relapse. Educate those around the ill person, and, if needed, help your ME/CFS friend create a safe boundary system in his/her home, as well as one that promotes well-being for all who live with him/her.

8   Should I challenge my friend or loved one to be more active so he/ she does not decondition too much?

Encourage whatever activity patients can manage without worsening their condition. You may not even associate what they are doing with activity because, for some, even the activities of daily living like showering are too much to tolerate. Once they are able to do more than the necessary daily activities, there are programs available that recommend exercise such as light stretching or mild strengthening. If they can walk short distances, walk with them and guard them from walking beyond their capabilities, and promote sitting down for periods during the walk. Start slowly and help them assess how much they can do over a week or month by charting the activity, along with the consequences. This is where tools like wheelchairs, walkers, canes, and even mobile chairs are useful to extend their energy and mobility.

9   How do I help my friend or loved one handle constant pain?

Some people with ME/CFS have pain as a symptom and also have fibromyalgia. They may have severe pain along with a host of other confusing symptoms. Be sympathetic and "acknowledge their pain" while working with them and their doctor to find solutions and monitor their response to any treatment they are trying. Understand "this pain is not mine" and keep yourself well and happy so you do not burn out as a carer for your loved one.

10   Can a person with ME/CFS find meaning and purpose in their life, even if they are homebound or only go out a couple times a week?

If patients are able to do so, reintegrating into the world of productive work, at home or outside the home, is important. As an example, although I have had severe ME/CFS, I have improved over the years and adapted my lifestyle so I can work part-time as a journalist. I am able to do almost all my work lying down. Not everyone with ME/CFS will be able to work, even part-time; and if the person you know is in this category, try to support him/her in other ways – for instance, find out if there are things he/she would like to do, like discussing a book or a television program. Listening to audio books may be more tolerable than reading paper books. Building meaningful relationships by phone or Internet can help to prevent isolation. A meaningful life can be attained regardless of the illness, but it may look very different than it did in good health.

This is a great opportunity to thank all of the people who care about, and for, someone with the illness. It is not always an easy task and often a long one, but you are heroes to us.

Ways to Support the Cause of ME/CFS

Valerie Free with Maureen MacQuarrie | August 2015 (partial update May 2016)

As you have just read, there are many ways to help individuals with ME/CFS. To broaden your reach into global progress, some ideas include donating time, expertise, or funds to a support organization, May Awareness events, or to research. Whatever you choose to do, your assistance will make a huge difference. Thank you for becoming part of the solution.

There are many fine patient support organizations across the globe including the U.S., U.K., Europe, Australia, Canada, New Zealand and Japan. Some of them have already been mentioned in this book. You can find them by browsing the web for ME and CFS organizations in your area. Another resource is an international newsletter, the **ME Global Chronicle**.[333]

#ME Action[334] was launched in spring 2015 as an exciting online platform[335] to help everyone become proactive for M.E. It has a detailed list of people and organizations from around the world who are participating in some way. You can create and post new initiatives there, and you can find current international advocacy actions to participate in.

May 12th International Awareness Day is an exciting way to get involved. One good source for learning about it is "**May 12th International ME/CFS & FM Awareness Day**",[336] which exists to bring awareness to Chronic Immunological and Neurological Diseases (or CINDs).[337]

What follows is a list of organizations that offer opportunities to support the cause. It is not an all-inclusive list. With the exception of the first two – National ME/FM Action Network, and IACFS/ME – the organizations listed are either solely devoted to research or have a large research component, and all of them have an easy-to-find DONATE button.

With the limited funding that ME/CFS receives from government health agencies, it is difficult to make the needed breakthroughs in research, so all of these organizations need additional private and corporate funding.

In this list, I introduce the organizations through quotes directly taken from their websites. I generally do not list specific studies or projects that they are undertaking because

---

333 let-me.be (accessed August 24, 2015). The ME Global Chronicle was started in 2014 as a way to share information.

334 www.meaction.net (accessed July 24, 2016).

335 #ME Action is "an international network of patients empowering each other to fight for health equality for Myalgic Encephalomyelitis," created by Jennifer Brea, Beth Mazur, and Rachael Korinek.

336 www.may12th.org (accessed May 26, 2016). You can also find them on Facebook at www.facebook.com/may12th. awareness (accessed May 26, 2016). This is a project run by www.actioncind.org, a new Canadian non-profit.

337 The term given to this family of illnesses by Tom Hennessy.

the studies are quite fluid; a specific study will come to an end and, with luck, a new one will begin.[338]

As I mentioned, the first two organizations listed differ from the research focus I have chosen due to their roles and importance to me personally and in the field:

National ME/FM Action Network – www.mefmaction.com.

"The National ME/FM Action Network became a Canadian charitable organization on June 18, 1993 dedicated to myalgic encephalomyelitis, also known as chronic fatigue syndrome (ME/CFS) and fibromyalgia (FM), through support, advocacy, education and research."

Nepean, ON, Canada
Phone: 613-829-6667
E-mail: mefminfo@mefmaction.com

The International Association for CFS/ME (IACFS/ME) – www.iacfsme.org.

"The mission of the non-profit IACFS/ME is to promote, stimulate and coordinate the exchange of ideas related to CFS, ME, and fibromyalgia (FM) research, patient care, and treatment. The IACFS/ME also conducts and/or participates in local, national, and international scientific conferences in order to promote and evaluate new research and to encourage future research ventures and cooperative activities to advance scientific and clinical knowledge of these illnesses."

Bethesda, MD, U.S.
Voice Mail: 301-634-7701
Email: membership@iacfsme.org

---

338 All of these research facilities have multiple studies ongoing and most websites will direct you to their current projects and fundraising ventures.

Organizations Involved In Fundraising and Research for ME and/or CFS

❧

AUSTRALIA

National Center for Neuroimmunolgy and Emerging Diseases (NCNED) – www. griffith.edu.au/health/national-centre-neuroimmunology-emerging-diseases.

(Professor Sonya Marshall-Gradisnik, PhD and Professor Donald Staines, MD)

From their February 2015 newsletter:

"The National Centre for Neuroimmunology and Emerging Diseases (NCNED) research team is located in Griffith Health Centre at Griffith University on the Gold Coast. Led by Professors Sonya Marshall-Gradisnik and Donald Staines, the team has a focus on Chronic Fatigue Syndrome/Myalgic Encephalomyelitis (CFS/ME).

"Our mission is to translate research findings into preventative medicine, social and clinical care and public health outcomes. By collaborating with local, national, and international research institutes, we aim to create sustained improvements in health and health care for not only sufferers of CFS/ME but also other immune disorders."

National Centre for Neuroimmunology and Emerging Diseases
(Mailbox 68)
Menzies Health Institute QLD
Griffith University, Parklands Drive, Gold Coast, QLD, Australia
email: ncned@griffith.edu.au
Phone number (inquiries re: research): (07) 5678 9283

Note: For those familiar with the Alison Hunter Memorial Foundation (AHMF) who are wondering what has happened to it – AHMF operated as a non-profit institution from 1998 to 2014, to advance scientific knowledge and medical care. The Board of AHMF announced that it has established a partnership with NCNED.

❧

JAPAN

RIKEN Institute – www.riken.jp/en/research/labs/clst.

(Professor Watanabe, MD, PhD)

Riken has released numerous studies seeking the potential causes for ME/CFS.

"RIKEN is Japan's only fully comprehensive research institute for the national sciences and a world leader in a wide range of different scientific fields. Since its founding in 1917, RIKEN has made innumerable scientific and technological breakthroughs...

"To support its research, RIKEN depends to a great extent on an operational budget from the Japanese government and competitive funds for strategic key national projects. These funding sources are not enough, however, to cover the broad and diverse range of activities conducted here. Your donations are invaluable in helping us to support the kind of creative, pioneering research that sows the seeds for innovative new applications.

"One of the labs at RIKEN is the Center for Life Science Technologies (CLST) where research on fatigue is taking place under Professor Watanabe, MD, PhD in the Imaging Application Group.[339] The CLST are developing technologies to measure and analyze the entire range of molecules functioning in our body at three levels – the atom, the cell, and the individual. To understand their real functions in the living body over time, we use a dynamic-comprehensive approach rather than a static and target-oriented approach."

Kobe, Hyogo, Japan
Tel: +81-(0)78-304-7138
How to Donate to Riken: www.riken.jp/en/about/support

NORWAY

ME-forskning – me-forskning.no/english/about-this-fundraising.

This fundraising initiative to support biomedical research projects into ME in Norway was started by ME patients, and relatives of ME patients, in collaboration with the Norwegian ME Association (www.me-foreningen.no).

"In 2014 we gave 1.5 million NOK (approximately 184,500 EUR, 237,000 USD) to a research project into medical treatment of ME with Rituximab.

---

339 For more information, www.riken.jp/en/research/labs/clst/biofunct_dyn_img/img_app/pathophysiol_health_sci; www.clst.riken.jp/en/science/labs/bdi/func/cfi; www.riken.jp/en/pr/press/2014/20140404_1 (accessed August 6, 2016).

"In 2015 we provided 200,000 NOK (approximately 12,000 EUR, 13,000 USD) to a research project on ME and genetics at Haukeland University Hospital in Bergen, Norway."

Oslo, Norway
Email: post@me-forskning.no
Donations: me-forskning.no/donations

❧

UNITED KINGDOM

Action for ME – www.actionforme.org.uk.
   "Action for ME supports high-quality, evidenced-based medical, social and economic research and invests in pilot research projects to help us learn more and to stimulate greater mainstream funding of ME research."

Keynsham, Bristol, England
Phone: 0117 927 9551
www.actionforme.org.uk
Donate: www.actionforme.org.uk/make-a-difference

CURE-ME (Creating clinical and biomedical Understanding through Research, Evidence – for the ethical study of ME/CFS) – www.meresearch.org.uk.
   CURE-ME is the ME/CFS research team at the London School of Hygiene & Tropical Medicine (LSHTM). The U.K. ME/CFS Biobank project is located at LSHTM and is overseen by a Steering Group.
   "Biomedical research into ME/CFS historically has been underfunded, although our research team has been very grateful for financial support from Action for ME, the ME Association, ME Research U.K. and a private donor, which has enabled us to launch the pioneering U.K. ME/CFS Biobank. We recognize that much of this funding originated from patients and their loved ones. Building on the successes of the U.K. ME/CFS Biobank, we are honoured to have secured funding from the U.S. National Institutes of Health (NIH) to continue our work, including expansion of the Biobank. However, significant need remains to fully fund our dedicated team members' time, to add a time-point to our longitudinal studies, and to enhance data collection and analysis. We are also fundraising for other biomedical research into ME/CFS."

To donate: www.lshtm.ac.uk/itd/crd/research/cure-me/donate/index.html
London School of Hygiene & Tropical Medicine

London, England

Tel: +44 (0) 20 7636 8636

Invest in ME (Research) – www.investinme.org/index.htm.

"Invest in ME (Research) IiME was set up with the objectives of making a change in how ME is perceived and treated in the media, by health departments and by healthcare professionals. We aim to do this by identifying three key areas to concentrate our efforts on – funding for biomedical research, education, and lobbying. Invest in ME aims to collaborate and coordinate events and activities in these areas in order to provide the focus and funding to allow biomedical research to be carried out."

IiME holds highly-anticipated conferences on ME annually in the U.K. The tenth such conference was held on May 29th, 2015. The 2016 Conference Events were June 1 – 3.

Current Invest in ME Research projects include topics such as the Microbiome, Rituximab (Clinical Trial and B-cell research), Autoimmunity and ME.

www.investinme.org/ResearchCurrentProjects.htm

Eastleigh, Hampshire, England

Phone: 02380 251719 or 07759 349743

Info@investinme.org

The ME Association – www.meassociation.org.uk.

(Charles Shepherd, MD, medical advisor) The goal of the ME Association is a big one – to help everyone with ME in the U.K. Part of their work relates to research, their Ramsay Research Fund, where (according to their website) all donations are ring-fenced for research-related activity. There are no payments for salaries or administrative costs as these are all covered by general funds.

In May 2015 they produced a report[340] with strong recommendations, aimed at changing the way Cognitive Behaviour Therapy (CBT), Graduated Exercise Therapy (GET), and Pacing are offered.

Gawcott Bucks, England

Tel: 01280 818964

Email: admin@meassociation.org.uk

ME Research U.K. – www.meresearch.org.uk.

"ME Research U.K., founded in 2000, is a national U.K. charity funding biomedical research into myalgic encephalomyelitis (also known as ME/CFS).

---

340 This report analyzes the 2012 ME/CFS Illness Management Survey, subtitled, "No decisions about me without me." www.meassociation.org.uk/wp-content/uploads/2015-ME-Association-Illness-Management-Report-No-decisions-about-me-without-me-30.05.15.pdf (accessed July 20, 2016).

"Its principal aim is to commission and fund high-quality scientific (biomedical) investigation into the causes, consequences and treatment of ME…"

Overview of funded research section –

"In early 2014, ME Research U.K. reached a milestone, topping the £1 million mark in grants awarded to researchers (approximately $1.5 million U.S.). This represents thirty-five specific biomedical projects, the results of which have now been published as fifty-eight research papers in peer-reviewed scientific journals."

ME Research U.K. is also home to **CureME** – www.mereasearch.org.uk/news/welcome-to-cureme. "CureME is a new site for listing research news about ME/CFS. Each post will be a stand-alone article, and the aim is to create a free 'one-stop portal' for research news about the disease. All you need to do is sign-up an email address, and thereafter you can access the list anytime using a password – dead simple."

Perth, Scotland
Telephone: 01738 451234
E-mail: meruk@pkavs.org.uk

~∾

UNITED STATES

Bateman Horne Center[341] – www.batemanhornecenter.org.

(Lucinda Bateman, MD)

"Empowering patients, advancing research, and improving clinical care for all those impacted by ME/CFS and Fibromyalgia.

"We envision a world where patients with ME/CFS and Fibromyalgia are readily diagnosed, effectively treated, and widely met with empathy and understanding. BHC is led by Dr. Lucinda Bateman and Suzanne D. Vernon, PhD, who bring more than 40 years of combined experience and leadership to treating patients and advancing research in the areas of ME/CFS and Fibromyalgia."

Salt Lake City, UT
Phone: (801) 359-7400 (clinic)

---

341 The Bateman Horne Center, a Utah-based non-profit organization, formerly called OFFER (conceived and co-founded by Dr. Lucinda Bateman in 2002) absorbed and expanded what was formerly the Fatigue Consultation Clinic (founded by Dr. Bateman in 2000). This merger has broadened their scope to encompass research, patient care, and education.

(801) 364-3528 (research)

DONATE at www.batemanhornecenter.org/donate

Center for Infection and Immunity – cii.columbia.edu/research.aspx?8Fo92f.

(Ian Lipkin, MD and Mady Hornig, MD)

The Center for Infection and Immunity (CII) is located in the Mailman School of Public Health at Columbia University.

"CII is the world's largest and most advanced academic center for basic and translational research in microbe surveillance, discovery and diagnosis.

"Columbia University is accepting donations, which can be directed to the Center for Infection and Immunity and designated for ME/CFS Research. Some very interesting discoveries relating to ME/CFS are being made at the Center for Infection and Immunity, including that profiled in March 31, 2015 'Scientists find Clues into Cognitive Dysfunction in Chronic Fatigue Syndrome.'" [342]

New York, NY

Phone: (212) 851-9608: General information about giving to Columbia University.

Institute for Neuro Immune Medicine (INIM) – www.nova.edu/nim.

Nova Southeastern University

(Nancy Klimas, MD)

"The Institute for Neuro Immune Medicine (INIM) strives to advance knowledge and care for people with complex neuro-inflammatory illnesses through the integration of research, clinical care, and education. Current research focus at the Institute for Neuro Immune Medicine (INIM) includes myalgic encephalomyelitis/chronic fatigue syndrome (ME/CFS) and Gulf War illness (GWI).

"Nancy Klimas, MD, and her team bring decades of experience in patient care, research, and education that have contributed to furthering the understanding of these conditions and have changed lives. This work takes significant resources. Private philanthropy can make the difference needed to uncover a new genetic link or therapeutic approach that will improve treatments."

Fort Lauderdale, FL

Phone: (305) 595-4300: Nick Lewis, Administrative Director INIM

---

342 www.mailman.columbia.edu/public-health-now/news/scientists-find-clues-cognitive-dysfunction-chronic-fatigue-syndrome (accessed July 24, 2016).

The National CFIDS Foundation – www.ncf-net.org.

The National CFIDS Foundation[343] is a national non-profit organization founded in 1997.

"The Foundation's objective is to fund research to find a cause, expedite treatments and eventually a cure, and provide information, education, and support to people who have CFIDS (chronic fatigue and immune dysfunction also known as chronic fatigue syndrome (CFS), myalgic encephalomyelitis (ME) and many other names."

The Foundation publishes a quarterly newsletter, *The National Forum*. They also maintain a memorial list of people with CFIDS/ME who have died.

Needham, MA
Phone: (781) 449-3535
E-mail: info@ncf-net.org

Neuro-Immune Disease Alliance, Incorporated[344] – www.nidalliance.org.

"The Neuro-Immune Disease Alliance (NIDA) is dedicated to improving the quality of life of people suffering from Myalgic Encephalomyelitis (ME/CFS) by accelerating collaborative research towards finding a cure and providing patient and family support. NIDA is supporting the efforts of the Open Medicine Foundation and Institute (OMF & OMI), as well as others, to move research fast forward.

"The Neuro-Immune Disease Alliance, Inc. has supported a number of important projects and is currently (December, 2015) raising funds to support the Open Medicine Foundation's End ME/CFS Project."

Agoura Hills, CA
Contact: www.nidalliance.org

Open Medicine Foundation – www.openmedicinefoundation.org.

(Linda Tannenbaum, CEO/President)

"The Open Medicine Foundation (OMF) is committed to helping people with ME/CFS/FM and Lyme with the #1 purpose to help as many patients as possible find symptom relief while continuing in the quest to find a cure.

"An OMF project is the End ME/CFS Project[345] (Ron Davis, PhD, project director) and has the goals of unlocking the mystery of myalgic encephalomyelitis/chronic fatigue syndrome (ME/CFS) and ending the suffering caused by the disease. The project's first

---

343 For people who have CFIDS; chronic fatigue and immune dysfunction syndrome also known as chronic fatigue syndrome (CFS), myalgic encephalomyelitis (ME) and many other names, as well as related illnesses such as Gulf War Illness (GWI) and multiple chemical sensitivity (MCS).

344 "Don and Linda Tannenbaum founded NIDA in 2011, five years after their daughter suddenly fell ill when she was only sixteen. Their daughter was finally diagnosed with ME/CFS. The quest for a diagnosis stopped and the search for a cure and symptom relief began..."

345 More information about this project appears in Chapter 12.

study is the ME/CFS Severely Ill, Big Data Study, a study designed to find a clinically useful diagnostic biomarker. The OMF is currently (2016) soliciting donations for this study. More information about the End ME/CFS Project can be found at www.open-medicinefoundation.org/the-end-mecfs-project."

Agoura Hills, CA
Phone: (650) 352-0310

Simmaron Research – www.simmaronresearch.com.
    (Scientific Advisory Board includes Daniel Peterson, MD)
    "Simmaron Research, Inc.[346] is a Nevada-based non-profit organization dedicated to advancing scientific research, potentially leading to the discovery of diagnostic markers and effective treatments that will ultimately improve the quality of life for people suffering from CFS/ME and related neuroimmune disorders."

Incline Village, NV
Phone: (775) 298-0030
Email: redefiningmecfs@gmail.com

Solve ME/CFS Initiative (formerly CFIDS Association of America) – www.solvecfs.org.
    "The Solve ME/CFS Initiative (SMCI) has been the leading organization focused on myalgic encephalomyelitis (ME) and Chronic Fatigue Syndrome (CFS) since being founded in 1987. SMCI envisions a world free of ME/CFS and works steadfastly to make this disease understood, diagnosable, and treatable. SMCI seeks to actively engage the entire ME/CFS community in research, works to accelerate the discovery of safe and effective treatments, and strives for an aggressive expansion of funding towards a cure."
    SMCI has established a Solve ME/CFS Biobank and Patient Registry.[347] Its Research 1st e-newsletter offers a concise digest of the latest research, policy, and organizational news, as well as information about media coverage and events of interest.

Los Angeles, CA
Phone: (704) 364-0016
E-mail: solvecfs@solvecfs.org

Stanford Myalgic Encephalomyelitis/Chronic Fatigue Syndrome Initiative
– www.med.stanford.edu/chronicfatiguesyndrome.html.
    (Jose Montoya, MD)

---

346 Simmaron has an ambitious international research collaboration between Dr. D. Peterson, Griffith University (Australia), Wisconsin Viral Research Group, Columbia University Mailman School of Public Health & Center for Infection and Immunity, George Washington University, Workwell Foundation, and Ohio State University.

347 The Solve ME/CFS Biobank started as an inventory of blood samples from ME/CFS patients as well as healthy controls. It has evolved to a Solve ME/CFS Biobank and Patient Registry. solvecfs.org/solvecfs-biobank-gets-retooled and solvecfs.org/biobank (accessed July 20, 2016).

Gift or donation: www.med.stanford.edu/chronicfatiguesyndrome/about/donation.html.

"Mission: To become a center of excellence that improves the health of patients with chronic diseases in which infection or its immune response plays a major etiologic role.

"To provide leadership, facilitate multidisciplinary collaboration, make new discoveries, and educate in the field of infection-associated chronic diseases."

The impressive work they are doing was profiled at a symposium[348] in March 2014 in conjunction with the IACFS/ME conference.

Stanford University School of Medicine
Stanford, CA
Phone: (650) 723-4000

Whittemore Peterson Institute for Neuro-Immune Disease – In 2016, it was renamed Nevada Center for Biomedical Research (NVCBR). www.wpinstitute.org.

"The Whittemore Peterson Institute for Neuro-Immune Disease exists to bring discovery, knowledge, and effective treatments to patients with illnesses that are caused by acquired dysregulation of both the immune system and the nervous system, often resulting in life-long disease and disability."

They have changed the name to reflect Nevada's significant contributions to NVCBR's medical research efforts and it emphasizes their innovative medical research program to include multiple sclerosis and autoimmunity.

University of Nevada, Reno, NV
Phone: (775) 682-8250
E-mail: info@wpinstitute.org

RELATED CONDITIONS:

I have included information on the two U.S. foundations below as they are doing work that is related and beneficial to research on ME/CFS.

Enterovirus Foundation – www.enterovirusfoundation.org.
(Board of Directors includes J. Chia, MD, Infectious Disease Specialist).

"The Enterovirus Foundation, founded in November 2008, is a non-profit organization created to fund research to discover the persistent effects of enteroviruses, to determine the role they play in both acute and chronic disease, and to develop treatments to cure and prevent these diseases."

---

348 An article about the symposium appeared at www.cortjohnson.org/blog/2014/03/20/tweeting-stanford-symposium-chronic-fatigue-syndrome (accessed July 25, 2016).

Phone: (415) 393-9558
E-mail: Info@EnterovirusFoundation.org

HHV-6 Foundation – www.hhv-6foundation.org.

(Dharam Ablashi, PhD, co-discoverer of the HHV-6 virus and co-founder of the IACFS/ME)

"The HHV-6 Foundation is a non-profit institution that encourages scientific exchange between investigators by holding conferences for virologists and clinical researchers, maintaining a repository of reagents to facilitate research, and offering pilot grants for promising research projects."

Phone: (805) 969-1174 Administrative Office
E-mail: info@hhv-6foundation.org

I hope that you have found this list interesting and informative, as well as an inspiration to take part in some of the projects that these organizations are spearheading. Your contribution will be valuable, regardless of its focus. With your participation and with donations to ME/CFS research, our future, as well as that of future generations, will be brighter, healthier, and stronger.

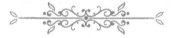

APPENDICES

APPENDICES A-I

APPENDIX A

CANADIAN CONSENSUS CRITERIA – CLINICAL WORKING CASE DEFINITION OF ME/CFS [1] AND APPLICATION NOTES [2]

A patient with ME/CFS will meet the criteria for fatigue, post-exertional malaise and/or fatigue, sleep dysfunction, and pain; have two or more neurological/cognitive manifestations, and one or more symptoms from two of the categories of autonomic, neuroendocrine, and immune manifestations; and adhere to item 7.

1. *Fatigue:* The patient must have a significant degree of new-onset, unexplained, persistent, or recurrent physical and mental fatigue that substantially reduces activity level.

2. *Post-Exertional Malaise and/or Fatigue:* There is an inappropriate loss of physical and mental stamina, rapid muscular and cognitive fatigability, post-exertional malaise and/or fatigue and/or pain, and a tendency for other associated symptoms within the patient's cluster of symptoms to worsen. There is a pathologically slow recovery period – usually 24 hours or longer.

3. *Sleep Dysfunction:** There is unrefreshed sleep, or sleep quantity or rhythm disturbances such as reversed or chaotic diurnal sleep rhythms.

4. *Pain:** There is a significant degree of myalgia. Pain can be experienced in the muscles, and/or joints, and is often widespread and

---

1 Carruthers BM, Jain AK, De Meirleir KL, Peterson DL, Klimas NG, Lerner AM, Bested AC, Flor-Henry P, Joshi P, Powles ACP, Sherkey JA, van de Sande MI "Myalgic Encephalomyelitis/Chronic Fatigue Syndrome: Clinical Working Case Definition, Diagnostic and Treatment Protocols." J CFS 11(1):7-115, 2003. www.mefmaction.com/images/stories/Medical/ME-CFS-Consensus-Document.pdf (accessed July 20, 2016).

2 Application Notes are from the Overview document. Carruthers BM, and van de Sande MI. 2005. "Myalgic Encephalomyelitis/Chronic fatigue syndrome: A Clinical Case Definition and Guidelines for Medical Practitioners: An Overview of the Canadian Consensus Document." Vancouver, BC: Carruthers and van de Sande. 3. One place to view the overviews is the website of the National ME/FM Action Network. www.mefmaction.com/images/stories/Overviews/ME-Overview.pdf (accessed July 20, 2016).

migratory in nature. Often there are significant *headaches* of new type, pattern, or severity.

5. *Neurological/Cognitive Manifestations:* <u>*Two or more*</u> of the following difficulties should be present: confusion, impairment of concentration and short-term memory consolidation, disorientation, difficulty with information processing, categorizing and word retrieval, and perceptual and sensory disturbances e.g., spatial instability and disorientation and inability to focus vision. Ataxia, muscle weakness, and fasciculations are common. There may be overload [3] phenomena: cognitive or sensory, e.g., photophobia and hypersensitivity to noise and/or emotional overload, which may lead to "crash" [4] periods and/or anxiety.

6. *At Least* <u>*One*</u> *Symptom from* <u>*Two*</u> *of the Following Categories*:

   a   *Autonomic Manifestations*: orthostatic intolerance – neurally mediated hypotension (NMH); postural orthostatic tachycardia syndrome (POTS); delayed postural hypotension; light-headedness; extreme pallor; nausea and irritable bowel syndrome; urinary frequency and bladder dysfunction; palpitations with or without cardiac arrhythmias; exertional dyspnea.

   b   *Neuroendocrine Manifestations*: loss of thermostatic stability – subnormal body temperature and marked diurnal fluctuation, sweating episodes, recurrent feelings of feverishness and cold extremities; intolerance of extremes of heat and cold; marked weight change – anorexia or abnormal appetite; loss of adaptability and worsening of symptoms with stress.

   c   *Immune Manifestations*: tender lymph nodes, recurrent sore throat, recurrent flu-like symptoms, general malaise, new sensitivities to food, medications, and/or chemicals.

7. *The illness persists for at least six months. It usually has a distinct onset, **although it may be gradual.* Preliminary diagnosis may be possible earlier. Three months is appropriate for children.

To be included, the symptoms must have begun or have been significantly altered after the onset of this illness. It is unlikely that a patient will suffer from all symptoms in criteria 5 and 6. The disturbances tend to form symptom clusters that may fluctuate and

---

3   "Overload" refers to hypersensitivities to stimuli that have changed from pre-illness status.
4   "Crash" refers to a temporary period of immobilizing physical and/or cognitive fatigue.

change over time. Children often have numerous prominent symptoms, but their order of severity tends to vary from day to day.

*There are a small number of patients who have no pain or sleep dysfunction, but no other diagnosis fits except ME/CFS. A diagnosis of ME/CFS can be entertained when this group has an infectious illness-type onset.

**Some patients have been unhealthy for other reasons prior to the onset of ME/CFS and lack detectable triggers at onset and/or have more gradual or insidious onset.

Exclusions: Exclude *active* disease processes that explain most of the major symptoms of fatigue, sleep disturbance, pain, and cognitive dysfunction. It is essential to exclude certain diseases, which would be tragic to miss: Addison's disease, Cushing's syndrome, hypothyroidism, hyperthyroidism, iron deficiency, other treatable forms of anemia, iron overload syndrome, diabetes mellitus, and cancer. It is also essential to exclude treatable sleep disorders such as upper airway resistance syndrome and obstructive or central sleep apnea; rheumatological disorders such as rheumatoid arthritis, lupus, polymyositis, and polymyalgia rheumatica; immune disorders such as AIDS; neurological disorders such as multiple sclerosis (MS), Parkinsonism, myasthenia gravis, and B12 deficiency; infectious diseases such as tuberculosis, chronic hepatitis, Lyme disease, etc.; primary psychiatric disorders; and substance abuse. Exclusion of other diagnoses, which cannot be reasonably excluded by the patient's history and physical examination, is achieved by laboratory testing and imaging. If a potentially confounding medical condition is under control, then the diagnosis of ME/CFS can be entertained if patients meet the criteria otherwise.

Co-morbid Entities: fibromyalgia syndrome (FMS), myofascial pain syndrome (MPS), temporomandibular joint syndrome (TMJ), irritable bowel syndrome (IBS), interstitial cystitis, irritable bladder syndrome, Raynaud's phenomenon, prolapsed mitral valve, depression, migraine, allergies, multiple chemical sensitivities (MCS), Hashimoto's thyroiditis, sicca syndrome, etc. Such co-morbid entities may occur in the setting of ME/CFS. Others such as IBS may precede the development of ME/CFS by many years, but then become associated with it. The same holds true for migraines and depression. Their association is thus looser than between the symptoms within the syndrome. ME/CFS and FMS often closely connect and should be considered to be "overlap syndromes."

Idiopathic Chronic Fatigue: If the patient has unexplained prolonged fatigue (6 months or more) but has insufficient symptoms to meet the criteria for ME/CFS, it should be classified as idiopathic chronic fatigue.

Application Notes:

- *Total illness burden* is determined by observing and obtaining a complete description of the patient's symptoms, their interactions, and their functional impact.

- *Variability and coherence of symptoms:* The cluster of symptoms exhibited will vary, however, they are connected by their temporal, coherent, and causal relationships.

- *Symptom severity and impact:* Symptom severity is significant if it substantially impacts the patient's *premorbid activity level* (by an approximate 50% reduction). Confirm symptom severity and impact by dialogue with the patient over time.

- *The hierarchy of symptom severity* will vary over time and among patients. Periodic ranking of the severity and hierarchy of symptom severity helps orient the treatment program and monitor its effectiveness.

- *Separate primary symptoms from secondary symptoms and aggravators.* Symptom dynamics and interactions, and the effects of aggravators should be noted.

APPENDIX B

2010 AND 2005 CANADIAN COMMUNITY HEALTH SURVEY RESULTS

Numbers of people who reported they were diagnosed with:
Myalgic Encephalomyelitis/Chronic Fatigue Syndrome (ME/CFS),[**]
Fibromyalgia (FM) and/or Multiple Chemical Sensitivities (MCS)
in Canada in 2010 with the 2005 totals

MCS = 800,500   note: 598,500 (2005)

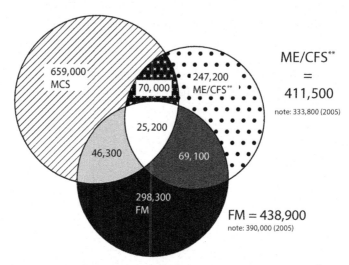

ME/CFS[**]
=
411,500
note: 333,800 (2005)

659,000 MCS
70,000
247,200 ME/CFS[**]
25,200
46,300
69,100
298,300 FM

FM = 438,900
note: 390,000 (2005)

Total reporting one or more diagnoses: 1,415,100[*]

[*]survey results rounded   note: 1,135,000 (2005)

MCS	MCS + FM	MCS + FM + ME/CFS[**]
FM	MCS + ME/CFS[**]	
ME/CFS[**]	FM + ME/CFS[**]	

ME/CFS, FM and MCS **CANADA**   Canadian Community Health Survey

[**]CCHS uses terminology CFS not ME/CFS

This diagram was created Oct. 6, 2011 by M. MacQuarrie
for the National ME/FM Action Network

(Redesigned for publication in 2016)

Appendix B Summary – The Appendix B Diagram demonstrates the prevalence and overlap of CFS, FM, and MCS derived from the 2010 Canadian Community Health Survey (CCHS). It also reflects the prevalence, but not the overlap, of the conditions from the 2005 CCHS.[1] The National ME/FM Action Network analyzed and published the results. (The numbers in the diagram have been rounded off for clarity.)

According to the 2005 CCHS, these are the numbers of people who reported they were diagnosed by a health professional with one or more of these chronic health conditions from a target population of 27,126,165:[2]

> Chronic Fatigue Syndrome (CFS) 333,816 – 1.2%;
>
> Fibromyalgia (FM) 389,782 – 1.4%;
>
> Multiple Chemical Sensitivities (MCS) 598,585 – 2.2%;
>
> One or more of CFS, FM, and MCS 1,135,225 – 4.2%. (Those with more than one of the conditions are counted as one person in this total.)

The CCHS does not always include questions on CFS, FM, or MCS, but they were included in 2010.

These are the 2010 prevalence results from a target population of 28,891,000:[3]

> Chronic fatigue syndrome 411,500 – 1.4%;
>
> Fibromyalgia 439,000 – 1.5%;
>
> Multiple Chemical Sensitivities 800,500 – 2.8%;
>
> One or more of CFS, FM, and MCS 1,415,000 – 4.9%. (Those with more than one of the conditions are counted as one person in this total.)

For both 2005 and 2010, the numbers for the three illnesses combined were well over 1 million people which is the population of some of our largest cities in Canada, such as Calgary or Edmonton.

Note: The overlap figures for 2010 in Diagram B were extracted from the CCHS Public Use Microdata File by National ME/FM Action Network.

---

1   According to the Statistics Canada website, "The CCHS is a cross-sectional survey done by Statistics Canada that collects information related to health status, health care utilization, and health determinants for the Canadian population."

2   These figures are from the 2005 CCHS. Quest 80 Newsletter, p.11, "Prevalence of Chronic Health Conditions." www.mefmaction.com/images/stories/quest_newsletters/Quest80springsummer2009.pdf (accessed August 6, 2016).

3   These figures are from the 2010 CCHS. Quest 88 Newsletter p. 3. www.mefmaction.com/images/stories/quest_newsletters/QUEST88Summer2011.pdf (accessed August 6, 2016).

APPENDIX C

QUALITY OF LIFE ISSUES AS SHOWN IN 2005 CANADIAN COMMUNITY HEALTH SURVEY (CCHS)

Summarized from the report *"Profile and Impact of 23 Chronic Conditions in the 2005 Canadian Community Health Survey."* [1]

The National ME/FM Action Network analyzed the 2005 CCHS results and prepared a report containing fact sheets comparing 23 chronic health conditions, as well as the national average, on issues such as impairment, socio-economic disadvantage, and health service delivery. In addition to CFS, some of the other chronic illnesses that were included were effects of stroke, FM, MCS, cancer, diabetes, heart disease, mood and anxiety disorders, and epilepsy.

(1) Social problems explored by the 2005 CCHS questions	(2) % of CFS cohort reporting problems under column (1)	(3) Ranking of **CFS** % compared to 22 other chronic health conditions. #1 indicates the highest percentage reporting the problem
Unmet medical care needs	30%	#1 is CFS
Unmet homecare needs	14%	#1 is CFS
Food insecurity	17%	#1 is CFS
Very weak sense of belonging to the community	19%	#1 is CFS
Needing help with tasks	60%	#2 is CFS (1 is effects of stroke)
Experiencing difficulty in social situations	27%	#2 is CFS (1 is effects of stroke)
Permanently unable to work	18%	#2 is CFS (1 is effects of stroke)
Personal income under $15,000	44%	#3 is CFS (1 is effects of stroke and 2 is epilepsy)

1   "Profile and Impact of 23 Chronic Conditions in the 2005 Canadian Community Health Survey." For the full report including the questions that were asked and how it was prepared, see www.mefmaction.com/images/stories/quest_newsletters/Quest80springsummer2009 pdf (accessed July 25, 2016). This summarized chart was prepared by Valerie Free and Maureen MacQuarrie.

APPENDIX D

WHAT AN ACCURATE DEFINITION WILL DO FOR IMPROVED PATIENT QUALITY OF LIFE[1]

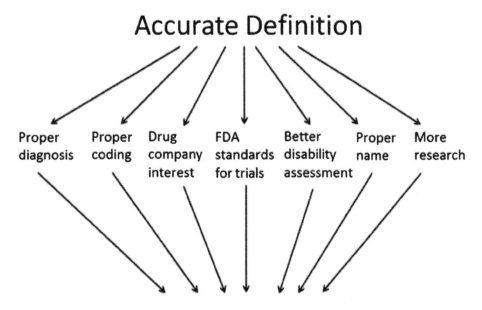

1   Presentation by Lori Chapo-Kroger, RN, PANDORA Org to the Institute of Medicine Committee on the Diagnostic Criteria for ME/CFS, Committee Meeting, January 27, 2014. iom.nationalacademies.org/~/media/Files/Activity%20 Files/Disease/MECFS/Chapo-Kroger%20IOM%20MECFS%20Presentation.pdf – Slide 7 of 8 – Diagnostic Criteria for ME/CFS.

APPENDIX E
SUMMARY OF THE PRIMARY CFS, ME/CFS, AND ME DEFINITIONS

Source: Dimmock M, and Lazell-Fairman M. "Thirty Years of Disdain (Background) How HHS and a Group of Psychiatrists Buried ME." December 2015. Appendix 1: Summary of the Primary CFS, ME/CFS and ME Definitions – http://bit.ly/The_Burial_of_ME_Background.

Definition Name	Label Used	Key Symptoms in the definition	Psychiatric Illness allowed?	PEM Required	Comment
1986 Ramsay[1]	ME	Muscle weakness and fatigability after trivial exertion, cognitive impairment, pain, circulatory issues/ temperature sensitivity, other autonomic signs	States ME is not mental illness but that there can be emotional lability	Yes as fatigability after exertion	PEM term not used but muscle fatigability after trivial exertion is central to PEM
1988 CDC Holmes[2]	CFS	6 months chronic fatigue plus any 8 symptoms out of eleven. No PEM, but e.g. muscle weakness, pain	Prior chronic psychiatric illness excluded but a 1989 clarification allowed	No	Replaced by Fukuda. Patients show more signs of infectious process than Fukuda[3]
1991 Oxford [4]	CFS	6 months severe fatigue that affects mental or physical function	No schizophrenia, manic-depressive illness. Anxiety, depression allowed	No	Myalgia, sleep, mood disturbance may be present but not required. PEM not mentioned
1994 CDC Fukuda[5]	CFS	6 months fatigue plus any 4 of memory impairment, sore throat, tender lymph nodes, muscle pain, joint pain, headaches of new type, unrefreshing sleep, PEM	Major depressive & bipolar disorder, schizophrenia excluded. Anxiety somatoform & other types of psych disorder allowed	No	PEM one of optional symptoms but not required. Fukuda includes more depressed and less symptomatic patients than CCC [6]
2003 Canadian Consensus Criteria (CCC)[7]	ME/ CFS	PEM plus two neurological/ cognitive plus 1 of autonomic, immunological & neuroendocrine symptoms	Primary psychiatric illness excluded	Yes	Requires PEM plus combination of these symptoms. 6 month wait

Definition Name	Label Used	Key Symptoms in the definition	Psychiatric Illness allowed?	PEM Required	Comment
2005 CDC Empirical (Reeves) Criteria [8]	CFS	Operationalization of Fukuda	Depression, anxiety, somatoform disorders not exclusionary	No	Led to ten-fold prevalence increase. Jason has shown 38 percent of patients with depression fit criteria.[9]
Pediatric Case Definition for ME & CFS (2006) Jason et al [10]	ME/ CFS	3 months of fatigue, PEM, unrefreshing sleep, neurocognitive, pain plus one of autonomic, neuroendocrine, or immune	Schizophrenia, bipolar, depressive disorders exclusionary. May have concomitant anxiety, depression, somatoform	Yes	3 month waiting period
NICE Clinical Guideline (2007)[11]	CFS	4 months chronic fatigue plus any one of 10 symptoms	Appears to allow primary psychiatric illness	Consider CFS if PEM exists	Pain, cognitive, and sleep difficulties considered key. 3 months duration in child
2011 ME International Consensus Criteria (ME-ICC)[12]	ME	PENE and neurological, plus immunological, GI/GU* plus energy metabolism/ transport GU* - genitourinary	Primary psychiatric illness excluded	Yes	Requires PENE (expansion of PEM) plus symptoms from each of other categories. No waiting period

Other less commonly used definitions can be found here: Brurberg, K., et al. Case definitions for chronic fatigue syndrome/myalgic encephalomyelitis (CFS/ME): a systematic review. BMJ Open 2014;4:e003973 doi:10.1136/bmjopen-2013-003973 bmjopen.bmj.com/content/4/2/e003973.long#T1.

1   **References:** Ramsay issued two articles on the definition, one in 1986 and one in 1988. Some sources indicate that Ramsay published the definition in 1981 but this author's research was unable to confirm that. Ramsay, M. "Myalgic Encephalomyelitis: A Baffling Syndrome With a Tragic Aftermath." Published 1986. www.meactionuk.org.uk/ ramsey.html and www.name-us.org/DefintionsPages/DefRamsay.htm#MYALGIC_ENCEPHALOMYELITIS_:_A_ Baffling_Syndrome_With_a_Tragic_Aftermath Ramsay, M. *Myalgic Encephalomyelitis and Postviral Fatigue States: The Saga of Royal Free Disease,* Gower Medical Publishing Corporation, London, 2nd ed. 1988. Extract provided by Connie Nelson to Mary Schweitzer who provided it on www.cfids-me.org/ramsay86.html Ramsay A.M., Rundle A. "Clinical and biochemical findings in ten patients with benign myalgic encephalomyelitis." *Postgraduate Medical Journal* December 1979; 55(654):856-7. The article states that one of the dominant clinical features of the disease is "Abnormal muscular fatigability and weakness. Muscular power was restored by a period of rest but recurred following further activity." The study findings are discussed with "particular reference to recent suggestions that the permeability of cell membranes may be impaired by changes in intracellular energy mechanisms."

2   Holmes G, Kaplan J, Gantz N, Komaroff A, Schonberger L, Straus S, Jones J, Dubois R, Cunningham-Rundles C, Pahwa S, Tosato G, Zegans L, Purtilo D, Brown N, Schooley R, Brus I. "Chronic Fatigue Syndrome: A Working Case Definition." *Annals of Internal Medicine.* March 1, 1988; 108(3): 387-389. PMID: 2829679.

dx.doi.org/10.7326/0003-4819-108-3-387   and   www.ncf-net.org/patents/pdf/Holmes_Definition.pdf   See also: Letter recommending preceding mood disorder not be considered exclusionary. Komaroff A, Straus S, Gantz N, Jones J. "The Chronic Fatigue Syndrome." Letter to *Ann Intern Med.* March 1, 1989; 110(5):407-408. dx.doi.org/10.7326/0003-4819-110-5-407.

Note that the 1991 NIH conference noted that the following were allowed. "Nonpsychotic depression: concurrent, 1 month post-onset or 6 months or more before onset: recurrent or non-recurrent, somatoform disorders, anxiety disorders: generalized or panic disorder."

Schluederberg A, Straus S, Peterson P, Blumenthal S, Komaroff A, Spring S, Landay A, Buchwald D. "NIH Conference. Chronic Fatigue Syndrome Research Definition and Medical Outcome Assessment." *Annals of Internal Medicine* August 1992; 117(4): 325-31. PMID: 1322076. annals.org/article.aspx?articleid=705740 (abstract) and annals.org/data/Journals/AIM/19757/AIME199208150-00010.pdf (full text).

3   Arpino C, Carrieri MP, Valesini G, Pizzigallo E, Rovere P, Tirelli U, Conti F, Dialmi P, Barberio A, Rusconi N, Bosco O, Lazzarin A, Saracco A, Moro ML, Vlahov D. "Idiopathic chronic fatigue and chronic fatigue syndrome: a comparison of two case-definitions." *Ann Ist Super Sanita.*1999; 35(3): 435-41. PMID: 10721210 www.ncbi.nlm.nih.gov/pubmed/10721210?dopt=Abstract The paper states "In conclusion, the 1994 criteria increased the number of patients classified as CFS (compared to Holmes); however, those who fit only the 1994 criteria were less likely to have an acute symptomatic onset and signs and symptoms suggestive of an infectious process."

4   Sharpe M, Archard L, Banatvala J, Borysiewicz L, Clare A, David A, Edwards R, Hawton K, Lambert H, Lane R, McDonald E, Mowbray J, Pearson D, Peto T, Preedy V, Smith A, Smith D, Taylor D, Tyrrell D, Wessely S, White P. "A report—chronic fatigue syndrome." *J Roy Soc Med* February 1991; 84(2): 118-121. PMID: 1999813. www.ncbi.nlm.nih.gov/pmc/articles/PMC1293107. The criteria for Oxford CFS are:

"A syndrome characterized by fatigue as the principal symptom,"

"A syndrome of definite onset that is not life long,"

"The fatigue is severe, disabling, and affects physical and mental functioning."

a)   "The symptom of fatigue should have been present for a minimum of 6 months during which it was present for more than 50% of the time"

b)   "Other symptoms may be present, particularly myalgia, mood, and sleep disturbance."

5   Fukuda K, Straus S.E., Hickie I, Sharpe M.C., Dobbins J.G., Komaroff A and the International Chronic Fatigue Syndrome Study Group. "The chronic fatigue syndrome: a comprehensive approach to its definition and study." *Ann Intern Med* 1994; 121(12): 953-9. PMID: 7978722. www.ncf-net.org/patents/pdf/Fukuda_Definition.pdf and dx.doi.org/10.7326/0003-4819-121-12-199412150-00009.

6   Jason, L, Torres-Harding, S, Jurgens, A, Helgerson, J. "Comparing the Fukuda et al. Criteria and the Canadian Case Definition for Chronic Fatigue Syndrome, Journal of Chronic Fatigue Syndrome 2004; 12(1): 37-52. informahealthcare.com/doi/abs/10.1300/J092v12n01_03?src=recsys and web.archive.org/web/20120216181206/www.cfids-cab.org/cfs-inform/CFS.case.def/jason.etal04.pdf.

Also see

• Jason, L. "Defining CFS: Diagnostic Criteria and Case Definition" Presented at CFIDS Association webinar, April 14, 2010. web.archive.org/web/20120425130843/www.cfids.org/webinar/jason-slides041410.pdf.

• On slide 12, Jason describes how fatigue plus 4 Fukuda symptoms are equivalent to the symptoms of depressed patients.

7   Carruthers B.M., Jain A.K., De Meirleir K.L., Peterson D.L., Klimas N.G., Lerner A.M., Bested A.C., Flor-Henry P., Joshi P., Powles A.C.P., Sherkey J.A., van de Sande M.I. "Myalgic Encephalomyelitis/Chronic Fatigue Syndrome: Clinical Working Case Definition, Diagnostic and Treatment Protocols." Journal of Chronic Fatigue Syndrome 2003; 11(1): 7-117. mefmaction.com/images/stories/Medical/ME-CFS-Consensus-Document.pdf. Also see the following overview of the CCC, produced in 2005.

• Carruthers B, van de Sande M. "Myalgic Encephalomyelitis/Chronic Fatigue Syndrome: A Clinical Case Definition and Guidelines for Medical Practitioners. An Overview of the Canadian Consensus Document." Published by Carruthers B, van de Sande M. 2005. www.name-us.org/DefintionsPages/DefinitionsArticles/ConsensusDocument%20Overview.pdf.

8   Reeves W, Wagner D, Nisenbaum R, Jones J, Gurbaxani B, Solomon L, Papanicolaou D, Unger E, Vernon S, Heim C. "Chronic Fatigue Syndrome – A clinically empirical approach to its definition and study." *BMC Medicine* December 2005; 3:19. PMID: 16356178. dx.doi.org/10.1186/1741-7015-3-19.

9   Jason L, Najar N, Porter N, Reh C. "Evaluating the Centers for Disease Control's Empirical Chronic Fatigue Syndrome Case Definition." *Journal of Disability Policy Studies* Published online October 2008, in print September 2009; 20(2): 93-100. dx.doi.org/10.1177/1044207308325995 and web.archive.org/web/20090816013354/www.co-cure.org/Jason-7.pdf.

10   Jason L, Jordan K, Miike T, Bell D.S., Lapp C, Torres-Harding S, Rowe K, Gurwitt A, DeMeirleir K, Van Hoof EA "A Pediatric Case Definition for Myalgic Encephalomyelitis and Chronic Fatigue Syndrome." *J Chronic Fatigue Syndr.* 2006; 13(2-3): 1-44. informahealthcare.com/doi/abs/10.1300/J092v13n02_01 and solvecfs.org/wp-content/uploads/2013/06/pediatriccasedefinitionshort.pdf.

11   U.K. National Institute for Health and Care Excellence (NICE). *Chronic fatigue syndrome/myalgic encephalomyelitis (or encephalopathy). Diagnosis and management of CFS/ME in adults and children.* (NICE clinical guideline 53). August 2007. guidance.nice.org.uk/CG53 and www.nice.org.uk/guidance/cg53/evidence NICE requires "fatigue with all of the following features: new or had a specific onset (that is, it is not lifelong); persistent and/or recurrent; unexplained by other conditions; has resulted in a substantial reduction in activity level; [and is] characterised by post-exertional malaise and/or fatigue (typically delayed, for example by at least 24 hours, with slow recovery over several days). The diagnosis of CFS/ME should be reconsidered if none of the following key features are present: post-exertional fatigue or malaise, cognitive difficulties, sleep disturbance, or chronic pain."

12   Carruthers B.M., van de Sande M.I., De Meirleir K.L., Klimas N.G., Broderick G., Mitchell T, Staines D., Powles A.C.P., Speight N., Vallings R., Bateman L., Baumgarten-Austrheim B., Bell D.S., Carlo-Stella N., Chia J, Darragh A., Jo D., Lewis D., Light A.R, Marshall-Gradisbik S., Mena I., Mikovits J.A., Miwa K., Murovska M., Pall M.L., Stevens S. "Myalgic Encephalomyelitis: International Consensus Criteria." Journal of Internal Medicine October 2011; 270(4): 327–338. PMID: 21777306. dx.doi.org/10.1111/j.1365-2796.2011.02428.x and onlinelibrary.wiley.com/doi/10.1111/j.1365-2796.2011.02428.x/full.

APPENDIX F

OVERLAP AND DIFFERENCES BETWEEN ME/CFS AND MAJOR DEPRESSION

ME/CFS	Major Depression
Clinical Presentation	
Infectious onset in majority of cases	Rarely follows infectious illness
Fatigue is necessary for diagnosis	Mood change is necessary for diagnosis
Muscle and/or joint pain and significant headaches	Not usually associated with pain symptoms
Afternoon and evening usually the worst time of day	Morning usually the worst time of day
Orthostatic intolerance, tachy-cardia, and other autonomic dysfunction are common	No association with autonomic symptoms
Immune manifestations including tender lymph nodes, sore throat, chemical and food sensitivities	No association with immune symptoms
Loss of temperature stability and intolerance to extremes of temperature	No association with temperature problems
Fatigue and other symptoms are worsened by physical or mental exercise	Fatigue and mood improve with exercise
Decreased positive affect (energy, enthusiasm, happiness)	Increased negative affect (apathy, hope-lessness, suicidal ideation, self reproach)
Children have a better prognosis than adults	Children have a worse prognosis than adults

Source: Stein E, MD, FRCP(C). "Let Your Light Shine Through – Strategies for Living with Myalgic Encephalomyelitis/ Chronic Fatigue Syndrome, Fibromyalgia and Multiple Chemical Sensitivity." 2012.
Session 8. Depression and Anxiety, page 8-13.

APPENDIX G
RESPONSE TO PHYSICAL OR MENTAL EXERTION – POST-EXERTIONAL MALAISE AND/OR FATIGUE

Source: Carruthers BM, and van de Sande MI. 2005. "Myalgic encephalomyelitis/chronic fatigue syndrome: A Clinical Case Definition and Guidelines for Medical Practitioners: An Overview of the Canadian Consensus Document." Vancouver, BC: Carruthers and van de Sande, page 4.

Physical or mental exertion often causes debilitating malaise and/or fatigue, generalized pain, deterioration of cognitive functions, and worsening of other symptoms that may occur immediately after activity or be delayed. Patients experience rapid muscle fatigue and lack endurance. These symptoms are suggestive of a pathophysiology which involves immune system activation, channelopathy with oxidative stress and nitric oxide related toxicity,[1] and/or orthostatic intolerance. Recovery time is inordinately long, usually a day or longer, and exercise may trigger a relapse. The following chart indicates some of the documented dysfunctional reactions to exercise that patients may exhibit:[2]

RESPONSE TO EXERCISE

Response to Exercise	Healthy People	ME/CFS Patients
Sense of well-being	Invigorating, anti-depressant effect	Feel malaise, fatigue, and worsening symptoms[3, 4]
Resting heart rate	Normal	Elevated[5, 6]
Heart rate at maximum workload	Elevated	Reduced heart rate[5, 6]
Maximum oxygen uptake	Elevated	Approximately ½ of sedentary controls[5]
Age-predicted target heart rate	Can achieve it	Often cannot achieve it and should not be forced[5, 6]
Cardiac output	Increased	Suboptimal level[5, 6]
Cerebral blood flow	Increased	Decreased[7, 8]

Response to Exercise	Healthy People	ME/CFS Patients
Cerebral oxygen	Increased	Decreased[7]
Body temperature	Increased	Decreased[9]
Respiration	Increased	Breathing irregularities: shortness of breath[9], shallow breathing
Cognitive processing	Normal, more alert	Impaired[10]
Recovery period	Short	Often 24 hours, but can last days or weeks[3, 4, 11]
Oxygen delivery to muscles	Increased	Impaired[5]
Gait kinematics	Normal	Gait abnormalities[12]

1 Snell C.F., VanNess J.M., Stayer D.R., Stevens S.R. "Exercise capacity and immune function in male and female patients with chronic fatigue syndrome." (CFS). In Vivo 19(2):387-90, Mar.-Apr. 2005.

2 van de Sande M.I. "ME/CFS and post-exertional malaise and exercise." #60, National ME/CFS Action Network, 2003.

3 Carruthers B.M., Jain A.K., De Meirleir K.L., Peterson D.L., Klimas N.G., Lerner A.M., Bested A.C,. Flor-Henry P, Joshi P, Powles A.C.P., Sherkey J.A. van de Sande M.I. "Myalgic Encephalomyelitis/Chronic Fatigue Syndrome: Clinical Working Case Definition, Diagnostic and Treatment Protocols." J CFS 11(1):7-115, 2003.

4 Fukuda K., Straus S.E., Hickie I., et al. "Chronic fatigue syndrome: a comprehensive approach to its definition and study." Annals Med 121:953-959, 1994.

5 De Becker P, Roeykens J, Reynders M, et al. "Exercise capacity in chronic fatigue syndrome." Arch Intern Med 160(21):3270-3277, Nov. 27, 2000.

6 Inbar O, Dlin R, Rotstein A, et al. "Physiological responses to incremental exercise in patients with chronic fatigue syndrome." Med Scie Sports Exer 33(9):1463-1470, Sept. 2001.

7 Goldstein J.A. "Chronic Fatigue Syndrome: The Limbic Hypothesis." Haworth Medical Press, Binghamton NY 1993, 116.

8 Streeten D.H. "Role of impaired lower-limb venous innervations in the pathogenesis of the chronic fatigue syndrome." Amer J Med Sci 321:163-167, Mar. 2001.

9 Goldstein J.A. "CFS and FMS: dysregulation of the limbic system." FM Network Oct. 1993, 10-11.

10 La Manca J.J., Sisto S.A., DeLuca J, et al. "Influence of exhaustive treadmill exercise on cognitive functioning in chronic fatigue syndrome." Am J Med 105(3A):59S-65S, Sept. 27, 1998.

11 De Becker P, McGregor N, De Meirleir K. "A definition-based analysis of symptoms in a large cohort of patients with chronic fatigue syndrome." J Inter Med 250:234-240, 2001.

12 Boda W.L., Natelson B.H., Sisto S.A., Tapp W.N. "Gait abnormalities in patients with chronic fatigue syndrome." J Neurol Sci 131(2):156-161, Aug. 1995.

APPENDIX H
GUIDELINES FOR MEASURING ENERGY

1. **Karnofsky Energy Rating Scale adapted for use in ME/CFS**
Source: Bell, D.S. (1995) *The Doctor's Guide to Chronic Fatigue Syndrome,* Da Capo Press. Boston, MA. Further adapted by Dr. Ellie Stein in the manual *Let Your Light Shine Through* under "Charts and Tools".

100% Totally well; no concerns about fatigue. You can think clearly and do several things at once. You can exercise to your maximum potential without any problems.

90% Energy good but you feel fatigued after hard exercise.

80% You feel well with respect to your energy but must monitor your energy through the day. Your thinking is good but not quite clear. Tasks are easy and you can still do multiple tasks at once. You are fatigued after moderate exercise. Full-time work is possible for most.

70% Your overall energy is OK but everything you do is much more difficult and your energy is easily shifted. Your thought processes are much slower and more difficult and memory is poor. Exercise tolerance is poor and any strenuous exercise will make you feel unwell while light activity is tolerable. You can achieve a full day (8 hours) of tasks, but it requires a high degree of effort. You are too tired to do anything additional such as socializing. Full-time work is possible only if you do not have to do any household tasks, errands or childcare. Part-time work is possible for most.

60% You are able to complete 1/2 day of tasks and feel tired during it. Your thinking and memory are poor. You must rest at some point in the day. Even with rest, there is no part of the day in which you feel normal with respect to energy or can think clearly. Part-time work is possible only if hours are flexible to coincide with your energy peaks and you do not have to do any household tasks, errands or childcare.

50% Your energy only allows you to do about 3 tasks per day (2-3 hours of activity). Your energy is easily drained. Thought processes are difficult. Your exercise tolerance is poor; walking up stairs is difficult.

40% You can only perform 2 light tasks per day. Physical exercise is not tolerable. Your thought processes are very slow and your memory is poor.

30% You can only perform one light task per day, any extra physical movement makes you feel unwell. You have difficulty reading and writing.

20% You are unable to perform any daily tasks; even going to the bathroom is tiring. The most physical exertion you can manage is to sit in a chair for short periods. Emotions are very unstable and fluctuate without warning.

10% You are in bed for most of the day and you have zero tolerance for anything extra. You are frequently too exhausted to even eat.

2. **Functional Capacity Scale as developed by Drs. Alison Bested & Lynn Marshall**
Source: IACFS/ME (International Association for Chronic Fatigue Syndrome/Myalgic Encephalomyelitis) "ME/CFS Primer for Clinical Practitioners." 2014. Chicago, IL: IACFS/ME. Appendix C p. 38.

FUNCTIONAL CAPACITY SCALE
The Functional Capacity Scale incorporates energy rating, symptom severity, and activity level. The description after each scale number can be used to rate functional capacity.

0 = No energy, severe symptoms including very poor concentration; bed-ridden all day; cannot do self-care (e.g. need bed bath to be given)

1 = Severe symptoms at rest, including very poor concentration; in bed most of the day; need assistance with self-care activities (bathing)

2 = Severe symptoms at rest, including poor concentration; frequent rests or naps; need some assistance with limited self-care activities (can wash face at the sink), and need rest afterwards for severe post-exertional fatigue

3 = Moderate symptoms at rest, including poor concentration; need frequent rests or naps; can do independent self-care (can wash standing at the sink for a few minutes) but have severe post-exertion fatigue and need rest

4 = Moderate symptoms at rest, including some difficulty concentrating; need frequent rests throughout the day; can do independent self-care (can take a shower) and limited activities of daily living (e.g. light housework, laundry); can walk for a few minutes per day

5 = Mild symptoms at rest with fairly good concentration for short periods (15 minutes); need a.m. and p.m. rest; can do independent self-care and moderate activities of daily living, but have slight post-exertion fatigue; can walk 10-20 minutes per day

6 = Mild or no symptoms at rest with fairly good concentration for up to 45 minutes; cannot multitask; need afternoon rest; can do most activities of daily living except vacuuming; can walk 20-30 minutes per day; can do volunteer work – maximum total time 4 hours per week, with flexible hours

7 = Mild or no symptoms at rest with good concentration for up to 1/2 day; can do more intense activities of daily living (e.g. grocery shopping, vacuuming), but may get post-exertion fatigue if 'overdoes'; can walk 30 minutes per day; can work limited hours, less than 25 hours per week; no or minimal social life

8 = Mild intermittent symptoms with good concentration; can do full self-care, work 40 hours per week, enjoy a social life, do moderate vigorous exercise three times per week

9 = No symptoms; very good concentration; full work and social life; can do vigorous exercise three to five times a week

10 = No symptoms; excellent concentration; overachiever (sometimes may require more sleep than average person)

Dr. Alison Bested © Dr. Lynn Marshall.

APPENDIX I

ADDITIONAL RESOURCES –
BOOKS, DOCUMENTARIES, VIDEOS, AND OTHER
MEDIA

Delivered through multiple mediums, these resources are a good reminder that the ME/CFS world is not hidden at all – when one is looking for it. People are speaking it, singing it, making it into film, and photographing it, in order to give it a broader context with a universal theme. This hidden world is very ready to be found: seen, heard, felt and understood.

Film-maker and ME advocate Jennifer Brea,[1] sums it up beautifully:

> ...We think that no one can understand what we go through unless they also have this illness. On a certain level, that's true. Yet, everyone at some point will face a difficult, confusing, or scary health issue; or it will happen to someone they love; or they will confront some other obstacle that will alter the course of their lives and destroy the image they once had of their personal future. To reach an audience outside of our community, I believe we need to tap into those universal themes.
>
> We learn by telling stories, and to quote Danny Cohen of the BBC, we learn by feeling the facts. I want people to walk away from the film [Canary in a Coal Mine] thinking not, "That was an interesting story about ME"...
>
> My goal is for people to say, "Wow! That was brilliant, heartbreaking, moving, exhilarating, terrifying." I want them to know what it's like to live with M.E., and then to never be able to feel the same way about "Chronic Fatigue Syndrome" again.

COLLECTIONS OF ME AND CFS STORIES FROM AROUND THE WORLD

- U.K. – *Lost Voices from a Hidden Illness*. Wild Conversations Press. Natalie Boulton ed. 2008.

---

1   October 23, 2013. phoenixrising.me/archives/20117 (accessed January 16, 2016). Jennifer Brea is an ME patient and the film-maker of the documentary "Canary in a Coal Mine" to be released soon.

– *From ME to You, With Love*. Louise Harding. CreateSpace. 2014.

- Sweden – *Trött är fel ord: Om att leva med den osynliga sjukdomen ME/CFS* – translates as Tired is the wrong word: About living with invisible illness ME/CFS. Britt-Marie Thurén. 2011.

- Italy – *Stanchi: Vivere con la Sindrome da Fatica Cronica* – translates as Tired: Living with Chronic Fatigue Syndrome. Giada Da Ros ed. 2012.

- Canada – Lydia Neilson, the founder of the National ME/FM Action Network, has launched a project called *Unheard Voices: My Story* which can be found at www.mefmaction.com.

- U.S. – *Stricken: Voices from the Hidden Epidemic of Chronic Fatigue Syndrome*. Peggy Munson ed. Routledge. 2000.
    – The Solve ME/CFS Initiative started a project in 2015 entitled *Humans of ME/CFS* which "was launched to help increase awareness of – and ultimately research funding for – the millions of people whose lives have been stolen by ME/CFS." www.homecfs. solvecfs.org.

RECENT BOOKS (including novels, about living with ME, CFS or other chronic illness)

- *The Sound of a Wild Snail Eating*. Elisabeth Tova Bailey. Algonquin Books. 2010.

- *Love and Fatigue in America*. Roger King. University of Wisconsin Press. 2012.

- *How to Be Sick: A Buddhist-inspired Guide for the Chronically Ill and their Caregivers*. Toni Bernhard. Wisdom Publications. Boston. 2010.

- *How to Wake Up: A Buddhist-inspired Guide to Navigating Joy and Sorrow*. Toni Bernhard. Wisdom Publications. 2013.

- *How to Live Well with Chronic Pain and Illness: A Mindful Guide*. Toni Bernhard. Wisdom Publications. 2015.

- *Verity Red's Diary: A story of surviving M.E.* Maria Mann. Janus Publishing Company. 2007. Maria has also written *Love and Best Witches* (a book, aimed at children, about a witch with M.E. first published by Epic Press in 2010; 2nd edition self-published in 2013 by easyBroom) and *Verity Writes Again* (self-published by easyBroom 2015). You can read an interview with Maria at mecfsghost.com/interview-with-maria-mann-author-of-verity-reds-diary.

- *Chronic Fatigue Syndrome: A Novel.* Carol Wolf. Second Revised Edition, 2015. Originally published in 2010, Caroline T. Anderson. It is, as the cover notes, "a tale of bureaucracy, money and health." The second revised edition has updated information about ME/CFS including the new name *SEID*. More about the novel can be found at: www.carolwolfmedia.com/#!chronic-fatigue-syndrome-a-novel/c1bxr.

- *The State of Me.* Nasim Marie Jafrey. The Friday Project, an imprint of Harper Collins. 2008.

- *Can I tell you about ME/Chronic Fatigue Syndrome? A Guide for Friends, Family & Professionals.* Jacqueline Rayner, illustrated by Jason Lythgoe-Hay. Jessica Kingsley Publishers. 2014. A short, illustrated book about what it is like to live with ME/CFS and how it affects family life.

- *Chronic Fatigue Syndrome/ME: Support for Family and Friends.* Elizabeth Turp. Jessica Kingsley Publishers. 2010.

- *M.E., Myself And I: An insider's view of Myalgic Encephalomyelitis & Chronic Fatigue Syndrome.* K.C. Finn/Createspace. 2014.

- *Falling Through the World.* Rachel Clarke. Lunette Publishing. 2012.

- *My A - Z of M.E. (Myalgic Encephalomyelitis).* Ros Lemarchand. 2013.

BOOKS OF RECOVERY

- *CFS Unravelled.* Dan Neuffer. Kindle Edition, Amazon Digital Services, Inc. 2013.

- *CFS is a Call for Soulwork.* Gretchen Brooks Nassar. Food for your Soul. 2005.

- *Recovery from CFS: 50 Personal Stories.* Alexandra Barton. Authorhouse. 2008.

- *Defeat Chronic Fatigue Syndrome: You Don't Have to Live with It – An Eight step Protocol.* Martha Kilkoyne. Triple Spiral Press. 2007.

ME CLASSICS (books/articles)

- *Osler's Web: Inside the Labyrinth of the Chronic Fatigue Syndrome Epidemic.* Hillary Johnson. Iuniverse, Inc. (10th year updated edition, 2006.) Original edition published in 1996.

- *Faces of CFS: Case Histories of Chronic Fatigue Syndrome* by Dr. David S. Bell. MZR Publishing. August 2000. It can be found

at web.archive.org/web/20140213014605/www.mecfs-vic.org.au/sites/
www.mecfs-vic.org.au/files/Resource-BellFacesOfCFS.pdf.

- *Encounters with the Invisible: Unseen Illness, Controversy and Chronic Fatigue Syndrome.* Dorothy Wall, afterword by Nancy Klimas M.D. Southern Methodist University Press. 2005. Dorothy explains more about the book, including how she came to write it in an informative YouTube video which you can watch at www.youtube.com/watch?v=2D9JfQZwxMs.

- *A Sudden Illness – How my Life Changed.* Laura Hillenbrand. *The New Yorker* July 7, 2003. www.kenwilber.com/Writings/PDF/A_Sudden_Illness.pdf.

- *Chronic Fatigue no longer seen as 'Yuppie Flu'.* David Tuller in *The New York Times.* July 17, 2007. www.nytimes.com/2007/07/17/science/17fatigue.html?_r=0.

- *Tuller Tells It Like It Is.* 2011, Kimberley McCleary, solvecfs.org/tuller-tells-it-like-it-is.

INTERNATIONAL NEWSLETTER

ME Global Chronicle, produced since January 2014. It is available for download and contains up-to-date information from various countries at let-me.be/download.php?list.1.

DOCUMENTARIES

Several documentaries that aim to raise public and professional awareness have just been released or are in the making.

United States:

- *Forgotten Plague: M.E. and the Future of Medicine,* a documentary from ME patient Ryan Prior and his co-director Nicole Castillo, was released in 2015 and is available for screenings. The film is about Ryan's personal journey with M.E. and about the medical and scientific context. It is chilling and at the same time hopeful about science's ability to transform medicine. Screenings can be held by anyone, and it is available in DVD as well as other mediums. More information about the film and its mission to educate and raise awareness about neuro-immune conditions can be found at www.forgottenplague.com.

- *Canary in a Coal Mine,* told through the lives of people living with ME, is from filmmaker Jennifer Brea, ME/CFS patient and PhD student at Harvard. The film has been gaining great interest with a release date anticipated in 2017. www.canaryinacoalminefilm.com.

- *I Remember Me.* Kim Snyder. An excellent documentary from 2000 at www.YouTube.com/watch?v=401--WCB5dc.

Lyme Disease

- *Under Our Skin*, director Andy Abraham Wilson. This is an award-winning film released in 2014. "*Under Our Skin* had a tremendous impact, raising awareness among patients, doctors and health authorities alike. Since the film's release in 2014, the CDC has raised its estimated prevalence of Lyme by 10 times, making it more prevalent than HIV and breast cancer combined in the U.S." www.mercola.com August 16, 2016.

- *Under Our Skin 2: Emergence*, director Andy Abrahams Wilson. "Around the world, controversy around Lyme disease is still brewing, and the film reveals medical collusion and conflicts of interest that keep Lyme patients suffering. The film ends on a hopeful note however, by showing how patients in the original film have managed to improve their health and reclaim their lives." www.mercola.com August 16, 2016.

United Kingdom:

- *Voices from the Shadows.* Josh Biggs and Natalie Boulton. 2011. "Voices from the Shadows" shows the brave and sometimes heartrending stories of five ME patients and their carers, along with input from Dr. Nigel Speight, Prof. Leonard Jason and Prof. Malcolm Hooper. It was filmed and edited between 2009 and 2011 by the brother and mother of an ME patient in the UK. The film shows the devastating consequences that occur when patients are disbelieved and the illness is misunderstood. A website with recent information is at voicesfromtheshadowsfilm.co.uk. This will direct you to view the film through Vimeo for free.

- *What about ME?* This documentary premiered in France, May 2016. It is a 90-minute documentary that takes the audience on a journey to investigate the debilitating condition of Myalgic Encephalomyelitis known as ME/CFS … It has been filmed in locations including the U.S., Sweden, and the U.K. "DoubleD Productions embarked on a seven-year journey to capture the revelation in our documentary to produce a story of intrigue, heartbreak, and hope." www.doubledproductions.co.uk/in-production.

- *Myalgic Encephalomyelitis: The Hidden Truth.* "The idea for *M.E.: The Hidden Truth* documentary was conceived by Kara Spencer, a severe M.E. patient. People with M.E. often wish that those sceptical of the condition...

could spend just one week in their shoes to gain some insight and understanding. We can't deliver that, but I think we did just about the next best thing. We spent 7 days and 7 nights filming around the clock to capture the parts of this illness that remain hidden." The filming was completed April 2016 and the trailers can be found at www.methehiddentruth.com.

Germany:

- *In engen Grenzen – Leben mit CFS* (translated as *"In Narrow Limits – Life with chronic fatigue syndrome"*). This film, a 50-minute documentary, is in German. It was released on August 12, 2012. It was uploaded to YouTube on April 14, 2014. www.youtube.com/watch?v=vjtoz4Ojdeo. The film webpage and supporting information (which can be translated) is at www.in-engen-grenzen.de. The film includes footage of Katharina Voss (who blogs on ME – meversuscfs.blogspot.ca) and her two children, both of whom have ME.

Norway:

- *Sykt Mørkt* (translated as *Perversely Dark*) was released on May 12, 2014, after six years of filming. This is director Päl Winsents' second ME/CFS film. His earlier film was the 2010 *Fä Meg Frisk* (translated as *Heal Me*). As the English information for *Sykt Mørkt* notes: "It is perverse that many formerly able-bodied persons have to lie in complete darkness and isolation. And, indefinitely so."

VIDEOS AND VIDEO SERIES

- *Science to Patients.* There is a very good ongoing series of YouTube videos: *Wetenschap voor Patiënten* (*Science to Patients*) by the ME/cvs Vereniging (the Dutch ME/CFS Association). They feature interviews with a number of prominent ME/CFS professionals including Dr. K. DeMeirleir, Dr. F.C. Visser, Dr. Nigel Speight, Dr. Charles Shepherd, Dr. Julia Newton, and Leonard Jason PhD. A list of the videos (and transcripts) can be found at www.me-cvsvereniging.nl/english-page.

- *ME/CFS Alert.* Journalist Llewellyn King teamed up with long-time patient and New York writer Deborah Waroff to create this series of videos promoting ME/CFS awareness. As of May 2016, 79 episodes in this series have been produced as well as a number of other videos, including a full episode (7044) of Mr. King's White House Chronicle entitled *Chronic Fatigue Syndrome: A Disease Looking for Doctors and Researchers.* www.youtube.com/user/MECFSAlert.

- *Get Well From ME.* Patient Giles Meehan has created a series of videos about ME/CFS exploring what it is, how to live with it, as well as ways to improve one's health. One of them from 2012, *This is M.E. – Myalgic Encephalomyelitis,* includes the faces and voices of 34 patients who explain M.E. www.getwellfromme.com.

- A patient, who goes by the name *SuddenOnset,* has created (and is working on) a number of videos dealing with ME/CFS, including some on emerging scientific evidence. www.youtube.com/user/SuddenOnset/videos.

- *Mom Needs to Lie Down: The Years and Lives Slept Away by ME/CFS.* In 2014, Taylor Cole, a creative communications student from Manitoba, Canada, made a short video about ME/CFS, told from the perspectives of four women (including Taylor's mother). www.youtube.com/watch?v=EvrU-ciEFcM.

- *Invisible Illness – Stories of Chronic Fatigue Syndrome.* www.youtube.com/watch?v=9_HwOUilmvw. Published on July 10, 2015. This mini documentary reveals 3 stories of people who have been impacted by Chronic Fatigue Syndrome …They share emotions of treating loved ones with the disease, their frustrations of being ignored by members of society and the healthcare industry and express hopes of treatment and research. Video by Veronica Weber/Palo Alto Online.

WEBSITES AND BLOGS

Many ME, CFS and other chronic illness organizations maintain websites with very good information about the conditions. In addition to organizational sites, there are many excellent websites with news and information about ME/CFS and other chronic conditions. A number of them have been mentioned or used as references in this book including:

- Health Rising (Cort Johnson) – www.cortjohnson.org.

- Paradigm Change – www.paradigmchange.me.

- Phoenix Rising – www.phoenixrising.me.

- ProHealth – www.prohealth.com.

- Stonebird: The Lived Experience of Severe ME – www.stonebird.co.uk.

Blogs tend to be more immediate, interactive and personal than websites. There are many excellent ones available. ProHealth has compiled a list of some of the blogs, grouped in categories of Advocacy, Coping, News and Information, Personal and Research. This book has benefited from many blogs, including, but not limited to, Cort Johnson's *Health Rising,* Jennie Spotila's *Occupy M.E. – formerly Occupy CFS,* Jeannette Burmeister's

Thoughts about M.E. and Erica Verrillo's *Onward through the Fog*. Prohealth's list can be found at www.prohealth.com/me-cfs/me-chronic-fatigue-syndrome-blogs.cfm.

Vincent Racaniello, PhD hosts *Virology Blog* which houses articles by journalist David Tuller and others including *Chronic fatigue syndrome and the CDC: A Long, Tangled Tale*, Nov. 23, 2011; and the *Trial by Error* series dealing with the PACE trial which can be found in a dedicated ME/CFS section of the blog – www.virology.ws/mecfs.

One of the articles in the *Trial by Error* series was co-written with Julie Rehemeyer. More articles by Julie, including *Massive Flaws in the Largest Treatment Trial in ME/CFS history*, December 4, 2015, can be found at julierehmeyer.com/articles-and-essays/chronic-fatigue-syndrome.

- On July 10, 2016, V. Racaniello interviewed D. Tuller about the flaws of the $8 million U.K. PACE study and they gave an update of the efforts made to demand an independent analysis of the study and a retraction of it from publication. www.microbe.tv/twiv/twiv-397.

- *ME-pedia.org* is a very recent and ambitious project. It is a wiki co-developed by #MEAction and the patient community. It is anticipated that it will be a knowledge base for the history, science and medicine of ME and CFS.

PHOTOGRAPHY AND MUSIC

- *Out of Darkness Comes Light.* Penny Clare Images. Mysterious beautiful photography from a bedbound sufferer. This includes some of Penny's ME/CFS story along with her amazing photographs. December 23, 2013. phoenixrising.me/archives/21305.

- *Patience.* Ren Gill. M.E. Published on March 18, 2015. Video by imperfection-project.com. www.youtube.com/watch?v=284ugnS_ruQ. Ren performs many songs on YouTube but this particular performance includes some of his chronic illness story and his determined strength.

ABOUT THE AUTHOR

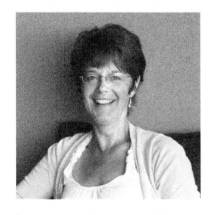

In 1990, Valerie Free was a happy, vibrant thirty-year-old woman – a court stenographer, a loving wife, and the mother of a precious baby girl. In July of that year, she came down with a sudden, flu-like illness, and after months of unrelenting and bizarre symptoms, was diagnosed with chronic fatigue syndrome (CFS), later to be understood as myalgic encephalomyelitis (ME) or ME/CFS. Valerie had entered a world that she could never have imagined, a world she still lives in to this day. Despite the challenges posed by her health, she went on to search for answers. *Lighting Up a Hidden World: CFS and ME* is the result, involving decades of research and outreach to the chronic illness community. Her natural curiosity, her love of people – as well as her interest in storytelling for social change – have allowed her to write this in-depth investigation into this mysterious illness. Valerie resides on an acreage with her family in Alberta, Canada.

www.valeriefree.org